Design and Synthesis of Novel Antibiotics

Design and Synthesis of Novel Antibiotics

Guest Editors

Katarzyna Turecka
Kenneth Ikenna Onyedibe

MDPI

Basel • Beijing • Wuhan • Barcelona • Belgrade • Novi Sad • Cluj • Manchester

Guest Editors
Katarzyna Turecka
Department of Pharmaceutical
Microbiology
Medical University of Gdańsk
Gdańsk
Poland

Kenneth Ikenna Onyedibe
Department of Chemistry
Purdue University
West Lafayette
USA

Editorial Office
MDPI AG
Grosspeteranlage 5
4052 Basel, Switzerland

This is a reprint of the Special Issue, published open access by the journal *Antibiotics* (ISSN 2079-6382), freely accessible at: https://www.mdpi.com/journal/antibiotics/special_issues/1E91M5A6DK.

For citation purposes, cite each article independently as indicated on the article page online and as indicated below:

Lastname, A.A.; Lastname, B.B. Article Title. *Journal Name* **Year**, *Volume Number*, Page Range.

ISBN 978-3-7258-5377-9 (Hbk)
ISBN 978-3-7258-5378-6 (PDF)
https://doi.org/10.3390/books978-3-7258-5378-6

Contents

antibiotics

MDPI

Article

A FtsZ Inhibitor That Can Utilize Siderophore-Ferric Iron Uptake Transporter Systems for Activity against Gram-Negative Bacterial Pathogens

Eric J. Bryan [1], Qi Qiao [2], Yuxuan Wang [1], Jacques Y. Roberge [2], Edmond J. LaVoie [3] and Daniel S. Pilch [1,*]

1 Department of Pharmacology, Rutgers Robert Wood Johnson Medical School, Piscataway, NJ 08854, USA; ejb236@dls.rutgers.edu (E.J.B.); yw782@rwjms.rutgers.edu (Y.W.)
2 Department of Molecular Design and Synthesis, Rutgers University Biomedical Innovation Cores, Piscataway, NJ 08854, USA; qq10@research.rutgers.edu (Q.Q.); jr1257@research.rutgers.edu (J.Y.R.)
3 Department of Medicinal Chemistry, Ernest Mario School of Pharmacy, Rutgers, The State University of New Jersey, Piscataway, NJ 08854, USA; elavoie@pharmacy.rutgers.edu
* Correspondence: pilchds@rwjms.rutgers.edu

Abstract: The global threat of multidrug-resistant Gram-negative bacterial pathogens necessitates the development of new and effective antibiotics. FtsZ is an essential and highly conserved cytoskeletal protein that is an appealing antibacterial target for new antimicrobial therapeutics. However, the effectiveness of FtsZ inhibitors against Gram-negative species has been limited due in part to poor intracellular accumulation. To address this limitation, we have designed a FtsZ inhibitor (**RUP4**) that incorporates a chlorocatechol siderophore functionality that can chelate ferric iron (Fe^{3+}) and utilizes endogenous siderophore uptake pathways to facilitate entry into Gram-negative pathogens. We show that **RUP4** is active against both *Klebsiella pneumoniae* and *Acinetobacter baumannii*, with this activity being dependent on direct Fe^{3+} chelation and enhanced under Fe^{3+}-limiting conditions. Genetic deletion studies in *K. pneumoniae* reveal that **RUP4** gains entry through the FepA and CirA outer membrane transporters and the FhuBC inner membrane transporter. We also show that **RUP4** exhibits bactericidal synergy against *K. pneumoniae* when combined with select antibiotics, with the strongest synergy observed with PBP2-targeting β-lactams or MreB inhibitors. In the aggregate, our studies indicate that incorporation of Fe^{3+}-chelating moieties into FtsZ inhibitors is an appealing design strategy for enhancing activity against Gram-negative pathogens of global clinical significance.

Keywords: *Klebsiella pneumoniae*; *Acinetobacter baumannii*; antibiotic-siderophore conjugate; antibiotic uptake; FtsZ inhibitor-antibiotic synergy

1. Introduction

The global spread of multidrug-resistant (MDR) bacterial pathogens represents a public health crisis [1–3]. Patients diagnosed with MDR infections suffer much worse prognoses, including extended hospital stays and higher mortality rates, than patients with drug-susceptible infections [1]. Globally, 1.3 million deaths per year are directly attributable to resistant bacterial infections [4], with this figure predicted to rise to 10 million annual deaths by 2050 in the absence of intervention [5]. Of particular concern are ESKAPE pathogens [6], bacterial strains that are typically associated with high rates of clinical resistance [7,8]. Two of the more resistant ESKAPE pathogens are the Gram-negative species *Klebsiella pneumoniae* and *Acinetobacter baumannii*, each of which is responsible for more than 100,000 deaths annually [2,4]. Current clinical antibiotics, including carbapenems, third generation cephalosporins, and fluoroquinolones, are becoming increasingly ineffective against these two pathogens, leaving clinicians with few treatment options [4,9,10].

The threat posed by highly resistant Gram-negative pathogens emphasizes the need to develop new and effective antibiotics with novel bacterial targets. One promising new antibacterial drug target is FtsZ, an essential and highly conserved bacterial divisome protein that is not targeted by any current clinical drug [11,12]. FtsZ is a GTPase that polymerizes into a structure known as the Z-ring at the midcell of a dividing bacterium [13]. The FtsZ Z-ring is a major factor in driving bacterial cytokinesis, acting as a scaffold for recruitment of essential cell division components, which include the cell wall-forming penicillin-binding proteins (PBPs) [11,14]. In addition, FtsZ acts in concert with the cell wall synthesis coordinator, MreB, in both septal cell wall synthesis and lateral cell wall synthesis at the poles of rod-shaped bacteria [15,16].

FtsZ is a highly druggable target, and benzamide-based FtsZ inhibitors (including PC190723, TXA707, and TXH9179, as well as their corresponding prodrugs TXY541, TXA709, and TXH1033, respectively) with potent bactericidal activity against clinically significant Gram-positive pathogens, such as methicillin- and vancomycin-resistant *S. aureus* (MRSA and VRSA, respectively), have been previously described by us and others [17–31]. However, these FtsZ-targeting drug candidates are typically associated with poor activity against Gram-negative bacteria [20,32]. One of the principal resistance mechanisms in Gram-negative bacteria is their outer membrane, a hydrophobic barrier that limits the intracellular accumulation of most antibiotics, including benzamide FtsZ inhibitors [33–35]. This barrier must be overcome to improve the intracellular uptake of FtsZ inhibitors by Gram-negative pathogens as well as their resultant antibacterial efficacy.

One appealing approach for enhancing antibiotic uptake by Gram-negative bacteria is the design of agents that incorporate iron-chelating siderophore functionalities into their structures [36]. Ferric iron (Fe^{3+}) is an essential nutrient for bacterial growth and survival, providing a critical redox factor for many important metabolic processes, including respiration, oxygen transport, and DNA synthesis [37,38]. However, Fe^{3+} availability is typically limited at sites of infection, due to restriction by the innate immune system in host environments [37–40]. To facilitate the scavenging of Fe^{3+} from the environment, bacteria synthesize and export molecules, termed siderophores, which chelate Fe^{3+} and are then internalized by the bacteria via dedicated uptake pathways [41,42]. Many clinically important Gram-negative pathogens, including *K. pneumoniae* and *A. baumannii*, rely on siderophores for Fe^{3+} acquisition and virulence [43,44]. Incorporation of Fe^{3+}-chelating siderophore functionalities in antibacterial drug structures offers the potential for drug uptake by endogenous siderophore uptake pathways. In support of this design approach, cefiderocol, a PBP-targeting cephalosporin analog containing an Fe^{3+}-chelating chlorocatechol moiety, has been recently approved for the treatment of complicated urinary tract infections caused by highly resistant Gram-negative pathogens [45–47].

In this study, we describe a novel oxazole-benzamide FtsZ inhibitor (**RUP4**) that, like cefiderocol, incorporates a Fe^{3+}-chelating chlorocatechol moiety. This chlorocatechol moiety contains hydroxyl groups at the 3- and 4-positions (Figure 1), which are designed to chelate Fe^{3+}. Significantly, **RUP4** is active against both *K. pneumoniae* and *A. baumannii*, in marked contrast to a corresponding negative control compound (**RUP5**) that lacks the hydroxyl group at the 3-position of the catechol moiety (Figure 1). We show that the antibacterial activity of **RUP4** against *K. pneumoniae* is due to its ability to chelate Fe^{3+} and that the compound utilizes endogenous *K. pneumoniae* siderophore-Fe^{3+} uptake transporters for entry into the bacteria. We also show that **RUP4** acts synergistically against *K. pneumoniae* when combined with select β-lactam antibiotics as well as a MreB inhibitor, with this bactericidal synergy being greatest upon combination with the PBP2-targeting antibiotic mecillinam and the MreB inhibitor TXH11106. Viewed as a whole, our results highlight **RUP4** as an appealing proof-of-concept agent for the design of next-generation benzamide FtsZ inhibitors with enhanced activity against Gram-negative bacterial pathogens.

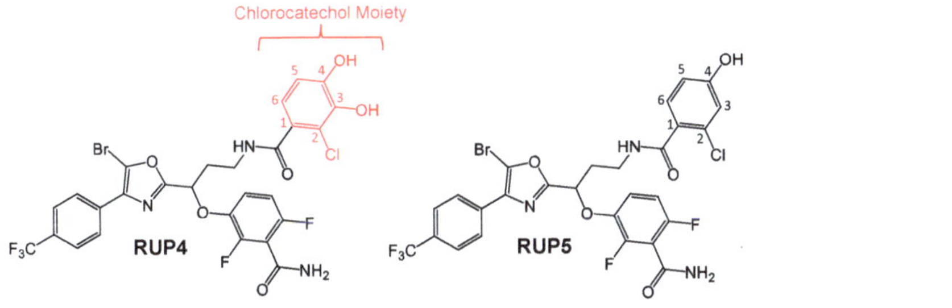

Figure 1. Chemical structures of **RUP4** and **RUP5**. The chlorocatechol siderophore moiety in **RUP4** is shown in red. The atomic numbering for the chlorocatechol moiety of **RUP4** and the equivalent ring of **RUP5** is also indicated.

2. Results

2.1. *Evaluation of **RUP4** and **RUP5** for Their Ability to Chelate* Fe^{3+}

We first sought to determine the potential for **RUP4** and **RUP5** to chelate Fe^{3+}. Nolan and co-workers have shown that catechol chelation of Fe^{3+} is associated with a ligand-to-metal charge transfer (LMCT) reaction that is manifested by the induction of a peak in the absorption spectrum of the catechol in the wavelength region of 400–750 nm [48]. In this connection, we measured the absorption spectra of 50 μM **RUP4** and **RUP5** in the absence or presence of an equimolar concentration of Fe^{3+}. The addition of Fe^{3+} to **RUP4** resulted in the induction of a broad absorbance peak in the region between 400 and 750 nm that was absent from the spectrum of either **RUP4** or Fe^{3+} alone (Figure 2A). This induced absorption peak is indicative of an LMCT reaction (denoted by the green arrow in Figure 2A). We observed the induction of similar LMCT peaks in the absorption spectra of our positive comparator control agents 3,4-dihydroxybenzoic acid (34DHBA) and cefiderocol (CEF) upon addition of Fe^{3+} (see spectra in Figure 2B and chemical structures of 34DHBA and CEF in Figure 2C). Note that the LMCT peak in the spectrum of **RUP5** in the presence of Fe^{3+} is markedly reduced in magnitude compared with the corresponding LMCT peak in the spectrum of **RUP4** (Figure 2A).

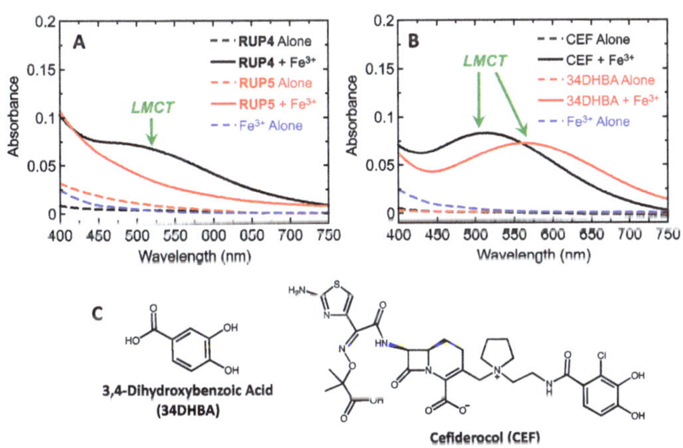

Figure 2. Absorption spectra of **RUP4** and **RUP5** (**A**) or 3,4-dihydroxybenzoic acid (34DHBA) and cefiderocol (CEF) (**B**) in the absence or presence of an equimolar concentration of added Fe^{3+}. All compounds were used at a concentration of 50 μM, and all absorbance spectra were acquired in 75 mM Tris-HCl (pH 8.0). The green arrows in (**A**) and (**B**) highlight absorption peaks representative of ligand-to-metal charge transfer (LMCT) reactions associated with compound chelation of Fe^{3+}. The chemical structures of 34DHBA and CEF are shown in (**C**).

2.2. Evaluation of **RUP4** and **RUP5** for Antibacterial Activity against *K. pneumoniae* and *A. baumannii*

We characterized the antibacterial activity of **RUP4** and **RUP5** against *K. pneumoniae* (ATCC 10031) and *A. baumannii* (ATCC 19606) in Fe^{3+}-limiting M9 media. In these studies, both compounds were assessed at concentrations up to their limits of solubility, with the resulting growth profiles being shown in Figure 3. **RUP4** inhibits the growth of both *K. pneumoniae* (Figure 3A) and *A. baumannii* (Figure 3B) with similar IC_{50} values of 25 ± 1 and 24 ± 2 μM, respectively, as well as corresponding minimal inhibitory concentration (MIC) values of 46 μM against *K. pneumoniae* and 185 μM against *A. baumannii* (Table 1). We also determined the minimal bactericidal concentration (MBC) of **RUP4** against *K. pneumoniae* to be 92 μM, a value twice the corresponding MIC of 46 μM, with the MBC of **RUP4** against *A. baumannii* being greater than the solubility limit of the compound (>185 μM). In marked contrast to **RUP4**, **RUP5** did not inhibit the growth of *K. pneumoniae* or *A. baumannii* to any significant degree (Figure 3), with associated IC_{50}, MIC, and MBC values all being greater than the solubility limit of the compound (>95 μM) (Table 1).

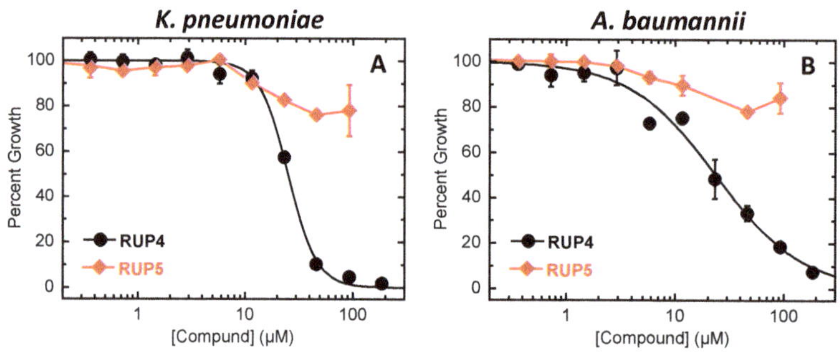

Figure 3. Impact of increasing concentrations of **RUP4** or **RUP5** on the percent growth of *K. pneumoniae* 10031 (**A**) or *A. baumannii* 19606 (**B**) in modified M9 media. Each experimental data point represents the average of three replicates, and the error bars reflect the standard deviation from the mean. The black curves represent nonlinear least squares fits of the experimental data points for **RUP4** using Equation (1).

Table 1. Antibacterial activities of **RUP4** and **RUP5** against *K. pneumoniae* and *A. baumannii*.

Strain	MIC (μM)		MBC (μM)	IC_{50} (μM)	
	RUP4	RUP5	RUP4	RUP4 *	RUP5
K. pneumoniae 10031	46	>95	92	25 ± 1	>95
A. baumannii 19606	185	>95	>185	24 ± 2	>95

MIC and MBC values were determined as described in Materials and Methods Section 4.3. * IC_{50} values for **RUP4** were determined from fits of the growth profiles shown in Figure 3 using Equation (1), with the indicated uncertainties reflecting the standard deviation of the fitted curves from the experimental data.

2.3. Impact of Added Exogenous Fe^{3+} on the Antibacterial Activity of **RUP4** against *K. pneumoniae*

We sought to determine whether the observed activity of **RUP4** against *K. pneumoniae* is sensitive to the concentration of exogenous Fe^{3+}. To this end, we explored the impact of adding 0, 2, 10, or 25 μM exogenous Fe^{3+} on the activity of **RUP4** against *K. pneumoniae* in modified M9 media. The resulting growth profiles are shown in Figure 4. Significantly, the addition of exogenous Fe^{3+} markedly reduced the activity of **RUP4**, as reflected by IC_{50} values that increased with increasing concentrations of added exogenous Fe^{3+} [with these IC_{50} values being 23 ± 1 μM with 0 μM added Fe^{3+}, 29 ± 1 μM with 2 μM added Fe^{3+}, 55 ± 6 μM with 10 μM added Fe^{3+}, and 73 ± 4 μM with 25 μM added Fe^{3+}] (Table 2).

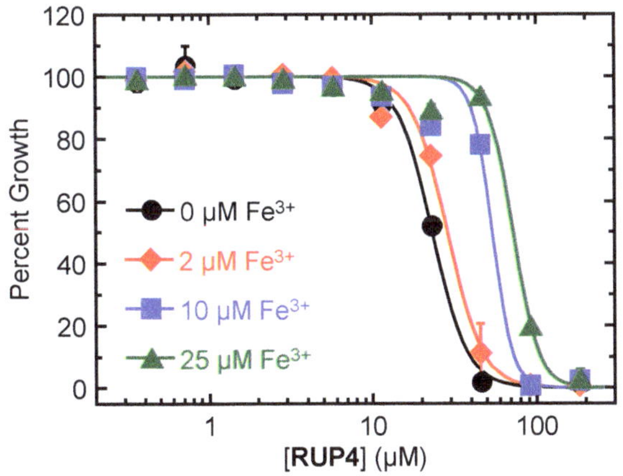

Figure 4. Impact of increasing concentrations of added exogenous Fe^{3+} on the antibacterial activity of **RUP4** against *K. pneumoniae* 10031 in modified M9 media. The media was supplemented with 0, 2, 10, or 25 μM Fe^{3+}. Each experimental data point represents the average of three replicates, and the error bars reflect the standard deviation from the mean. The solid curves represent nonlinear least squares fits of the experimental data points using Equation (1).

Table 2. Impact of added exogenous Fe^{3+} on the activity of **RUP4** against *K. pneumoniae* 10031.

Added [Fe^{3+}] (μM)	IC_{50} (μM)
0	23 ± 1
2	29 ± 1
10	55 ± 6
25	73 ± 4

IC_{50} values were determined from fits of the growth profiles shown in Figure 4 using Equation (1), with the indicated uncertainties reflecting the standard deviation of the fitted curves from the experimental data.

2.4. Expression of Siderophore Biosynthesis, Exporter, and Uptake Transporter Genes by K. pneumoniae in Nutrient-Rich CAMH Media Versus Fe^{3+}-Limiting M9 Media

As an initial step toward determining whether **RUP4** can utilize the native siderophore-Fe^{3+} uptake machinery of target bacteria, we first explored how Fe^{3+} restriction affects the expression of native siderophore uptake, biosynthesis, and exporter genes in *K. pneumoniae*. To this end, we used RT-qPCR to compare the expression of key siderophore uptake, biosynthesis, and exporter genes in nutrient-rich CAMH media versus Fe^{3+}-limiting M9 media. For siderophore uptake transporter genes, we evaluated the expression of the enterobactin outer membrane transporter *fepA*, the catecholate outer membrane transporters *cirA* and *fiu*, the ferrichrome outer membrane transporter *fhuA*, the enterobactin ABC inner membrane transporter components *fepD* and *fepG* (channel components) as well as *fepC* (ATPase), and the ferrichrome ABC inner membrane transporter components *fhuB* (channel) and *fhuC* (ATPase). For siderophore biosynthesis genes, we evaluated the expression of the catecholate synthesis pathway component *entB* and the enterobactin synthesis pathway component *entF*. For siderophore exporter genes, we evaluated expression of the enterobactin exporter *entS*. The expression of the bacterial transcription factor *rho* was used as an endogenous control for all comparisons.

Expression of all siderophore genes was significantly upregulated in M9 media relative to CAMH media (Figure 5). Among the outer membrane uptake transporters, *cirA* was upregulated to the greatest extent (82.1-fold), followed by *fhuA*, *fepA*, and *fiu* at 10.4-, 6.3-, and 4.5-fold, respectively. Among the inner membrane uptake transporters, *fepD* was upregulated to the greatest extent (9.7-fold), followed by *fhuB* and *fepG* at 2.8- and 2.5-fold, respectively. The inner membrane uptake transporter ATPases *fepC* and *fhuC* were upregulated by 16.1- and 5.9-fold, respectively. Finally, the catecholate siderophore synthesis genes *entF* and *entB* as well as the siderophore exporter gene *entS* were upregulated by 44.8-, 12.0-, and 30.1-fold, respectively.

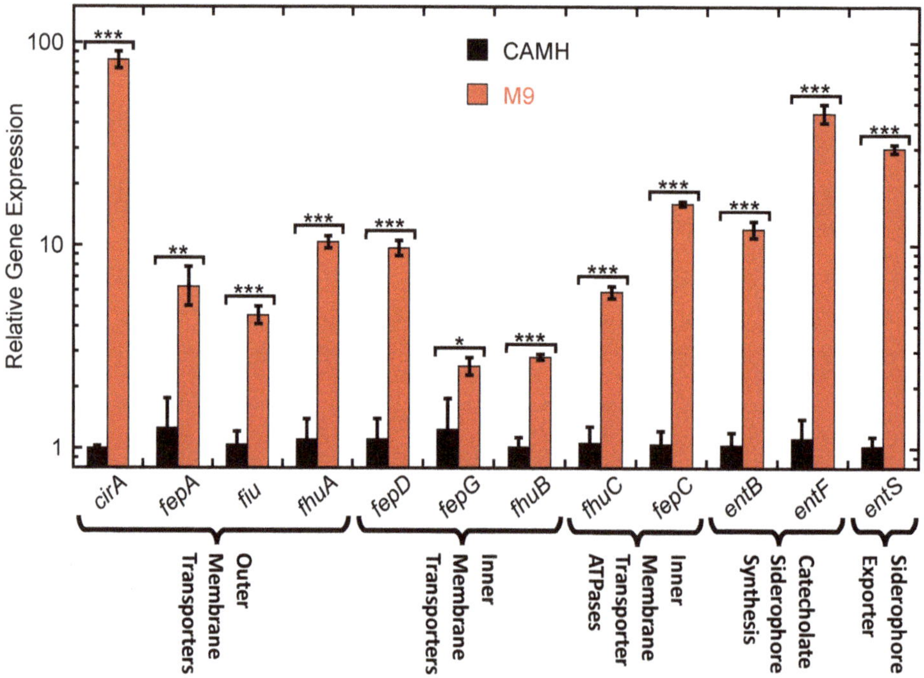

Figure 5. Relative expression of Fe^{3+} uptake outer membrane transporter, inner membrane transporter, inner membrane transporter ATPase, catecholate siderophore synthesis, and siderophore exporter genes in *K. pneumoniae* 10031 cells grown in either cation-adjusted Mueller Hinton (CAMH) or modified M9 media. Each bar represents an average of five replicates, and the error bars reflect the standard error from the mean. The statistical differences between gene expression levels in CAMH and M9 were determined by a Student's *t*-test. ***, $p \leq 0.001$; **, $0.01 \geq p > 0.001$; *, $0.05 \geq p > 0.01$.

*2.5. Impact of Deleting Select Siderophore-Fe^{3+} Uptake Transporter Genes on **RUP4** Activity against K. pneumoniae*

Towards the goal of elucidating the specific uptake pathway of **RUP4**, we generated mutant strains of *K. pneumoniae* containing a deletion of the siderophore-Fe^{3+} outer membrane transporter *fepA*, *fiu*, or *cirA*. We then compared the activity of **RUP4** against each of these deletion mutant strains (Δ*fepA*, Δ*fiu*, or Δ*cirA*) relative to the activity against the wild-type (WT) *K. pneumoniae* strain, with the corresponding growth profiles comparing Δ*fepA* and Δ*cirA* versus WT being shown in Figure 6A. The activity of **RUP4** was attenuated by approximately 4-fold against the Δ*fepA* mutant and 2-fold against the Δ*cirA* mutant, as reflected by IC_{50} values of 75 ± 5 μM for the Δ*fepA* strain and 35 ± 5 μM for the Δ*cirA* strain relative to 18 ± 1 μM for WT (Table 3). By contrast, the activity of **RUP4** against the Δ*fiu* strain (IC_{50} = 22 ± 4 μM) was comparable to the activity versus WT (Table 3).

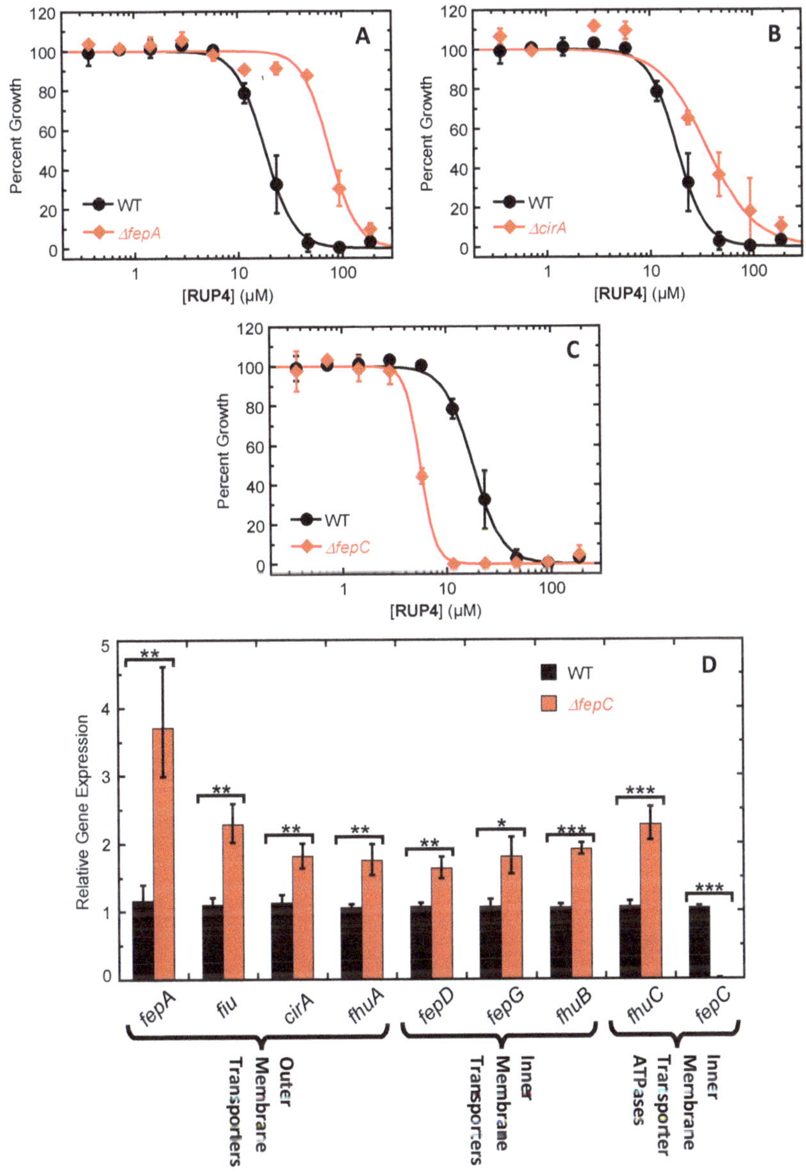

Figure 6. (**A**–**C**) Impact of deleting the *fepA* (**A**), *cirA* (**B**), or *fepC* (**C**) gene on the antibacterial activity of **RUP4** against *K. pneumoniae* 10031 in modified M9 media. Each experimental data point represents the average of five replicates, and the error bars reflect the standard error from the mean. The solid curves represent nonlinear least squares fits of the experimental data points using Equation (1). (**D**) Relative expression of Fe^{3+} uptake outer membrane transporter, inner membrane transporter, and inner membrane transporter ATPase genes in wild-type (WT) versus Δ*fepC* *K. pneumoniae* 10031 cells grown in modified M9 media. Each bar represents an average of five replicates, and the error bars reflect the standard error from the mean. The statistical differences between relative gene expression levels in WT versus Δ*fepC* cells were determined by a Student's *t*-test. ***, $p \leq 0.001$; **, $0.01 \geq p > 0.001$; *, $0.05 \geq p > 0.01$.

Table 3. Impact of deleting specific siderophore-Fe^{3+} uptake transporters on the activity of **RUP4** against *K. pneumoniae* 10031.

Strain	IC_{50} (μM)
WT	18 ± 1
Δ*fepA*	75 ± 5
Δ*cirA*	35 ± 5
Δ*fiu*	22 ± 4
Δ*fepC*	5.6 ± 0.1

IC_{50} values were determined from fits of growth profiles represented by those shown in Figure 6 using Equation (1), with the indicated uncertainties reflecting the standard deviation of the fitted curves from the experimental data.

We also generated a mutant strain of *K. pneumoniae* containing a deletion of the siderophore-Fe^{3+} inner membrane transporter ATPase *fepC*, with the corresponding growth profiles comparing Δ*fepC* versus WT being shown in Figure 6C. Unlike the attenuated activity exhibited by **RUP4** versus the Δ*fepA* and Δ*cirA* mutant strains relative to WT, the corresponding activity of the compound versus the Δ*fepC* mutant strain was enhanced by approximately 3-fold (IC_{50} = 5.6 ± 0.1 μM) relative to WT (Figure 6C, Table 3). To further explore the basis for the increased activity of **RUP4** against the Δ*fepC* mutant, we used RT-qPCR to compare the expression of the siderophore outer membrane uptake genes *fepA*, *fiu*, *cirA*, and *fhuA* as well as the inner membrane uptake genes *fepD*, *fepG*, *fhuB*, and *fhuC* in the Δ*fepC* mutant strain relative to WT. The expression of all the tested genes was significantly upregulated (Figure 6D). Among the outer membrane uptake genes, expression of *fepA* was upregulated to the greatest extent (3.7-fold), followed by *fiu*, *cirA*, and *fhuA* at 2.3-, 1.8-, and 1.7-fold, respectively. Expression of the inner membrane uptake genes *fepD*, *fepG*, *fhuB*, and *fhuC* was upregulated by 1.6-, 1.8-, 1.9-, and 2.3-fold, respectively.

2.6. Direct Binding of **RUP4** to Purified K. pneumoniae FtsZ (KpFtsZ)

As an initial step towards the validation of FtsZ as the antibacterial target of **RUP4**, we sought to demonstrate that **RUP4** can directly interact with purified KpFtsZ. To this end, we leveraged the intrinsic fluorescence properties of **RUP4**, whose excitation and emission spectra are shown in Figure S1. Specifically, we monitored the impact of added KpFtsZ on the fluorescence anisotropy of **RUP4** at 25 °C. The addition of KpFtsZ induced an increase in fluorescence anisotropy with increasing protein concentration (Figure 7A), indicative of a direct binding reaction. The resulting binding profile was fit with Equation (2) to yield a K_d value of 49 ± 5 μM.

2.7. Impact of **RUP4** on Cell Division and FtsZ Localization in K. pneumoniae

To further establish FtsZ as the antibacterial target of **RUP4**, we explored the impact of **RUP4** treatment on cell morphology and FtsZ localization in *K. pneumoniae* grown in Fe^{3+}-limiting M9 media. In these studies, *K. pneumoniae* cells were treated for 3 h with either DMSO vehicle or **RUP4** at 185.3 μM (4× MIC) and then labeled with 0.1 μM BOFP. Differential interference contrast (DIC) and fluorescence micrographs of the treated cells are shown in Figure 7B–E. Treatment with vehicle results in normal cell morphology and size, with approximately 3–8% of cells actively undergoing cell division. An actively dividing cell with FtsZ localized to the septum at the midcell is highlighted by the white arrow in Figure 7C. In non-dividing vehicle-treated cells, FtsZ often appears to localize in punctate regions at the cell poles (Figure 7C). In contrast to vehicle treatment, **RUP4** treatment results in enlarged and elongated cells with no defined septa and FtsZ more diffusely localized to foci throughout the cell as well as along the cell periphery (Figure 7D,E). This pattern of behavior is similar to that previously observed in rod-shaped bacteria that have been treated with a FtsZ inhibitor or in which FtsZ has been depleted [20,49,50].

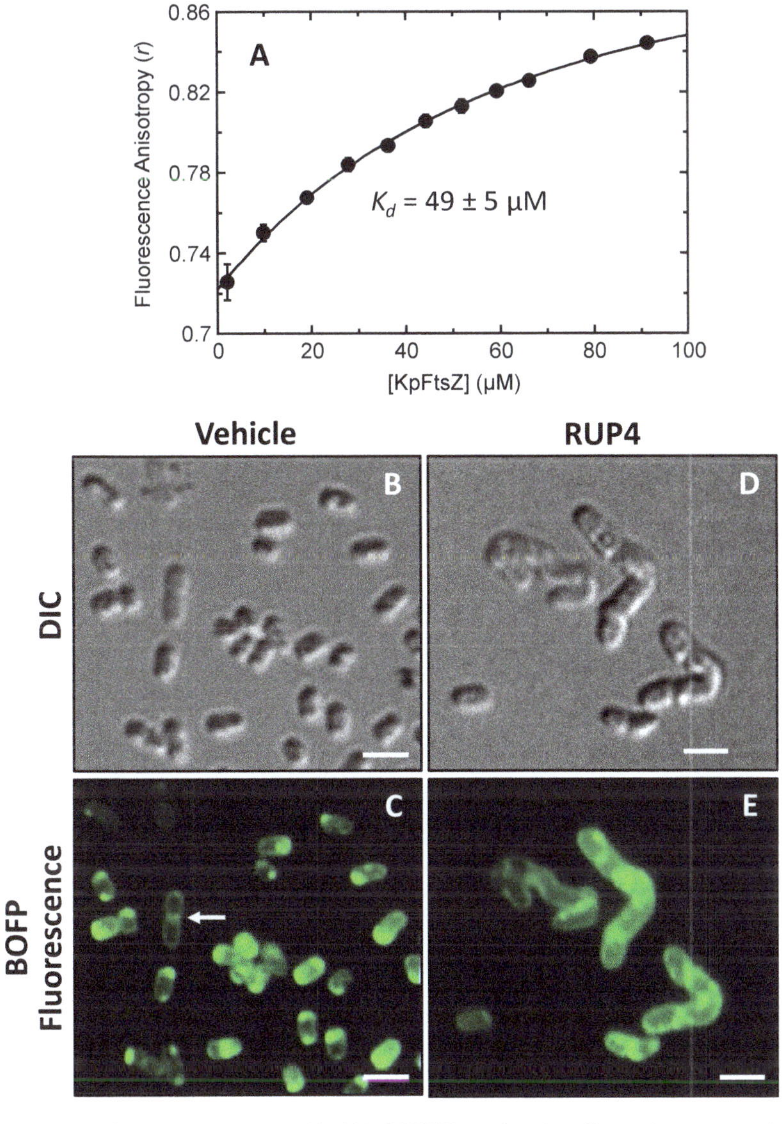

Figure 7. (**A**) Fluorescence anisotropy (r) of 20 μM RUP4 as a function of increasing concentrations of *K. pneumoniae* FtsZ (KpFtsZ). The titration experiment was conducted at 25 °C in a solution containing 50 mM Tris-HCl (pH 7.6) and 50 mM KCl. The solid curve represents a nonlinear least squares fit of the experimental data points using Equation (2), with the indicated dissociation constant (K_d) value being derived from this fit. (**B–E**) Differential interference contrast (DIC) and fluorescence micrographs of *K. pneumoniae* 10031 cells treated for 3 h with either DMSO vehicle (**B**,**C**) or 185.3 μM (4× MIC) **RUP4** (**D**,**E**). The fluorescence micrographs in (**C**,**E**) depict cells labeled with BOFP just prior to visualization. The white arrow in (**C**) highlights an actively dividing cell with FtsZ localized to the septum at midcell. Scale bars reflect 1 μm.

*2.8. Bactericidal Synergy of **RUP4** in Combination with Select PBP-Targeting β-Lactam Antibiotics and an MreB-Targeting Agent against K. pneumoniae*

We assessed the potential of **RUP4** to act synergistically in combination with various PBP-targeting β-lactam antibiotics [mecillinam (MEC), amoxicillin (AMX), piperacillin (PIP), cefazolin (CFZ), imipenem (IMI), and meropenem (MER)] as well as an MreB-targeting agent TXH11106 (TXH) we have previously developed [51]. In this connection, we evaluated the intrinsic activities of the test agents against *K. pneumoniae*, with the resulting MIC values being listed in Table S1. We then used a checkerboard assay to define the fractional inhibitory concentration (FIC) of each test agent and **RUP4** when used in combination against *K. pneumoniae*. For each combination, synergy is indicated when the FIC values for both agents are ≤0.25. Figure 8 shows the isobolograms plotting the FICs for **RUP4** as a function of the FICs for MEC (Figure 8A), PIP (Figure 8B), IMI (Figure 8C), or TXH (Figure 8D). All four test agents act synergistically with **RUP4**, as indicated by the presence of combination FICs in the lower left quadrant of the isobolograms (on or to the left of the black dashed line in each plot). The corresponding isobolograms for the combinations of **RUP4** and CFZ, AMX, or MER are plotted in Figure S2, with these plots revealing additive behavior (with combination FICs falling to the right of the black dashed line and on or to the left of the gray dashed line).

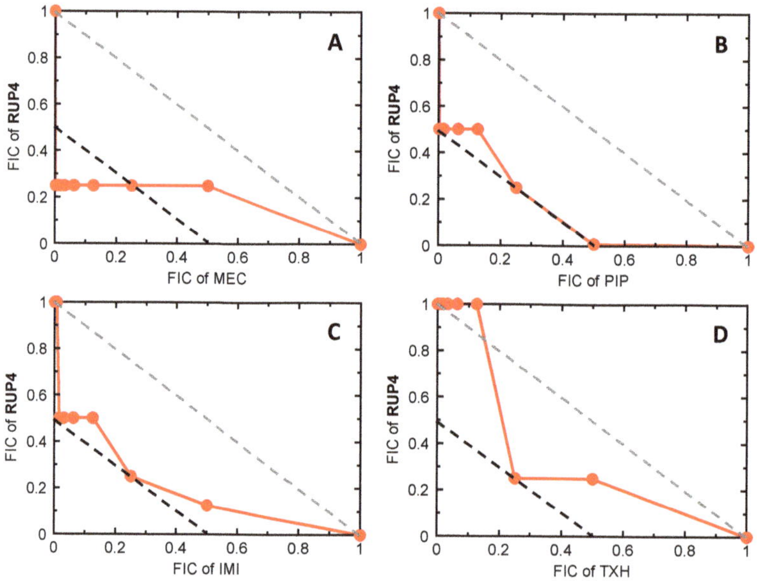

Figure 8. Isobolograms for *K. pneumoniae* 10031 treated with a combination of **RUP4** and either mecillinam (MEC) (**A**), piperacillin (PIP) (**B**), imipenem (IMI) (**C**), or TXH11106 (TXH) (**D**). In each plot, the black dashed line indicates the upper boundary for a synergistic combination, while the gray dashed line indicates the upper boundary for an additive combination. FIC denotes the fractional inhibitory concentration, as defined in Materials and Methods (Section 4.8.1.).

Another indication of synergistic versus additive activity is provided by the FIC index (FICI), defined as the sum of the FICs of the two agents being tested in combination. A FICI ≤ 0.5 is indicative of synergy, while a FICI > 0.5 but ≤1 is reflective of additivity. The synergistic actions of **RUP4** in combination with MEC are reflected by a FICI of 0.251 (Table 4), with those of **RUP4** in combination with PIP, IMI, or TXH being reflected by FICI values of 0.5. The additive behavior of **RUP4** in combination with CFZ, AMX, or MER is reflected by FICI values of 0.508, 0.531, and 0.531, respectively (Table 4).

Table 4. Combinatorial activities **RUP4** and select PBP-targeting β-lactam antibiotics or an MreB-targeting agent against *K. pneumoniae* 10031.

Test Agent (TA)	FIC_{TA}	FIC_{RUP4}	FICI
MEC	0.0005	0.25	0.2505
PIP	0.25	0.25	0.5
IMI	0.25	0.25	0.5
TXH	0.25	0.25	0.5
CFZ	0.008	0.5	0.508
AMX	0.031	0.5	0.531
MER	0.031	0.5	0.531

MEC = Mecillinam; PIP = Piperacillin; IMI = Imipenem; TXH = TXH11106; CFZ = Cefazolin; AMX = Amoxicillin; MER = Meropenem. FIC_{TA} and FIC_{RUP4} reflect the fractional inhibitory concentrations of the indicated antibacterial test agent and **RUP4**, respectively. The fractional inhibitory concentration index (FICI) reflects the sum of FIC_{TA} + FIC_{RUP4}. Synergistic combinations are indicated by a FICI $\leq$ 0.5 (denoted in red), while additive combinations are indicated by a FICI > 0.5 but $\leq$1.

In addition to checkerboard assays for synergy, we also performed time–kill assays of **RUP4** in combination with MEC, PIP, IMI, or TXH against *K. pneumoniae*. In these assays, cells were treated with DMSO vehicle, 0.5× MIC test agent alone, 0.5× MIC **RUP4** alone, or a combination of 0.5× MIC test agent and 0.5× MIC **RUP4,** and the number of colony-forming units (CFUs) was assessed after 0, 3, 6, 9, and 24 h of treatment. The resulting time–kill curves are shown in Figure 9. Treatment with either the test agent alone or **RUP4** alone resulted in growth at 24 h comparable to that of the vehicle. By contrast, the combination of each test agent with **RUP4** resulted in bactericidal behavior. In this connection, complete kill was observed after 6 h of treatment with the combination of MEC and **RUP4**, and after 9 h of treatment with the combination of TXH and **RUP4** (Figure 9A,D). Combination of **RUP4** and IMI or PIP resulted in 5-logs of kill within 24 h of treatment (Figure 9B,C).

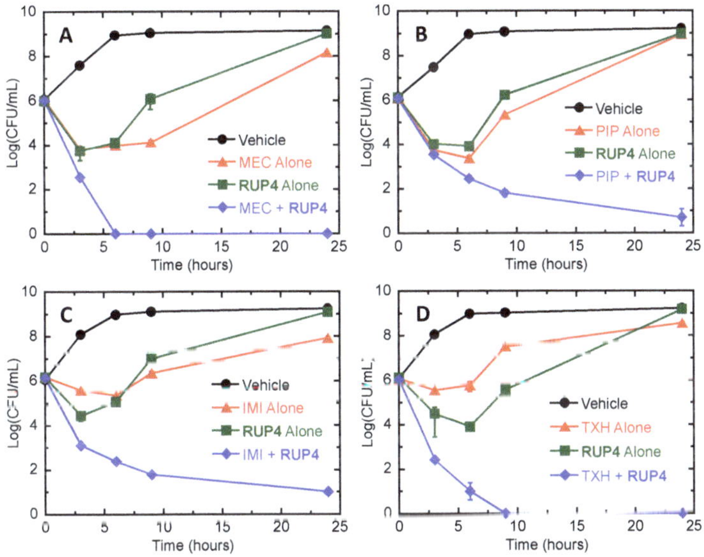

Figure 9. Time–kill curves for *K. pneumoniae* 10031 showing bactericidal synergy between **RUP4** and mecillinam (MEC) (**A**), piperacillin (PIP) (**B**), imipenem (IMI) (**C**), or TXH11106 (TXH) (**D**). Bacteria were treated with DMSO vehicle (black), test agent alone at 0.5× MIC (red), **RUP4** alone at 0.5× MIC (green), or a combination of test agent at 0.5× MIC and **RUP4** at 0.5× MIC (blue). Each experimental data point represents the average of two replicates, with the error bars reflecting the standard deviation from the mean.

3. Discussion

Gram-negative bacterial pathogens are often more difficult to treat than Gram-positive pathogens due to the presence of an outer membrane barrier that limits the intracellular accumulation of many antibiotics [33,35]. In this connection, benzamide-based FtsZ inhibitors have been associated with potent activity against Gram-positive pathogens like *S. aureus* while exhibiting poor or no activity against Gram-negative pathogens [17–31,34]. Here, we describe a strategy for overcoming this limitation by developing an oxazole-benzamide FtsZ inhibitor (**RUP4**) that incorporates a chlorocatechol siderophore moiety (Figure 1) and can utilize endogenous siderophore-Fe^{3+} uptake pathways to facilitate entry into the target bacterial cells. Significantly, **RUP4** is active against both *K. pneumoniae* and *A. baumannii* (Figure 3, Table 1), two Gram-negative pathogens of acute clinical importance. As indicated by MIC, the observed activity of **RUP4** is approximately 4-fold greater against *K. pneumoniae* (MIC = 46.3 μM) than against *A. baumannii* (MIC = 185.3 μM), though **RUP4** exhibited a similar IC_{50} value of approximately 25 μM against both pathogens (Table 1).

3.1. *Importance of the Catechol Siderophore Functionality for the Antibacterial Activity of* ***RUP4***

Our design strategy is premised on the hypothesis that the catechol siderophore moiety plays an important role in promoting the observed antibacterial activity of **RUP4**. To this end, we first sought to establish that the two hydroxyl groups at positions 3 and 4 of the **RUP4** catechol functionality (Figure 1) can chelate Fe^{3+}. Catechol chelation of Fe^{3+} is associated with a ligand-to-metal charge transfer (LMCT) reaction that is measurable by the induction of an absorption peak between 400 and 750 nm [48]. Consistent with such an Fe^{3+} chelation reaction, **RUP4** exhibits a robust LMCT peak in the presence of Fe^{3+} that is absent in the absorption spectra of either **RUP4** or Fe^{3+} alone (Figure 2A). The Fe^{3+}-chelating capability of **RUP4** is further supported by the corresponding spectra of the positive control molecules cefiderocol and 34DHBA, which exhibit similar LMCT peaks in the presence of Fe^{3+} (Figure 2B). By contrast, the spectrum of the negative control compound **RUP5**, which lacks the 3-hydroxyl on the catechol ring, has a markedly reduced LMCT peak (Figure 2A), indicative of an attenuated ability to chelate Fe^{3+}.

Armed with the knowledge that **RUP4** chelates Fe^{3+} to a significantly greater extent than **RUP5**, we determined if this differential capability manifested in a corresponding difference in antibacterial activity. Significantly, in striking contrast to **RUP4**, **RUP5** exerts a minimal impact on the growth of either *K. pneumoniae* or *A. baumannii* at concentrations up to its solubility limit of approximately 95 μM (Figure 3, Table 1). The absence of significant **RUP5** activity implies that the antibacterial activity of **RUP4** is linked to its ability to chelate Fe^{3+}. Consistent with this notion, we show that the activity of **RUP4** against *K. pneumoniae* is systematically reduced in the presence of increasing concentrations of added exogenous Fe^{3+} (Figure 4), with IC_{50} values ranging from 23 μM in the absence of added Fe^{3+} to 73 μM in the presence of 25 μM added Fe^{3+} (Table 2). In addition, the expression of siderophore-Fe^{3+} uptake transporter, catecholate siderophore biosynthesis, and siderophore exporter genes in *K. pneumoniae* is significantly upregulated under Fe^{3+}-limiting conditions (Figure 5). These collective results are indicative of **RUP4** utilizing endogenous siderophore-Fe^{3+} uptake pathways for its activity against *K. pneumoniae*.

We next sought to determine the specific siderophore-Fe^{3+} uptake transporters that **RUP4** can utilize for entry into *K. pneumoniae*. To this end, we generated deletion mutant strains of three different outer membrane transporters (Δ*fepA*, Δ*cirA*, and Δ*fiu*) in *K. pneumoniae* 10031 and compared the activity of **RUP4** against each deletion mutant strain relative to WT. The activity of **RUP4** was reduced against both the Δ*fepA* and Δ*cirA* strains compared to WT (Figure 6A,B), with the extent of this reduction being approximately 4-fold for the Δ*fepA* strain and 2-fold for the Δ*cirA* strain, as reflected by IC_{50} values (Table 3). By contrast, **RUP4** exhibited similar activity against the Δ*fiu* strain relative to WT (Table 3). These results suggest that **RUP4** crosses the outer membrane through both the FepA and CirA transporters, with FepA being the predominant transporter (schematically depicted in Figure 10).

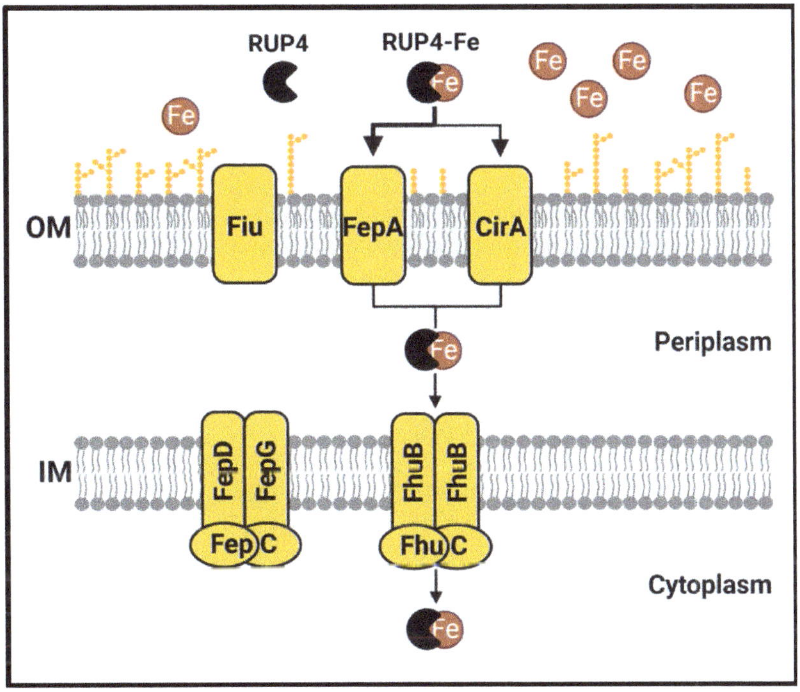

Figure 10. Putative mechanism for the uptake of **RUP4** into *K. pneumoniae* by endogenous outer membrane (OM) and inner membrane (IM) siderophore-Fe^{3+} uptake transporters.

We also generated a deletion mutant strain of the inner membrane transporter ATPase *fepC*. Surprisingly, the activity of **RUP4** against the Δ*fepC* strain was improved by approximately 3-fold compared to WT (Figure 6C, Table 3), suggesting that the enterobactin inner membrane transporter FepCDG is not the principal transporter through which **RUP4** crosses the inner membrane. To better understand the enhanced activity of **RUP4** against the Δ*fepC* strain, we measured the expression of all siderophore-Fe^{3+} uptake transporter genes in the Δ*fepC* strain relative to WT. Significantly, expression of the outer membrane transporter genes *fepA* and *fiu*, as well as the ferrichrome inner membrane transporter genes *fhuB* and *fhuC*, was among the most upregulated (Figure 6D), with *fepA* expression being upregulated to the greatest extent of all (approximately 3.7-fold). As previously noted, FepA appears to be the principle outer membrane transporter utilized by **RUP4**. Furthermore, aside from FepCDG, FhuBC is the only other inner membrane uptake transporter present in *K. pneumoniae* 10031. These collective results suggest that **RUP4** utilizes the FhuBC transporter for crossing the inner membrane, and the increased activity of **RUP4** against the Δ*fepC* strain relative to WT is primarily due to the increased expression of genes encoding the FepA and FhuBC transporters. Viewed as a whole, our genetic studies in *K. pneumoniae* are consistent with a putative uptake pathway (depicted in Figure 10) in which **RUP4** utilizes predominantly FepA but also CirA for crossing the outer membrane while utilizing FhuBC for crossing the inner membrane.

3.2. Validation of FtsZ as the Antibacterial Target of **RUP4**

As important as establishing the importance of the catechol siderophore moiety for the antibacterial activity of **RUP4** is verifying that incorporation of the catechol functionality does not hinder the ability of the compound to target FtsZ. In this connection, we first sought to confirm that **RUP4** can directly interact with FtsZ. To assay **RUP4** binding, we monitored changes in the fluorescence anisotropy of **RUP4** as a function of added KpFtsZ. We found that KpFtsZ increased the fluorescence anisotropy of **RUP4** in a concentration-dependent manner (Figure 7A), indicative of a direct binding reaction. Analysis of the resulting binding profile revealed that the binding interaction is associated with a K_d of 49 μM, a value similar in magnitude to the observed IC_{50} (25 μM) and MIC (46 μM) of **RUP4** against wild-type *K. pneumoniae* (Table 1).

To further establish FtsZ as the antibacterial target of **RUP4**, we explored the impact of **RUP4** on morphology and FtsZ localization in live *K. pneumoniae* cells. Previous studies have shown that FtsZ inhibition or depletion in rod-shaped Gram-negative bacteria results in elongated cells that lack septa, with FtsZ being more diffusely localized throughout the elongated cell [49,50]. Consistent with this behavior, treatment of *K. pneumoniae* with **RUP4** results in elongated cells that lack septa and exhibit a pattern of dispersed FtsZ localization (Figure 7D,E). This behavior markedly contrasts that observed in vehicle-treated cells, which exhibit normal size and shape as well as FtsZ localization either to the poles of non-dividing cells or to the septa of actively dividing cells (Figure 7B,C).

A third observation consistent with FtsZ being the antibacterial target of **RUP4** is the bactericidal action of the compound, as revealed by an MBC/MIC ratio of 2 against *K. pneumoniae* (Table 1). This type of behavior agrees with numerous previous studies demonstrating that FtsZ inhibitors act in a bactericidal fashion [17–22,25,27,29]. In the aggregate, the collective studies described above are fully consistent with **RUP4** acting as a FtsZ inhibitor.

3.3. Synergistic Drug Combinations with **RUP4**

Synergistic antibiotic combinations offer the potential for enhancing potency, reducing the potential for both toxicity and resistance, and repurposing existing drugs [52]. We therefore explored if the activity of **RUP4** against *K. pneumoniae* could be enhanced by a synergistic combination with other antibiotics. To this end, we probed for potential synergy when combining **RUP4** with select β-lactam antibiotics as well as a MreB inhibitor. **RUP4** exhibited bactericidal synergy in combination with the PBP2-targeting antibiotic mecillinam, the PBP3-targeting antibiotic piperacillin, the carbapenem antibiotic imipenem (which primarily targets PBP2 and PBP4), and the MreB-targeting agent TXH11106 (Figures 8 and 9, Table 4). The strongest bactericidal synergy was observed with mecillinam and TXH11106, with complete bacterial kill observed after 6–9 h of combination treatment (Figure 9A,D). Both PBP2 and MreB are critical components of the bacterial elongasome complex that synthesizes the lateral cell wall in rod-shaped bacteria and are known to transiently localize to the early divisome at the septum [15,53,54]. These results suggest that combining FtsZ inhibitors with agents that target the bacterial elongasome complex, including PBP2 and MreB, is an especially appealing strategy for enhancing the activity of FtsZ inhibitors against Gram-negative pathogens. In addition, mecillinam is associated with very poor intrinsic activity against *K. pneumoniae* 10031, with an associated MIC of 3147 μM (Table S3). However, combination with **RUP4** strongly activates mecillinam, as reflected by an FIC of 0.0005 (Table 4). Thus, combination with FtsZ inhibitors can also repurpose β-lactam antibiotics for use against Gram-negative pathogens that were previously resistant to those drugs. Future studies will be directed at further optimizing the antibacterial activity of **RUP4** both through chemical modification and in combination with other antibiotics.

4. Materials and Methods

4.1. Bacterial Strains, Growth Media, and Reagents

K. pneumoniae ATCC 10031 and *A. baumannii* ATCC 19606 were acquired from the American Type Culture Collection (ATCC, Manassas, VA, USA). Strains of *K. pneumoniae* 10031 containing the Δ*fepA*, Δ*fiu*, Δ*cirA*, and Δ*fepC* deletions were generated as described in the Supplementary Materials (Section 2). Unless otherwise noted, bacterial strains were grown in modified M9 minimal growth media (6.8 g/L Na_2HPO_4, 3 g/L KH_2PO_4, 0.5 g/L NaCl, 1 g/L NH_4Cl) supplemented with 0.4% glucose, 2 mM $MgSO_4$, 0.1 mM $CaCl_2$,

0.2% low-iron casein amino acids, and 16.5 μg/mL thiamine hydrochloride [48]. Agar, casein amino acids, cation-adjusted Mueller-Hinton (CAMH) media, Luria-Bertani (LB) media, and trypticase soy agar (TSA) were obtained from Becton Dickinson (Franklin Lakes, NJ, USA). Phosphate-buffered saline (PBS) was obtained from Lonza (Walkersville, MD, USA), and Tris-acetate-EDTA (TAE) buffer was obtained from Thermo Fisher Scientific (Waltham, MA, USA. Imipenem was obtained from LKT Labs (St. Paul, MN, USA), mecillinam was obtained from RPI (Mount Prospect, IL, USA), and meropenem was obtained from Toku-E (Bellingham, WA, USA). Amoxicillin, piperacillin, cefazolin, pentamidine isethionate, D-(+)-glucose, and thiamine hydrochloride were obtained from Sigma-Aldrich (St. Louis, MO, USA).

4.2. Compound Synthesis and *K. pneumoniae* FtsZ Protein Expression and Purification

RUP4 and **RUP5** were synthesized as detailed in the Supplementary Materials. BOFP was synthesized as described previously [49] and is also available from Millipore-Sigma (#SCT090). TXH11106 was synthesized as described previously [51]. *K. pneumoniae* FtsZ (KpFtsZ) was expressed and purified as described previously [49].

4.3. Antibacterial Assays

Two-fold serial dilutions of **RUP4** and **RUP5** were prepared in microtiter plates containing M9 media following Clinical and Laboratory Standards Institute (CLSI) protocols for broth microdilution assays [55]. The final volume in each well was 100 μL, and each test concentration was present in triplicate. Log-phase bacteria were added to the microtiter plates at a final concentration of 5×10^5 CFU/mL. All plates were incubated with shaking at 37 °C for 18 h. Bacterial growth in each well was determined by measuring the optical density at 600 nm (OD_{600}) using a VersaMax plate reader (Molecular Devices, San Jose, CA, USA). The percent growth of bacteria in each well corresponding to the associated OD_{600} value was then determined by normalization with the OD_{600} value associated with the bacterial growth in the absence of the test compound (100% growth) and the background value in M9 media alone (0% growth). These percent growth values were then plotted versus compound concentration (C), and IC_{50} values were derived from non-linear least squares fits of the resulting plots with the following relationship:

$$\text{Percent Growth} = \frac{100}{1 + \left(\frac{C}{IC_{50}}\right)^m} \quad (1)$$

In this relationship, m is the Hill slope.

Values of MBC for **RUP4** were determined by plating (in triplicate) on TSA plates 50 μL of solution from the wells corresponding to 1×, 2×, and 4× MIC. These plates were incubated at 37 °C for 24 h and counts of CFU/mL were then determined. MBC values were defined as the lowest compound concentration that yielded ≥3 logs of kill relative to the initial inoculum of 5×10^5 CFU/mL.

For assays determining the effect of added exogenous Fe^{3+} on **RUP4** activity, separate tubes containing 5 mL of M9 media were supplemented with 0, 2, 10, or 25 μM $FeCl_3$. The tubes were then inoculated with *K. pneumoniae* 10031 and incubated with shaking at 37 °C overnight. The overnight cultures were then diluted 1:10 in M9 media supplemented with the appropriate concentration of $FeCl_3$ and incubated with shaking at 37 °C to mid-log phase. Microtiter plates containing two-fold serial dilutions of **RUP4** were prepared as described above. The M9 media in each plate was supplemented with 0, 2, 10, or 25 μM $FeCl_3$. Each microtiter plate was then inoculated with 5×10^5 CFU/mL of log-phase bacteria grown in the corresponding concentration of $FeCl_3$, and the microtiter plates were then incubated with shaking at 37 °C for 18 h. Bacterial growth in each well was determined as described above.

4.4. Absorption Spectroscopy

All absorption experiments were conducted at 25 °C using an AVIV model 14DS spectrophotometer (Aviv Biomedical, Lakewood, NJ, USA) equipped with thermoelectric temperature control. Solutions containing 50 μM of either **RUP4**, **RUP5**, 3,4-dihydroxybenzoic acid (34DHBA), or cefiderocol (CEF) were prepared in 75 mM Tris-HCl (pH 8.0), and an absorbance spectrum of each solution was acquired from 750 to 400 nm in 1-nm increments (with an averaging time of 0.5 s for each reading). Furthermore, 50 μM of $FeCl_3$ was added directly to each compound solution, and an absorbance spectrum was obtained as described above. Corresponding absorbance spectra of buffer alone and buffer with 50 μM $FeCl_3$ were acquired as background controls.

4.5. Fluorescence Spectroscopy

Fluorescence spectroscopy experiments were conducted at 25 °C using an AVIV Model ATF105 spectrofluorometer (Aviv Biomedical, Lakewood, NJ, USA), with bandwidths set to 5 nm in both the excitation and emission directions. Excitation and emission spectra of 20 μM RUP4 (in buffer consisting of 50 mM Tris-HCl, pH 7.6, and 50 mM KCl) were acquired in 1-nm increments with an averaging time of 1 s for each reading. The excitation spectrum was acquired with the emission wavelength set at 508 nm, and the emission spectrum was acquired with the excitation wavelength set at 319 nm. For these experiments, a quartz cell (Hellma, Plainview, NY, USA) was used with a path length of 1 cm in both the excitation and emission directions.

For the fluorescence anisotropy measurements, the excitation and emission wavelengths were set to 319 and 508 nm, respectively. KpFtsZ was titrated into a solution containing 20 μM **RUP4** in the same buffer used for the acquisition of the excitation and emission spectra, with the final concentrations of KpFtsZ ranging from 2–91 μM. After each protein addition, the samples were equilibrated for 5 min, and the fluorescence anisotropy (r) was recorded, with each r value being the average of 5 readings. For these experiments, a quartz ultra-micro cell (Hellma, Plainview, NY, USA) was used with a 2 mm × 5 mm aperture and a 15 mm center height. The path lengths in the excitation and emission directions were 1 and 0.2 cm, respectively.

Values of r were plotted as a function of KpFtsZ concentration, and the K_d value for the binding reaction was derived from the non-linear least squares fit of the resulting plot with the following 1:1 binding formalism:

$$r = r_0 + \left(\frac{r_\infty - r_0}{2[P]_{tot}}\right) \times ([C]_{tot} + [P]_{tot} + K_d) - \sqrt{([C]_{tot} + [P]_{tot} + K_d)^2 - 4[C]_{tot}[P]_{tot}} \quad (2)$$

In this relationship, r_0 is the fluorescence anisotropy in the absence of KpFtsZ, r_∞ is the fluorescence anisotropy in the presence of an infinite concentration of KpFtsZ, $[C]_{tot}$ is the total concentration of **RUP4**, and $[P]_{tot}$ is the total concentration of KpFtsZ.

4.6. Differential Interference Contrast (DIC) and Fluorescence Microscopy

Log-phase *K. pneumoniae* 10031 bacteria were diluted to 0.1 OD_{600} and treated (with shaking) for 3 h at 37 °C with **RUP4** at 4× MIC (185 μM) or an equal volume of DMSO. The cells were then washed, labeled with BOFP, and imaged by DIC and fluorescence microscopy as described previously [49].

4.7. RNA Extraction and Reverse Transcription-Quantitative Polymerase Chain Reaction (RT-qPCR) Assays

RT-qPCR assays comparing expression levels of siderophore-Fe^{3+} uptake genes (*fepA*, *cirA*, *fiu*, *cirA*, *fhuA*, *fepD*, *fepG*, *fhuB*, *fepC*, and *fhuC*), enterobactin synthesis genes (*entB* and *entF*), and an enterobactin exporter gene (*entS*) in *K. pneumoniae* 10031 cells grown in either CAMH or M9 media were performed using a Luna Universal One-Step RT-qPCR Kit (New England Biolabs, Ipswich, MA, USA). The bacterial transcription termination factor gene *rho* was used as an endogenous control for all assays. Briefly, RNA was extracted from five different replicates of log-phase *K. pneumoniae* 10031 cells grown in either CAMH or M9 media using a RNeasy Mini Kit (Qiagen, Germantown, MD, USA), and contaminating DNA was removed using a TURBO DNA-free Kit (Thermo Fisher Scientific, Waltham, MA, USA). Samples containing 1× Luna Universal One-Step Reaction Mix, 1× Luna WarmStart RT Enzyme Mix, 0.4 μM forward primer, 0.4 μM reverse primer, and 25 ng of total RNA were prepared in nuclease-free water. The primers used for each gene are listed in Table S2. The samples were then transferred to a MicroAmp Optical 96-Well Reaction Plate (Applied Biosystems, Waltham, MA, USA). Each sample was added in triplicate, and the final volume in each reaction well was 20 μL. The plate was then affixed with a MicroAmp Optical Adhesive Film (Applied Biosystems, Waltham, MA, USA) and centrifuged at maximum speed in a VWR plate centrifuge for 2 min. The reaction plate was then inserted into a QuantStudio 5 real-time PCR system (Applied Biosystems, Waltham, MA, USA) affixed with a 96-well 0.2 mL block. A comparative C_T ($\Delta\Delta C_T$) experiment was run with the SYBR Green Reagents chemistry setting, utilizing the standard Luna Universal One-Step RT-qPCR thermocycling protocol. The protocol consisted of: (a) reverse transcription, 1 cycle of 55 °C for 1 min; (b) initial denaturation, 1 cycle of 95 °C for 1 min; (c) 40 cycles of denaturation at 95 °C for 10 s followed by extension at 60 °C for 30 s with plate read; and (d) 1 cycle of a three-step melt curve consisting of (i) 95 °C for 15 s, (ii) 60 °C for 1 min, and (iii) 95 °C for 15 s. The resulting amplification plots were visualized and analyzed using the QuantStudio Design and Analysis Software (v1.5.2). The statistical significance of differences in relative gene expression was analyzed with a Student's *t*-test. Assays comparing the gene expression levels of *fepA*, *cirA*, *fiu*, *fhuA*, *fepD*, *fepG*, *fhuB*, *fepC*, and *fhuC* in WT versus Δ*fepC* *K. pneumoniae* 10031 cells were performed as described above.

4.8. Antibacterial Synergy Assays

4.8.1. Checkerboard Assays

The checkerboard assay [56] was used to evaluate the synergy between **RUP4** and the test agents mecillinam, piperacillin, imipenem, TXH11106, amoxicillin, meropenem, and cefazolin against *K. pneumoniae* 10031. These assays were performed as described previously [57]. The fractional inhibitory concentration for each test agent (FIC_{TA}) was determined from the ratio of the MIC of the test agent in combination with **RUP4** to the MIC of the test agent alone. The fractional inhibitory concentration for **RUP4** (FIC_{RUP4}) was determined from the ratio of the MIC of **RUP4** in combination with each test agent to the MIC of **RUP4** alone. The values of FIC_{TA} and FIC_{RUP4} were then used to determine the corresponding FIC index (FICI) using the relationship $FICI = FIC_{TA} + FIC_{RUP4}$. A FICI ≤ 0.5 is indicative of a synergistic RUP4-test agent combination, while a FICI > 0.5 but $\leq$1.0 is indicative of an additive combination.

4.8.2. Time–Kill Assays

Overnight cultures of *K. pneumoniae* 10031 were diluted to 10^6 CFU/mL in four separate culture tubes containing 5 mL of M9 media. DMSO vehicle was added to the first tube, **RUP4** at 0.5× MIC (23 μM) alone was added to the second tube, test agent alone at 0.5× MIC (1574 μM mecillinam, 7.4 μM piperacillin, 0.8 μM imipenem, or 16 μM TXH11106) was added to the third tube, and a combination of 0.5× MIC **RUP4** and 0.5× MIC test agent was added to the final tube. Time-dependent kill assays were then conducted at 37 °C over a period of 24 h, as described previously [57].

5. Conclusions

Here we describe **RUP4** as a novel oxazole-benzamide FtsZ inhibitor that incorporates a chlorocatechol siderophore moiety and exhibits antibacterial activity against the clinically important Gram-negative pathogens *K. pneumoniae* and *A. baumannii*. Fe^{3+} chelation and addback studies establish that the catechol siderophore functionality plays a key role in the activity of **RUP4**. In this connection, **RUP4** is able to utilize endogenous siderophore uptake transporters for entry into *K. pneumoniae*, crossing the bacterial outer membrane through the FepA and CirA transporters and the inner membrane through the FhuBC transporter system. We validate FtsZ as the antibacterial target of **RUP4** by demonstrating the direct interaction of the compound with KpFtsZ as well as the induction of changes in morphology and FtsZ localization in treated *K. pneumoniae* cells consistent with FtsZ inhibition. Finally, synergy studies reveal that combinations of **RUP4** with select PBP- and MreB-targeting agents are associated with bactericidal synergy against *K. pneumoniae*, with combinations involving agents that target PBP2 and MreB being the most synergistic. Viewed as a whole, our results highlight the incorporation of Fe^{3+}-chelating siderophore moieties into FtsZ inhibitors as a promising design strategy for enhancing activity against Gram-negative pathogens of acute clinical significance.

Supplementary Materials: The following supporting information can be downloaded at: https://www.mdpi.com/article/10.3390/antibiotics13030209/s1. Figure S1: Excitation and emission spectra of **RUP4** at 25 °C; Figure S2: Isobolograms for *K. pneumoniae* treated with a combination of **RUP4** and either cefazolin (CFZ), amoxicillin (AMX), or meropenem (MER); Table S1: Intrinsic activities of test β-lactam antibiotics and a MreB-targeting agent against *K. pneumoniae*; Table S2: Sequences of the oligonucleotide primers used in the qPCR studies of the *K. pneumoniae* wild-type and deletion mutant strains; Table S3: Sequences of the oligonucleotide primers used for deleting and sequencing ferric iron transporter genes in *K. pneumoniae*; Supplementary Methods: Compound synthesis and generation of Δ*fepA*, Δ*fiu*, Δ*cirA*, and Δ*fepC* mutant strains of *K. pneumoniae*. References [24,58,59] are cited in the Supplementary Materials.

Author Contributions: E.J.B. contributed to the conceptualization and performance of the experiments, interpretation of the results, and writing and editing of the paper. Q.Q. contributed to the conceptualization and performance of the experiments and the interpretation of the results. Y.W. contributed to the conceptualization of the experiments and the interpretation of the results. J.Y.R. contributed to the conceptualization of the experiments, interpretation of the results, and writing and editing of the paper. E.J.L. contributed to the conceptualization of the experiments, interpretation of the results, and editing of the paper. D.S.P. contributed to the conceptualization of the experiments, interpretation of the results, writing and editing of the paper, and funding acquisition. All authors have read and agreed to the published version of the manuscript.

Funding: This research was funded by grant # PC 154-23 from the New Jersey Health Foundation (to D.S.P.), a Busch Biomedical Grant from Rutgers University (to D.S.P.), and a Rutgers University Core Facilities Utilization Grant (to D.S.P.).

Institutional Review Board Statement: Not applicable.

Informed Consent Statement: Not applicable.

Data Availability Statement: Data are contained within the article and Supplementary Materials.

Conflicts of Interest: The authors declare no conflicts of interest.

References

1. World Health Organization. *Global Action Plan on Antimicrobial Resistance*; World Health Organization: Geneva, Switzerland, 2015.
2. Centers for Disease Control and Prevention. *Antibiotic Resistance Threats in the United States, 2019*; Centers for Disease Control and Prevention: Atlanta, GA, USA, 2019.
3. Ventola, C.L. The Antibiotic Resistance Crisis: Part 1: Causes and Threats. *Pharm. Ther.* **2015**, *40*, 277–283.
4. Murray, C.J.L.; Ikuta, K.S.; Sharara, F.; Swetschinski, L.; Robles Aguilar, G.; Gray, A.; Han, C.; Bisignano, C.; Rao, P.; Wool, E.; et al. Global Burden of Bacterial Antimicrobial Resistance in 2019: A Systematic Analysis. *Lancet* **2022**, *399*, 629–655. [CrossRef] [PubMed]
5. O-Neill, J. *Antimicrobial Resistance: Tackling a Crisis for the Health and Wealth of Nations*; Wellcome Collection: London, UK, 2014.
6. Oliveira, D.M.P.D.; Forde, B.M.; Kidd, T.J.; Harris, P.N.A.; Schembri, M.A.; Beatson, S.A.; Paterson, D.L.; Walker, M.J. Antimicrobial Resistance in ESKAPE Pathogens. *Clin. Microbiol. Rev.* **2020**, *33*, e00181-19. [CrossRef] [PubMed]
7. Breijyeh, Z.; Jubeh, B.; Karaman, R. Resistance of Gram-Negative Bacteria to Current Antibacterial Agents and Approaches to Resolve It. *Molecules* **2020**, *25*, 1340. [CrossRef]
8. Morris, S.; Cerceo, E. Trends, Epidemiology, and Management of Multi-Drug Resistant Gram-Negative Bacterial Infections in the Hospitalized Setting. *Antibiotics* **2020**, *9*, 196. [CrossRef]

9. Kyriakidis, I.; Vasileiou, E.; Pana, Z.D.; Tragiannidis, A. *Acinetobacter baumannii* Antibiotic Resistance Mechanisms. *Pathogens* **2021**, *10*, 373. [CrossRef] [PubMed]
10. Navon-Venezia, S.; Kondratyeva, K.; Carattoli, A. *Klebsiella pneumoniae*: A Major Worldwide Source and Shuttle for Antibiotic Resistance. *FEMS Microbiol. Rev.* **2017**, *41*, 252–275. [CrossRef]
11. Margolin, W. FtsZ and the Division of Prokaryotic Cells and Organelles. *Nat. Rev. Mol. Cell Biol.* **2005**, *6*, 862–871. [CrossRef] [PubMed]
12. Silber, N.; Opitz, C.L.M.d.; Mayer, C.; Sass, P. Cell Division Protein FtsZ: From Structure and Mechanism to Antibiotic Target. *Future Microbiol.* **2020**, *15*, 801–831. [CrossRef]
13. Adams, D.W.; Errington, J. Bacterial Cell Division: Assembly, Maintenance and Disassembly of the Z Ring. *Nat. Rev. Microbiol.* **2009**, *7*, 642–653. [CrossRef]
14. Erickson, H.P.; Anderson, D.E.; Osawa, M. FtsZ in Bacterial Cytokinesis: Cytoskeleton and Force Generator All in One. *Microbiol. Mol. Biol. Rev.* **2010**, *74*, 504–528. [CrossRef]
15. Fenton, A.K.; Gerdes, K. Direct Interaction of FtsZ and MreB is Required for Septum Synthesis and Cell Division in *Escherichia coli*. *Embo J.* **2013**, *32*, 1953–1965. [CrossRef]
16. Varma, A.; Pedro, M.A.d.; Young, K.D. FtsZ Directs a Second Mode of Peptidoglycan Synthesis in *Escherichia coli*. *J. Bacteriol.* **2007**, *189*, 5692–5704. [CrossRef]
17. Bryan, E.; Ferrer-González, E.; Sagong, H.Y.; Fujita, J.; Mark, L.; Kaul, M.; LaVoie, E.J.; Matsumura, H.; Pilch, D.S. Structural and Antibacterial Characterization of a New Benzamide FtsZ Inhibitor with Superior Bactericidal Activity and In Vivo Efficacy against Multidrug-Resistant *Staphylococcus aureus*. *ACS Chem. Biol.* **2023**, *18*, 629–642. [CrossRef]
18. Chiodini, G.; Pallavicini, M.; Zanotto, C.; Bissa, M.; Radaelli, A.; Straniero, V.; Bolchi, C.; Fumagalli, L.; Ruggeri, P.; De Giuli Morghen, C.; et al. Benzodioxane–Benzamides as New Bacterial Cell Division Inhibitors. *Eur. J. Med. Chem.* **2015**, *89*, 252–265. [CrossRef]
19. Deng, J.; Zhang, T.; Li, B.; Xu, M.; Wang, Y. Design, Synthesis and Biological Evaluation of Biphenyl-Benzamides as Potent FtsZ Inhibitors. *Eur. J. Med. Chem.* **2022**, *239*, 114553. [CrossRef]
20. Haydon, D.J.; Stokes, N.R.; Ure, R.; Galbraith, G.; Bennett, J.M.; Brown, D.R.; Baker, P.J.; Barynin, V.V.; Rice, D.W.; Sedelnikova, S.E.; et al. An Inhibitor of FtsZ with Potent and Selective Anti-Staphylococcal Activity. *Science* **2008**, *321*, 1673–1675. [CrossRef] [PubMed]
21. Kaul, M.; Mark, L.; Zhang, Y.; Parhi, A.K.; LaVoie, E.J.; Pilch, D.S. An FtsZ-Targeting Prodrug with Oral Antistaphylococcal Efficacy In Vivo. *Antimicrob. Agents Chemother.* **2013**, *57*, 5860–5869. [CrossRef] [PubMed]
22. Kaul, M.; Mark, L.; Zhang, Y.; Parhi, A.K.; Lyu, Y.L.; Pawlak, J.; Saravolatz, S.; Saravolatz, L.D.; Weinstein, M.P.; LaVoie, E.J.; et al. TXA709, an FtsZ-Targeting Benzamide Prodrug with Improved Pharmacokinetics and Enhanced In Vivo Efficacy against Methicillin-Resistant *Staphylococcus aureus*. *Antimicrob. Agents Chemother.* **2015**, *59*, 4845–4855. [CrossRef] [PubMed]
23. Stokes, N.R.; Baker, N.; Bennett, J.M.; Berry, J.; Collins, I.; Czaplewski, L.G.; Logan, A.; Macdonald, R.; Macleod, L.; Peasley, H.; et al. An Improved Small-Molecule Inhibitor of FtsZ with Superior In Vitro Potency, Drug-Like Properties, and In Vivo Efficacy. *Antimicrob. Agents Chemother.* **2013**, *57*, 317–325. [CrossRef] [PubMed]
24. Stokes, N.R.; Baker, N.; Bennett, J.M.; Chauhan, P.K.; Collins, I.; Davies, D.T.; Gavade, M.; Kumar, D.; Lancett, P.; Macdonald, R.; et al. Design, Synthesis and Structure–Activity Relationships of Substituted Oxazole–Benzamide Antibacterial Inhibitors of FtsZ. *Bioorg. Med. Chem. Lett.* **2014**, *24*, 353–359. [CrossRef] [PubMed]
25. Straniero, V.; Pallavicini, M.; Chiodini, G.; Zanotto, C.; Volontè, L.; Radaelli, A.; Bolchi, C.; Fumagalli, L.; Sanguinetti, M.; Menchinelli, G.; et al. 3-(Benzodioxan-2-ylmethoxy)-2,6-Difluorobenzamides Bearing Hydrophobic Substituents at the 7-Position of the Benzodioxane Nucleus Potently Inhibit Methicillin-Resistant *Sa* and *Mtb* Cell Division. *Eur. J. Med. Chem.* **2016**, *120*, 227–243. [CrossRef] [PubMed]
26. Fujita, J.; Maeda, Y.; Mizohata, E.; Inoue, T.; Kaul, M.; Parhi, A.K.; LaVoie, E.J.; Pilch, D.S.; Matsumura, H. Structural Flexibility of an Inhibitor Overcomes Drug Resistance Mutations in *Staphylococcus aureus* FtsZ. *ACS Chem. Biol.* **2017**, *12*, 1947–1955. [CrossRef] [PubMed]
27. Kaul, M.; Mark, L.; Zhang, Y.; Parhi, A.K.; LaVoie, E.J.; Pilch, D.S. Pharmacokinetics and In Vivo Antistaphylococcal Efficacy of TXY541, a 1-Methylpiperidine-4-Carboxamide Prodrug of PC190723. *Biochem. Pharmacol.* **2013**, *86*, 1699–1707. [CrossRef]
28. Tan, C.M.; Therien, A.G.; Lu, J.; Lee, S.H.; Caron, A.; Gill, C.J.; Lebeau-Jacob, C.; Benton-Perdomo, L.; Monteiro, J.M.; Pereira, P.M.; et al. Restoring Methicillin-Resistant *Staphylococcus aureus* Susceptibility to β-Lactam Antibiotics. *Sci. Transl. Med.* **2012**, *4*, 126ra135. [CrossRef] [PubMed]
29. Song, D.; Bi, F.; Zhang, N.; Qin, Y.; Liu, X.; Teng, Y.; Ma, S. Design, Synthesis of Novel 4,5-Dihydroisoxazole-Containing Benzamide Derivatives as Highly Potent FtsZ Inhibitors Capable of Killing a Variety of MDR *Staphylococcus aureus*. *Bioorg. Med. Chem.* **2020**, *28*, 115729. [CrossRef] [PubMed]
30. Bi, F.; Song, D.; Qin, Y.; Liu, X.; Teng, Y.; Zhang, N.; Zhang, P.; Zhang, N.; Ma, S. Discovery of 1,3,4-Oxadiazol-2-One-Containing Benzamide Derivatives Targeting FtsZ as Highly Potent Agents of Killing a Variety of MDR Bacteria Strains. *Bioorg. Med. Chem.* **2019**, *27*, 3179–3193. [CrossRef]
31. Suigo, L.; Margolin, W.; Ulzurrun, E.; Hrast Rambaher, M.; Zanotto, C.; Sebastián-Pérez, V.; Campillo, N.E.; Straniero, V.; Valoti, E. Benzodioxane–Benzamides as FtsZ Inhibitors: Effects of Linker's Functionalization on Gram-Positive Antimicrobial Activity. *Antibiotics* **2023**, *12*, 1712. [CrossRef]

32. Kaul, M.; Zhang, Y.; Parhi, A.K.; LaVoie, E.J.; Pilch, D.S. Inhibition of RND-Type Efflux Pumps Confers the FtsZ-Directed Prodrug TXY436 With Activity against Gram-Negative Bacteria. *Biochem. Pharmacol.* **2014**, *89*, 321–328. [CrossRef]
33. Delcour, A.H. Outer Membrane Permeability and Antibiotic Resistance. *Biochim. Biophys. Acta* **2009**, *1794*, 808–816. [CrossRef]
34. Khare, S.; Hsin, J.; Sorto, N.A.; Nepomuceno, G.M.; Shaw, J.T.; Shi, H.; Huang, K.C. FtsZ-Independent Mechanism of Division Inhibition by the Small Molecule PC190723 in *Escherichia coli*. *Adv. Biosyst.* **2019**, *3*, 1900021. [CrossRef] [PubMed]
35. Miller, S.I. Antibiotic Resistance and Regulation of the Gram-Negative Bacterial Outer Membrane Barrier by Host Innate Immune Molecules. *mBio* **2016**, *7*, e01541-16. [CrossRef] [PubMed]
36. Negash, K.H.; Norris, J.K.S.; Hodgkinson, J.T. Siderophore–Antibiotic Conjugate Design: New Drugs for Bad Bugs? *Molecules* **2019**, *24*, 3314. [CrossRef]
37. Andrews, S.; Norton, I.; Salunkhe, A.S.; Goodluck, H.; Aly, W.S.M.; Mourad-Agha, H.; Cornelis, P. Control of Iron Metabolism in Bacteria. In *Metallomics and the Cell*; Banci, L., Ed.; Springer: Dordrecht, The Netherlands, 2013; pp. 203–239.
38. Andrews, S.C.; Robinson, A.K.; Rodríguez-Quiñones, F. Bacterial Iron Homeostasis. *FEMS Microbiol. Rev.* **2003**, *27*, 215–237. [CrossRef]
39. Finkelstein, R.A.; Sciortino, C.V.; McIntosh, M.A. Role of Iron in Microbe-Host Interactions. *Rev. Infect. Dis.* **1983**, *5*, S759–S777. [CrossRef]
40. Schaible, U.E.; Kaufmann, S.H.E. Iron and Microbial Infection. *Nat. Rev. Microbiol.* **2004**, *2*, 946–953. [CrossRef] [PubMed]
41. Chu, B.C.; Garcia-Herrero, A.; Johanson, T.H.; Krewulak, K.D.; Lau, C.K.; Peacock, R.S.; Slavinskaya, Z.; Vogel, H.J. Siderophore Uptake in Bacteria and the Battle for Iron with the Host; A Bird's Eye View. *BioMetals* **2010**, *23*, 601–611. [CrossRef]
42. Miethke, M.; Marahiel, M.A. Siderophore-Based Iron Acquisition and Pathogen Control. *Microbiol. Mol. Biol. Rev.* **2007**, *71*, 413–451. [CrossRef]
43. Paczosa, M.K.; Mecsas, J. *Klebsiella pneumoniae*: Going on the Offense with a Strong Defense. *Microbiol. Mol. Biol. Rev.* **2016**, *80*, 629–661. [CrossRef]
44. Sheldon, J.R.; Skaar, E.P. *Acinetobacter baumannii* Can Use Multiple Siderophores for Iron Acquisition, but Only Acinetobactin is Required for Virulence. *PLoS Pathog.* **2020**, *16*, e1008995. [CrossRef]
45. Hackel, M.A.; Tsuji, M.; Yamano, Y.; Echols, R.; Karlowsky, J.A.; Sahm, D.F. In Vitro Activity of the Siderophore Cephalosporin, Cefiderocol, against Carbapenem-Nonsusceptible and Multidrug-Resistant Isolates of Gram-Negative Bacilli Collected Worldwide in 2014 to 2016. *Antimicrob. Agents Chemother.* **2018**, *62*, e01968-17. [CrossRef] [PubMed]
46. Shortridge, D.; Streit, J.M.; Mendes, R.; Castanheira, M. In Vitro Activity of Cefiderocol against U.S. and European Gram-Negative Clinical Isolates Collected in 2020 as Part of the SENTRY Antimicrobial Surveillance Program. *Microbiol. Spectr.* **2022**, *10*, e0271221. [CrossRef] [PubMed]
47. Yamano, Y. In Vitro Activity of Cefiderocol against a Broad Range of Clinically Important Gram-Negative Bacteria. *Clin. Infect. Dis.* **2019**, *69*, S544–S551. [CrossRef] [PubMed]
48. Neumann, W.; Sassone-Corsi, M.; Raffatellu, M.; Nolan, E.M. Esterase-Catalyzed Siderophore Hydrolysis Activates an Enterobactin–Ciprofloxacin Conjugate and Confers Targeted Antibacterial Activity. *J. Am. Chem. Soc.* **2018**, *140*, 5193–5201. [CrossRef] [PubMed]
49. Ferrer-González, E.; Fujita, J.; Yoshizawa, T.; Nelson, J.M.; Pilch, A.J.; Hillman, E.; Ozawa, M.; Kuroda, N.; Al-Tameemi, H.M.; Boyd, J.M.; et al. Structure-Guided Design of a Fluorescent Probe for the Visualization of FtsZ in Clinically Important Gram-Positive and Gram-Negative Bacterial Pathogens. *Sci. Rep.* **2019**, *9*, 20092. [CrossRef] [PubMed]
50. Sánchez-Gorostiaga, A.; Palacios, P.; Martínez-Arteaga, R.; Sánchez, M.; Casanova, M.; Vicente, M. Life without Division: Physiology of *Escherichia coli* FtsZ-Deprived Filaments. *mBio* **2016**, *7*, e01620-16. [CrossRef]
51. Bryan, E.J.; Sagong, H.Y.; Parhi, A.K.; Grier, M.C.; Roberge, J.Y.; LaVoie, E.J.; Pilch, D.S. TXH11106: A Third-Generation MreB Inhibitor with Enhanced Activity against a Broad Range of Gram-Negative Bacterial Pathogens. *Antibiotics* **2022**, *11*, 693. [CrossRef]
52. CLSI. *Methods for Dilution Antimicrobial Susceptibility Tests for Bacteria That Grow Aerobically*, 11th ed.; Clinical and Laboratory Standards Institute: Wayne, PA, USA, 2018.
53. Orhan, G.; Bayram, A.; Zer, Y.; Balci, I. Synergy Tests by E test and Checkerboard Methods of Antimicrobial Combinations against *Brucella melitensis*. *J. Clin. Microbiol.* **2005**, *43*, 140–143. [CrossRef]
54. Kaul, M.; Mark, L.; Parhi, A.K.; LaVoie, E.J.; Pilch, D.S. Combining the FtsZ-Targeting Prodrug TXA709 and the Cephalosporin Cefdinir Confers Synergy and Reduces the Frequency of Resistance in Methicillin-Resistant *Staphylococcus aureus*. *Antimicrob. Agents Chemother.* **2016**, *60*, 4290–4296. [CrossRef]
55. Roemer, T.; Boone, C. Systems-Level Antimicrobial Drug and Drug Synergy Discovery. *Nat. Chem. Biol.* **2013**, *9*, 222–231. [CrossRef]
56. Figge, R.M.; Divakaruni, A.V.; Gober, J.W. MreB, the Cell Shape-Determining Bacterial Actin Homologue, Co-ordinates Cell Wall Morphogenesis in *Caulobacter crescentus*. *Mol. Microbiol.* **2004**, *51*, 1321–1332. [CrossRef] [PubMed]
57. Den Blaauwen, T.; De Pedro, M.A.; Nguyen-Distèche, M.; Ayala, J.A. Morphogenesis of Rod-Shaped Sacculi. *FEMS Microbiol. Rev.* **2008**, *32*, 321–344. [CrossRef] [PubMed]

58. Gao, C.; Fisher, Z.B.; Edgar, K.J. Azide Reduction by DTT or Thioacetic Acid Provides Access to Amino and Amido Polysaccharides. *Cellulose* **2019**, *26*, 445–462. [CrossRef]
59. Huang, T.-W.; Lam, I.; Chang, H.-Y.; Tsai, S.-F.; Palsson, B.O.; Charusanti, P. Capsule Deletion Via a λ-Red Knockout System Perturbs Biofilm Formation and Fimbriae Expression in *Klebsiella pneumoniae* MGH 78578. *BMC Res. Notes* **2014**, *7*, 13. [CrossRef] [PubMed]

antibiotics MDPI

Article

Activity of Cinnamic Acid Derivatives with 4-Chloro-2-mercaptobenzenesulfonamide Moiety against Clinical HLAR and VRE *Enterococcus* spp.

Rafał Hałasa [1,*], Anita Bułakowska [2], Jarosław Sławiński [2], Magdalena Smoktunowicz [1], Aleksandra Rapacka-Zdończyk [1] and Urszula Mizerska [3]

1 Department of Pharmaceutical Microbiology, Medical University of Gdansk, Al. Gen. J. Hallera 107, 80-416 Gdansk, Poland; magdalena.smoktunowicz@gumed.edu.pl (M.S.); a.rapacka-zdonczyk@gumed.edu.pl (A.R.-Z.)
2 Department of Organic Chemistry, Medical University of Gdansk, Al. Gen. J. Hallera 107, 80-416 Gdansk, Poland; anita.bulakowska@gumed.edu.pl (A.B.); jaroslaw.slawinski@gumed.edu.pl (J.S.)
3 Centre of Molecular and Macromolecular Studies, Department of Polymeric Nano-Materials, Polish Academy of Sciences, ul. Sienkiewicza 112, 90-363 Lodz, Poland; urszula.mizerska@cbmm.lodz.pl
* Correspondence: rafal.halasa@gumed.edu.pl

Abstract: The rapid increase in strains that are resistant to antibiotics requires new active compounds to be found whose mechanism of action on bacteria is different to those that are currently known. Of particular interest are compounds that occur in plants as secondary metabolites. The focus of this study concerns the examination of the effects of synthetic cinnamic acid derivatives, with 4-chloro-2-mercaptobenzenesulfonamide moiety on *Enterococcus* spp. with HLAR (high-level aminoglycoside resistance) and VRE (vancomycin-resistant *Enterococcus*) mechanisms. The minimum inhibitory concentration (MIC) values of the tested compounds were determined using the serial dilution method for *Enterococcus* spp. groups, and the most active compounds were as follows: **16d**, **17c**, **16a**, **16c** and **16f** (2–4 μg/mL). These compounds, at a concentration of 4 × MIC, inhibited the biofilm formation of HLAR strains (70 to 94%). At concentrations of 2 × MIC and 4 × MIC, they also inhibited the growth of VRE strains (42 to 96%). The best effect produced on the formed biofilm was demonstrated by compound **16f** (from 62% MIC concentration to 89% 4 × MIC concentration) on the tested HLAR strains. In vitro studies, using the peripheral blood of domestic sheep, demonstrated the stable bacteriostatic activity of the tested compounds against *Enterococcus* spp. The compounds **16a**, **16c**, **16d**, **16f** and **17c** showed synergism and additivity with ampicillin, streptomycin, gentamicin and vancomycin against resistant strains of *Enterococcus* spp. The tested compounds, when combined, reduce the MIC for antibiotics by 800 to 10,000 times for HLAR strains and by 8 to 10,000 times for VRE strains. The MIC of the tested compounds, in combination with antibiotics, is reduced 2–16-fold for HLAR strains and 2–32-fold for VRE strains. These studies demonstrate the potential for the therapeutic use of synthetic, cinnamic acid derivatives, with 4-chloro-2-mercaptobenzenesulfonamide moiety, to work against clinical strains of *Enterococcus* spp.

Keywords: 2-mercaptobenzenesulfonamide; antibiofilm; checkerboard assay; cinnamic acid derivatives; *Enterococcus* spp.; synergism

1. Introduction

The genus *Enterococcus* comprises Gram-positive, catalase negative cocci, usually facultative anaerobic bacteria, that grow in 6.5% NaCl, 40% bile salts, 0.1% methylene blue milk, and at pH 9.6. They also grow at 10 and 45 °C and can survive for 30 min at 60 °C [1]. Enterococci belong to the phylum *Firmicutes* of the *Enterococcaceae* family, which includes many different species, and they are a natural component of the human microbiota. They colonize the lower gastrointestinal tract, oral cavity, and genitals [2]. *E. faecalis* and *E.*

faecium are the main enterococci found in the human intestine. *E. cecorum* and *E. durans* are also frequently isolated, whereas *E. casseliflavus*, *E. hirae*, *E. gallinarum*, and *E. avium* are occasionally detected [3].

Enterococci can cause a wide range of clinical diseases. One of the factors causing the high infectivity of enterococci is biofilm formation ability. This property makes the treatment of the infection difficult [4]. *Enterococcus* spp. cause infections of the urinary tract, cardiovascular system, abdominal cavity, pelvis, central nervous system, and postoperative wounds. Asymptomatic bacteriuria is the most common clinical condition, but many of these cases are caused by colonization rather than infection. Other frequent causes of infection are bacteremia without endocarditis, which is followed by endocarditis [5]. *Enterococcus* spp. are frequently cited as one of the three most likely etiologies of both uncomplicated and complicated urinary tract infections (UTIs), especially healthcare-associated UTIs. Of these, the bacteria that most commonly cause these infections are *E. faecalis*, although *E. faecium* predominates among vancomycin-resistant isolates. It is usually associated with indwelling urinary catheters and instruments. The severity of the disease can range from uncomplicated cystitis to complicated cystitis, or it may cause pyelonephritis, a perinephric abscess, or prostatitis. All these cases result in the introduction of antibiotics to work against the enterococci [6].

Additionally, enterococci have the ability to obtain genetic material from other bacteria and to quickly adapt to the environment [3]. It is well established that enterococci are resistant to many antibiotics, including the following: β-lactams, aminoglycosides, trimethoprim/sulfamethoxazole, clindamycin, and some species of glycopeptides [7]. This requires combinations of glycopeptides or β-lactams with aminoglycosides to be used [5]. The application of antibiotics in hospitals, and for the treatment of animals, has led to the existence of resistant strains. Currently, drug-resistant enterococci that are isolated in hospitals include the following: high level of resistance to ampicillin; high-level aminoglycoside resistance (HLAR); resistance to glycopeptides (VRE; vancomycin and teicoplanin) and oxazolidinone resistant (LRE—linezolid-resistant *Enterococcus*) [3].

The World Health Organization (WHO) reports that antibiotics are becoming increasingly ineffective as drug resistance spreads around the world, thus causing difficult or 'impossible to control' infections. In its reports, the WHO lists microorganisms of particular concern, which require the discovery of new active compounds to work against them; among them are *E. faecium* VRE strains [8,9]. There is a constant need to search for new compounds with antibacterial properties.

In the light of these issues, research on new drugs to work against resistant bacteria strains is ongoing. An increasing number of studies are being conducted on combination therapies which could potentially reduce the MIC values of administered antibacterial drugs, improve pharmacokinetic/pharmacodynamic (PK/PD) parameters (e.g., bind a hydrophilic drug to a lipophilic drug), and increase activity against bacteria present in biofilm [10]. Examples of such combinations are as follows: omadacycline and oritavancin, or fosfomycin with either daptomycin or rifampicin [11,12].

Secondary plant metabolites (phytochemicals, including cinnamic acid) are a good source of active compounds, including those with antibacterial properties [13]. The broad biological activity of cinnamic acid, and its synthetic derivatives, has been demonstrated by several research teams [9,13–18]. Cinnamic acid can occur in nature in both *cis* and *trans* forms with the *trans* form being more stable than the *cis* form. Its antimicrobial activity is low against Gram-positive and Gram-negative bacteria [10]; however, synthetic derivatives (cinnamic acids, esters, amides) have a stronger antimicrobial effect on bacteria; moreover, cinnamic aldehydes inhibit the development of fungi. Cinnamic acid derivatives with phenolic groups have been classified as antioxidants. The chemical structure of cinnamic acid, which contains both a benzene ring and a carboxylic group, enables the modification and procurement of synthetic derivatives. Synthetic compounds that combine two pharmaceutical entities in one molecule may be a successful strategy since these molecules could be more effective than their individual components. Research has been conducted on the conjugation of several hydroxy- and phenyl-substituted derivatives of *trans*-cinnamic acids with an antimicrobial pharmacophore like carvacrol on ESKAPE pathogens [10]. *Trans*-cinnamaldehyde is a phenylpropanoid, which practically occurs in cinnamon essential oil, and it is Generally Recognized as Safe (GRAS) by the US Food and Drug Administration (US FDA) [19].

Sulfonamides and sulfamates are mainly known as synthetic compounds, but several were also discovered as secondary metabolites produced by actinomycetes, e.g., nucleocidin and dealanylascamycin. Sulfonamides and sulfamates constitute a diverse group of highly pharmacologically active compounds, and many clinically used drugs contain the signature sulfamoyl structural motif. Sulfonamides are widely known as synthetic "sulfa drugs", and these were the first chemotherapeutically used antibacterial compounds. They are applied to other diseases such as Alzheimer's disease and other central nervous system (CNS) disorders, diabetes, psychosis, and various cancers and tumors [20].

In this work, we examined the activity of synthetic derivatives of cinnamic acid with 4-chloro-2-mercaptobenzenesulfonamide moiety [17] against clinical strains of *Enterococcus* spp. The measure of the activity of compounds is their limit concentration value; for this purpose, we determined minimum inhibitory concentrations. From a clinical point of view, it is important to know: at what concentrations the tested compounds inhibit bacterial biofilm formation, whether they are able to penetrate the already formed biofilm and affect the bacteria or whether they are able to inhibit the further development of the existing biofilm. We examined the activity of new derivatives on enterococcal biofilm. Testing the bioavailability and pharmacodynamics of compounds in body fluids in vitro is one of the important elements showing the stable structure and activity of compounds as well as the influence of the elements of these fluids on the compounds and the impact of the compounds on the components of the higher organism. Therefore, we determined In vitro the stability and influence of blood elements on the antibacterial activity of the tested compounds. Combination therapy of two or three compounds with different targets in a bacterial cell is a common element of antibiotic therapy for infections with multi-resistant strains, including VRE HLAR strains. We investigated the interactions that may occur between the tested compounds and the antibiotics used in the antibiotic therapy of enterococcal infections.

2. Results

2.1. Synthesis and Chemical Characterization of Cinnamic Acid Derivatives with 4-Chloro-2-mercaptobenzenesulfonamide Moiety

The synthesis and chemical characterization of cinnamic acid derivatives with 4-chloro-2-mercaptobenzenesulfonamide moiety was described by Bułakowska et al. [18]. The structures of the tested derivatives are presented in Figure 1.

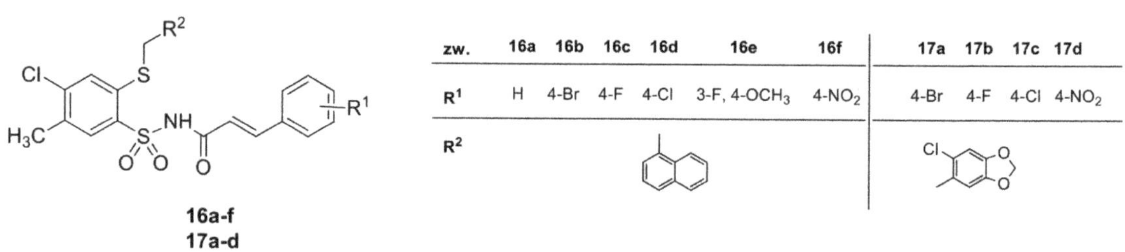

Figure 1. The stuctures of *N*-{[4-chloro-5-methyl-2-(naphthalen-1-ylmethylthio)phenyl]sulfonyl} cinnamamide derivatives (**16a–16f**) and *N*-{[4-chloro-2-(6-chlorobenzo[*d*][1,3]dioxol-5-yl)-methylthio-5-methylphenyl]sulfonyl}cinnamamide derivatives (**17a–17d**) [18].

2.2. Antibacterial Activity of Cinnamic Acid Derivatives

In this work, we decided to test the activity of cinnamic acid derivatives against *Enterococcus* characterized by VRE. We preceded the study activity by determining the resistance pattern of all our strains. The studies were performed using the disc diffusion method. The results are presented in Table 1.

Table 1. Phenotypic characterization of resistance of *Enterococcus* strains. Inhibition zone diameters around antibiotic discs (mm).

Full Strain Name, and Specific Resistance Mechanism	Ampicillin	Imipenem	Vancomicin	Teicoplanin	Co-trimoxazole	Norfloxacin	Gentamicin	Streptomycin	Doxycycline	Linezolid
Enterococcus faecium 12835 HLAR	6 ± 0.00	6 ± 0.00	15 ± 0.00	20 ± 0.50	6 ± 0.00	6 ± 0.00	6 ± 0.00	6 ± 0.00	6 ± 0.00	22 ± 0.0
Enterococcus faecium 12848 HLAR	6 ± 0.00	6 ± 0.00	17 ± 0.50	18 ± 0.50	6 ± 0.00	6 ± 0.00	6 ± 0.00	6 ± 0.00	6 ± 0.00	25 ± 0.00
Enterococcus faecalis 12214 HLAR	11 ± 0.50	21 ± 0.00	15 ± 0.00	20 ± 0.50	40 ± 1.00	6 ± 0.00	6 ± 0.00	6 ± 0.00	6 ± 0.00	19 ± 0.00
Enterococcus faecalis 12245 HLAR	12 ± 0.50	22 ± 0.00	15 ± 0.00	18 ± 0.50	40 ± 1.00	6 ± 0.00	6 ± 0.00	6 ± 0.00	6 ± 0.00	25 ± 0.00
Enterococccus faecium 12961 HLAR	6 ± 0.00	6 ± 0.00	12 ± 0.00	20 ± 0.50	41 ± 1.00	6 ± 0.00	6 ± 0.00	6 ± 0.00	20 ± 0.00	26 ± 0.00
Enterococcus faecalis 12338 HLAR	12 ± 0.50	21 ± 0.00	15 ± 0.00	19 ± 0.00	35 ± 1.00	6 ± 0.00	6 ± 0.00	6 ± 0.00	6 ± 0.00	25 ± 0.50
nterococcus faecium 16247 HLAR	6 ± 0.00	6 ± 0.00	12 ± 0.00	20 ± 0.50	6 ± 0.00	6 ± 0.00	6 ± 0.00	6 ± 0.00	6 ± 0.00	26 ± 0.00
Enterococcus faecalis 3937152 HLAR, VRE	14 ± 0.50	22 ± 0.00	6 ± 0.00	20 ± 0.00	6 ± 0.00	6 ± 0.00	6 ± 0.00	6 ± 0.00	6 ± 0.00	25 ± 0.50
Enterococcus faecium 3934825 HLAR, VRE	6 ± 0.00	6 ± 0.00	6 ± 0.00	16 ± 0.00	6 ± 0.00	6 ± 0.00	6 ± 0.00	6 ± 0.00	6 ± 0.00	25 ± 0.50
Enterococcus faecium 773081 HLAR, VRE	6 ± 0.00	6 ± 0.00	6 ± 0.00	17 ± 0.00	6 ± 0.00	6 ± 0.00	6 ± 0.00	6 ± 0.00	6 ± 0.00	25 ± 0.00
Enterococcus faecium 895612 HLAR, VRE	6 ± 0.00	6 ± 0.00	6 ± 0.00	15 ± 0.00	35 ± 0.50	20 ± 0.00	6 ± 0.00	6 ± 0.00	20 ± 0.00	26 ± 0.00
Enterococcus faecium 508171 HLAR, VRE	6 ± 0.00	6 ± 0.00	6 ± 0.00	15 ± 0.00	40 ± 0.50	6 ± 0.00	6 ± 0.00	6 ± 0.00	6 ± 0.00	24 ± 0.00
Enterococcus faecium 830981 HLAR, VRE	6 ± 0.00	6 ± 0.00	6 ± 0.00	6 ± 0.00	6 ± 0.00	6 ± 0.00	6 ± 0.00	6 ± 0.00	6 ± 0.00	25 ± 0.50
Enterococcus faecium 264281 HLAR, VRE	6 ± 0.00	6 ± 0.00	6 ± 0.00	6 ± 0.00	6 ± 0.00	6 ± 0.00	6 ± 0.00	6 ± 0.00	6 ± 0.00	25 ± 0.00
Enterococcus faecium 967321 HLAR, VRE	6 ± 0.00	6 ± 0.00	6 ± 0.00	15 ± 0.00	35 ± 0.50	6 ± 0.00	6 ± 0.00	6 ± 0.00	6 ± 0.00	25 ± 0.00
Enterococcus faecium 966351 HLAR, VRE	6 ± 0.00	6 ± 0.00	6 ± 0.00	16 ± 0.00	6 ± 0.00	6 ± 0.00	6 ± 0.00	6 ± 0.00	6 ± 0.00	26 ± 0.00
Enterococcus faecium 576181 HLAR, VRE	6 ±0.00	6 ± 0.00	6 ± 0.00	18 ± 0.00	40 ± 0.50	18 ± 0.00	6 ± 0.00	6 ± 0.00	6 ± 0.00	25 ± 0.50
Enterococcus faecium 885041 HLAR, VRE	6 ±0.00	6 ± 0.00	6 ± 0.00	6 ± 0.00	6 ± 0.00	6 ± 0.00	6 ± 0.00	6 ± 0.00	6 ± 0.00	24 ± 0.00

The results are presented as mean values ± standard deviation (±SD) from three independent experiments. Error bars represent standard deviation. HLAR (high-level aminoglycoside resistance), VRE (vancomycin-resistant *Enterococcus*).

It has been observed that all the tested strains were sensitive to linezolid (inhibition zone ≥ 20 mm), and 14 out of 17 bacterial strains were susceptible to teicoplanin (inhibition zone ≥ 16 mm). In turn, 100% HLAR strains were sensitive to vancomycin (inhibition zone ≥ 12 mm). Only one strain showed sensitivity to tetracycline (inhibition zone ≥ 20 mm). However, 100% of the strains tested were resistant to streptomycin (zone of inhibition ≤ 14 mm) and gentamicin (zone of inhibition ≤ 8 mm). Susceptibility to ampicillin (susceptible strain zone ≥ 10 mm; resistant strain ≤ 8 mm), imipenem (susceptible strain zone ≥ 21; resistant strain ≤ 20 mm) and co-trimoxazole (susceptible strain zone ≥ 23 mm) was variable.

The MIC values of the cinnamic acid derivatives with 4-chloro-2-mercaptobenzenesulfonamide moiety against the *Enterococcus* spp. VRE group are shown in Table 2.

Table 2. MIC values of cinnamic acid derivatives against *Enterococcus* spp. VRE.

Compd	MIC [µg/mL]							
	Enterococcus sp. 773081	*Enterococcus* sp. 508171	*Enterococcus* sp. 830981	*Enterococcus* sp. 264281	*Enterococcus* sp. 967321	*Enterococcus* sp. 966351	*Enterococcus* sp. 576181	*Enterococcus* sp. 885041
16a	4 ± 0.21	4 ± 0.18	4 ± 0.20	4 ± 0.15	4 ± 0.22	4 ± 0.30	4 ± 0.30	4 ± 0.33
16b	8 ± 0.30	8 ± 0.50	16 ± 0.48	8 ± 0.18	8 ± 0.25	4 ± 0.30	16 ± 0.38	8 ± 0.42
16c	4 ± 0.22	4 ± 0.38	4 ± 0.41	4 ± 0.24	4 ± 0.38	4 ± 0.31	4 ± 0.35	4 ± 0.30
16d	2 ± 0.10	2 ± 0.10	2 ± 0.10	2 ± 0.05	2 ± 0.15	2 ± 0.10	2 ± 0.22	2 ± 0.10
16e	16 ± 0.15	8 ± 0.50	16 ± 0.50	16 ± 0.50	16 ± 0.50	31.25 ± 0.50	8 ± 0.41	8 ± 0.50
16f	8 ± 0.45	4 ± 0.25	4 ± 0.18	8 ± 0.50	4 ± 0.25	4 ± 0.28	4 ± 0.28	4 ± 0.35
17a	8 ± 0.45	16 ± 0.50	16 ± 0.52	8 ± 0.50	16 ± 0.56	16 ± 0.50	16 ± 0.50	4 ± 0.20
17b	>125	>125	>125	>125	>125	>125	>125	>125
17c	2 ± 0.18	4 ± 0.25	4 ± 0.25	4 ± 0.19	2 ± 0.05	4 ± 0.25	2 ± 0.25	4 ± 0.25
17d	>125	>125	>125	>125	>125	>125	>125	>125
co-trimoxazole	>2000:400	2000:400 ± 0.50	>2000:400	>2000: 400	>2000:400	1250:250 ± 0.50	>2000:400	>2000:400

The results are presented as mean values ± standard deviation (±SD).

The most active compounds turned out to be **16d** and **17c** with MICs within the range of 2 ± 0.05–4 ± 0.38 µg/mL. Compounds **16a** and **16c** showed an MIC of 4 µg/mL. The least active compounds were **17b** and **17d** (MIC > 125 µg/mL). The most resistant strain turned out to be *Enterococcus* sp. 966351, and the most sensitive was *Enterococcus* sp. 885041. The majority of the compounds showed bacterial inhibitory activity, while bactericidal concentrations were equal to or greater than 125 µg/mL. The compounds **16d** and **17c** were the most active against *Enterococcus* spp. VRE.

2.3. *Effect of Derivatives on the Biofilm Produced by* Enterococcus *spp.*

The next step of our study was an evaluation of whether the tested cinnamic acid derivatives act on the biofilm produced by *Enterococcus* spp. It is known from the literature data that *Enterococcus* spp. are capable of producing a biofilm, but this is not a permanent feature of the species. Therefore, we decided to verify which of the tested strains exhibit this ability. Based on the literature reports, we chose to test biofilm formation by *Enterococcus* spp., using the following broths: tryptic soy broth medium (TSB), brain–heart infusion broth (BHI) supplemented with 2% glucose, and BHI supplemented with 5% bovine serum. The results of the effect of substrates on biofilm formation are shown in Figure 2.

The results presented in Figure 2 show that the ability to produce biofilm is diversified in the pool of *Enterococcus* spp. strains used for testing in the current study. The strains used include strong biofilm producers, e.g., *E. faecalis* 12245 HLAR and *E. faecalis* 3937152 HLAR and VRE; and those that form a weak biofilm regardless of the substrate used, e.g., *E. faecium* 12835 HLAR and *E. faecium* 12848 HLAR. To the best of our knowledge, it is the first study that differentiates *Enterococcus* according to its ability to form biofilm in different media. The bacteria that generate the strongest biofilm in TSB supplemented with 2% glucose medium are *Enterococcus* spp. HLAR: *E. faecalis* 12214, *E. faecalis* 12245, and *E. faecalis* 12338 ($p < 0.05$). However, in the BHI supplemented with 2% glucose medium, the strongest biofilm is formed by *Enterococcus* spp. VRE: *E. faecium* 3934825, *E. faecium* 967321, and *E. faecium* 264281 ($p < 0.05$). Surprisingly, all the tested strains produced biofilm at a very low level in the presence of bovine serum in the BHI medium ($p < 0.05$). For further research, which concerned the activity of the tested compounds against biofilm, we chose both media and the strains producing the strongest biofilm. The most active derivatives were used in concentrations of 0.5 MIC, MIC, 2 × MIC and 4 × MIC.

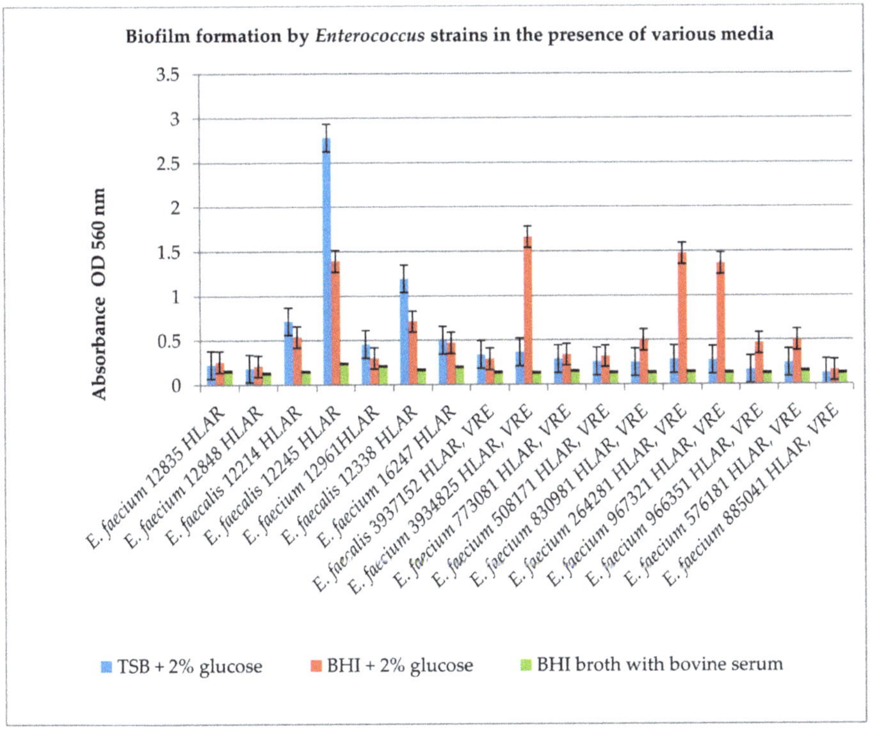

Figure 2. Biofilm formation by *Enterococcus* spp. strains in the presence of various media. The results are presented as mean values ± standard deviation (±SD) from three independent experiments. Error bars represent standard deviation. HLAR (high-level aminoglycoside resistance), VRE (vancomycin-resistant *Enterococcus*) TSB (tryptic soy broth) medium, BHI (brain–heart infusion broth) medium supplemented with 2% glucose and BHI supplemented 5% bovine serum. $p < 0.05$ was considered statistically significant.

Figure 3 shows the effect of the tested derivatives on biofilm formation by *Enterococcus* spp. HLAR strains. The most active compound was **16f**. In the tested concentration range, it significantly inhibited biofilm formation by the *Enterococcus* spp. HLAR strains from 89 to 94% ($p < 0.05$) compared to the control. For the remaining compounds tested, a concentration of 4 × MIC was the most active, as this inhibited biofilm formation from 69% (compound **16a** against *E. faecalis* 12338; $p < 0.05$) to 90% (compound **16d** against *E. faecalis* 12338; $p < 0.05$). The concentrations of 0.5 MIC and MIC turned out to be the least active in inhibiting biofilm formation with the effectiveness of significant effects ranging from 8% (compound **16a** for *E. faecalis* 12214; $p < 0.05$) to 60% (compound **16a** for *E. faecalis* 12245; $p < 0.05$).

Figure 4 shows the effect of the tested derivatives on biofilm formation by *Enterococcus* spp. VRE strains. The anti-biofilm activity of the tested compounds varied and depended on the concentration. The inhibition levels of compounds at 0.5 MIC and MIC ranged from 0.78% (compound **16c** at 0.5 MIC against *E. faecium* 3934825; $p < 0.05$) to 95% (compound **16d** at MIC against *E. faecium* 967321; $p < 0.05$). The concentrations of 2 × MIC and 4 × MIC were found to be more effective and inhibited biofilm formation from 42% (compound **16a** at 2 × MIC against *E. faecium* 3934825, $p < 0.05$) to 96% (compound **16d** at 4 × MIC against *E. faecium* 967321; $p < 0.05$) in comparison to the control samples. Comparing the results presented in Figures 2 and 3, it can be concluded that the tested derivatives inhibit the formation of biofilm by the VRE strains more efficiently than by the HLAR strains.

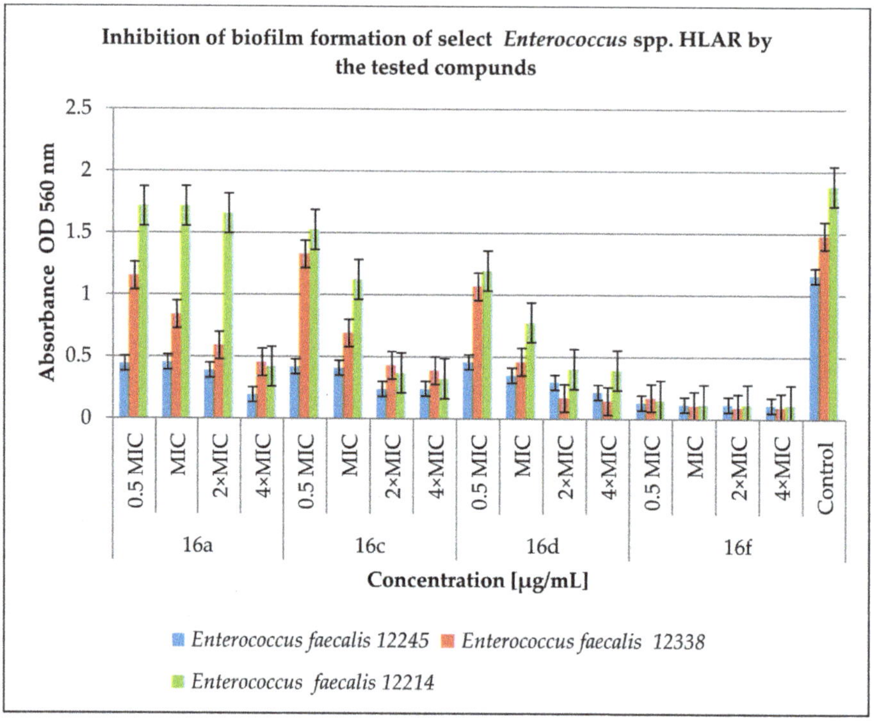

Figure 3. Inhibition of biofilm formation of the selected *Enterococcus* spp. HLAR strains by the tested compounds. A control group was bacterial sample without compounds. Half of the minimum inhibitory concentration—0.5 MIC, double the minimum inhibitory concentration—2 × MIC, quadruple the minimum inhibitory concentration—4 × MIC. The results are presented as mean values ± standard deviation (±SD) from three independent experiments. Error bars represent standard deviation. HLAR (high-level aminoglycoside resistance), VRE (vancomycin-resistant *Enterococcus*). $p < 0.05$ was considered as statistically significant.

The next step of our work was to test the antimicrobial effect of our derivatives on already formed enterococcal biofilm. The results are presented in Figures 5 and 6.

Figure 5 shows the effect of the tested compounds on biofilm already formed by *Enterococcus* spp. HLAR strains. Compounds **16a, 16c** and **16d** show a low effect on the already formed biofilm and the degree of reduction in the tested strains in biofilm ranged from 0.8% (compound **16a** at a concentration of 0.5 MIC against *E. faecalis* 12214; $p < 0.05$) to 38% (compound **16d** at a concentration of 4 × MIC against *E. faecalis* 12245; $p < 0.05$) when compared to the control. In contrast, compound **16f** turned out to most actively reduce the number of bacteria in the biofilm from 62% (0.5 MIC concentration against *E. faecalis* 12245; $p < 0.05$) to 89% (4 × MIC concentration against *E. faecalis* 12338; $p < 0.05$) compared to the control samples.

Nevertheless, the tested compounds had no significant effect on the inhibition of further biofilm formation by the *Enterococcus* spp. VRE strains (Figure 6). Inhibitory activities ranged from 0.16% (compound **16a** at MIC concentration against *E. faecium* 3934825; $p < 0.05$) to 23% (compound **17c** at MIC concentration against *E. faecium* 967321; $p < 0.05$) compared to the control.

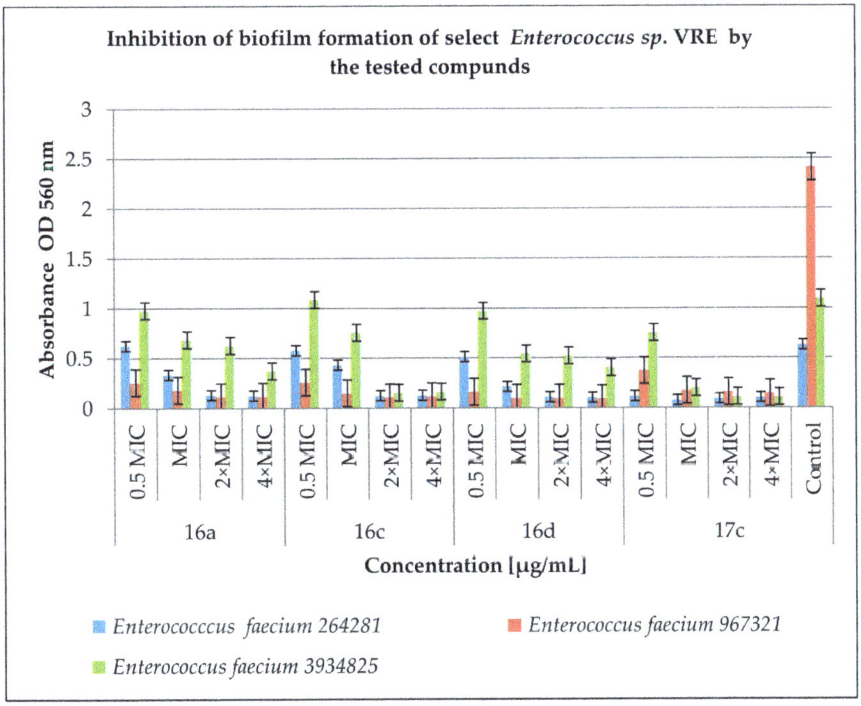

Figure 4. Inhibition of biofilm formation by selected *Enterococcus* spp. VRE by the tested compounds. A control group was bacterial sample without compounds. Half of the minimum inhibitory concentration—0.5 MIC, double the minimum inhibitory concentration—2 × MIC, quadruple the minimum inhibitory concentration—4 × MIC. The results are presented as mean values ± standard deviation (±SD) from three independent experiments. Error bars represent standard deviation. HLAR (high-level aminoglycoside resistance), VRE (vancomycin-resistant *Enterococcus*). $p < 0.05$ was considered as statistically significant.

The most active compounds were **16f** and **17c**. However, the activity of the tested compounds on the already formed biofilm was low in both groups of bacteria with the exception of compound **16f** acting on *Enterococcus* spp. HLAR, which inhibits the formation of the biofilm to about 90% when compared to the control.

2.4. Blood Bacteriostatic Activity Tests

The compounds we tested exhibited a bacteriostatic effect on *Enterococcus* spp. in the culture medium. We wanted to answer the question of whether this property is retained in the presence of blood components, as it was in the case of *Staphylococcus* spp. [18]. For this purpose, we selected two species of bacteria: *E. faecium* 264281 (Table 3) and *E. faecalis* 12245 (Table 4).

The initial number of bacteria at time t_0 was (2.00 ± 0.69) × 10^8 CFU/mL for *E. faecalis* 12245 and (7.30 ± 0.67) × 10^8 for *E. faecium* 264281. Bacteria in appropriate numbers were added to blood samples containing the tested compounds in the concentration range of 0.5–16 µg/mL and then incubated for 24 h at 37 °C. Controls consisted of samples of bacteria incubated in pure blood, without supplements, the number of which after 24 h incubation was (1.44 ± 0.47) × 10^8 CFU/mL for *E. faecalis* 12245 and (1.30 ± 0.48) × 10^8 CFU/mL for *E. faecium* 264281. There is a relationship here: the higher the concentration of the active compound in the sample, the lower the number of live bacteria. In the samples with compounds **16c** and **16d** (16 µg/mL), there is a significant decrease in the number of viable bacteria: **16c**—(7.00 ± 0.71) × 10^6 CFU/mL, **16d**—(1.20 ± 0.55) × 10^6 CFU/mL ($p <$ 0.05) compared to the control.

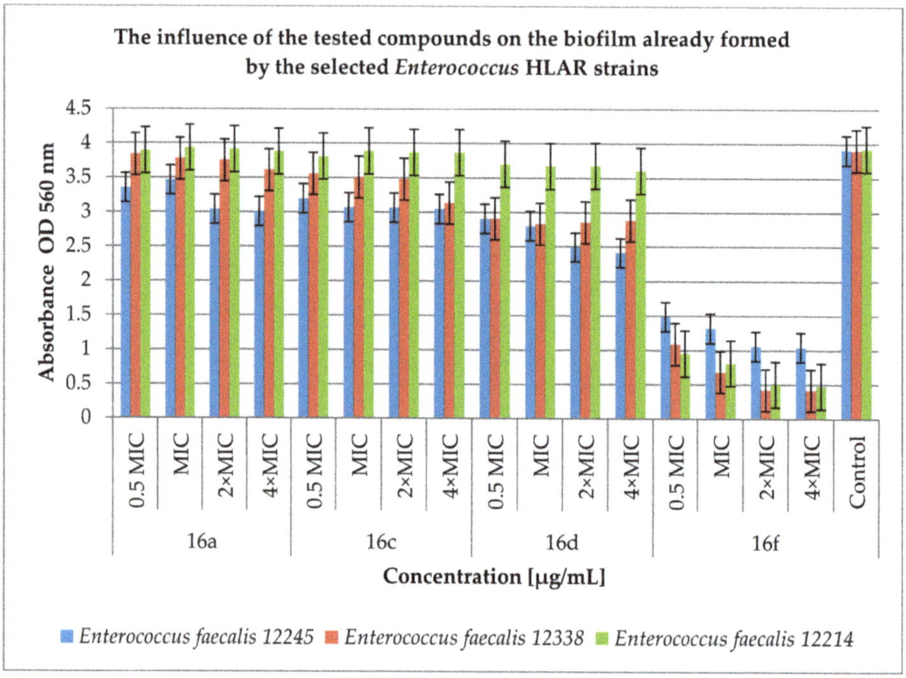

Figure 5. The effect of the tested compounds on the biofilm already formed by selected *Enterococcus* spp. HLAR strains. A control group was bacterial sample without compounds. Half of the minimum inhibitory concentration—0.5 MIC, double the minimum inhibitory concentration—2 × MIC, quadruple the minimum inhibitory concentration—4 × MIC. The results are presented as mean values ± standard deviation (±SD) from three independent experiments. Error bars represent standard deviation. HLAR (high-level aminoglycoside resistance), VRE (vancomycin-resistant *Enterococcus*. $p < 0.05$ was considered as statistically significant.

Table 3. The results of the bacteriostatic effect of the tested compounds in different concentrations on *Enterococcus faecalis* 12245. Bacterial density is given in CFU/mL of sample.

Concentration (μg/mL)	**0.5**	**1**	**2**	**4**	**8**	**16**
16a	[1.08 ± 0.65] × 10^8	[9.00 ± 0.35] × 10^7	[7.00 ± 0.14] × 10^7	[6.50 ± 0.10] × 10^7	[5.00 ± 0.21] × 10^7	[5.10 ± 0.35] × 10^7
16c	[2.00 ± 0.35] × 10^8	[9.30 ± 0.14] × 10^7	[8.30 ± 0.14] × 10^7	[5.90 ± 0.21] × 10^7	[5.90 ± 0.24] × 10^7	[4.10 ± 0.35] × 10^7
16d	[1.80 ± 0.10] × 10^8	[8.20 ± 0.10] × 10^7	[8.16 ± 0.13] × 10^7	[4.20 ± 0.14] × 10^7	[3.90 ± 0.42] × 10^7	[3.50 ± 0.77] × 10^7
16f	[1.59 ± 0.17] × 10^8	[1.27 ± 0.30] × 10^8	[5.70 ± 0.14] × 10^7	[4.40 ± 0.21] × 10^7	[2.60 ± 0.20] × 10^7	[2.00 ± 0.45] × 107

t_0 = (2.00 ± 0.69) × 10^8; t_{24} = (1.44 ± 0.47) × 10^8. The results are presented as mean values ± standard deviation (±SD) from three independent experiments. $p < 0.05$ was considered as statistically significant.

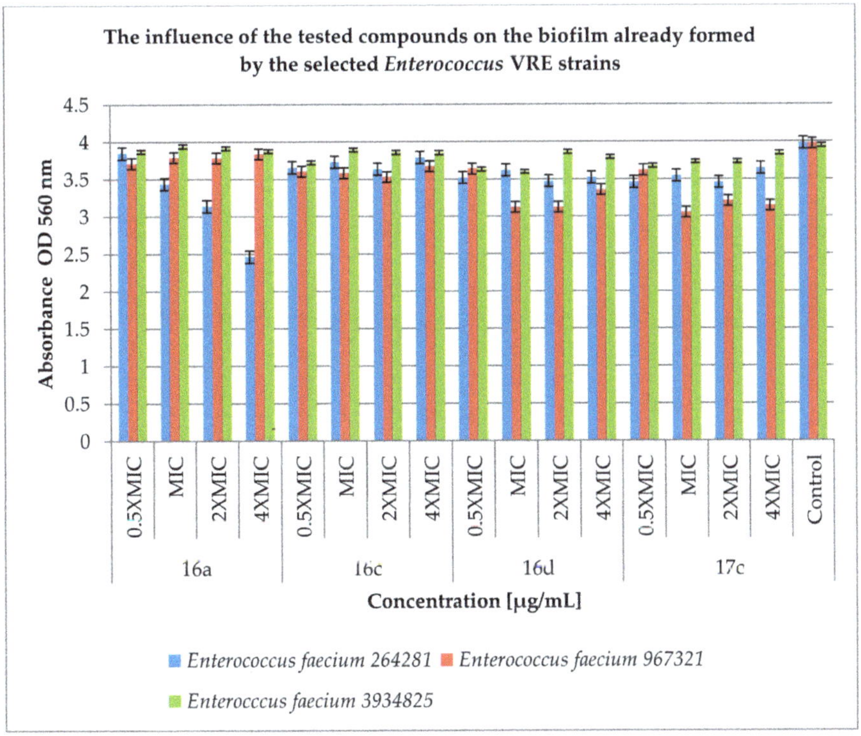

Figure 6. The effect of the tested compounds on the biofilm already formed by selected *Enterococcus* spp. VRE strains. A control group was bacterial sample without compounds. Half of the minimum inhibitory concentration—0.5 MIC, double the minimum inhibitory concentration—2 × MIC, quadruple the minimum inhibitory concentration—4 × MIC. The results are presented as mean values ± standard deviation (±SD) from three independent experiments. Error bars represent standard deviation HLAR (high-level aminoglycoside resistance), VRE (vancomycin-resistant *Enterococcus*. $p <$ 0.05 was considered as statistically significant.

Table 4. The results of the bacteriostatic effect of the tested compounds in different concentrations on *Enterococcus faecium* 264281. Bacterial density is given in CFU/mL of sample.

Concentration (µg/mL)	0.5	1	2	4	8	16
16a	[1.80 ± 0.28] × 10^8	[1.30 ± 0.85] × 10^7	[1.30 ± 0.41] × 10^7	[1.30 ± 0.70] × 10^7	[1.20 ± 0.70]× 10^7	[3.07 ± 0.64] × 10^7
16c	[1.90 ± 0.23] × 10^8	[3.00 ± 0.35] × 10^7	[3.00 ± 0.71] × 10^7	[3.10 ± 084] × 10^7	[8.00 ± 0.21] × 10^6	[7.00 ± 0.71] × 10^6
16d	[1.50 ± 0.56] × 10^8	[1.10 ± 0.60] × 10^7	[7.00 ± 0.77] × 10^6	[6.00 ± 0.71] × 10^6	[5.40 ± 0.42] × 10^6	[1.20 ± 0.55] × 10^6
17c	[2.27 ± 0.16] × 10^8	[1.59 ± 0.43] × 10^8	[1.15 ± 0.58] × 10^8	[4.40 ± 0.41] × 10^7	[2.60 ± 0.35] × 10^7	[2.00 ± 0.62] × 10^7

t_0 = (7.30 ± 0.67) × 10^8; t_{24} = (1.30 ± 0.48) × 10^8. The results are presented as mean values ± standard deviation (±SD) from three independent experiments. $p < 0.05$ was considered as statistically significant.

2.5. Study of Interactions of Cinnamic Acid Derivatives with Antibiotics on Resistant Strains of Enterococcus spp.

The most interesting interactions between antibacterial compounds relate to synergy. The synergy of compounds is based on increasing effectiveness, reducing toxicity, reducing undesirable side effects, increasing bioavailability, lowering the required dose and limiting the emergence of resistance to the tested preparations. New therapeutic combinations that include a connection with natural products have become a research priority.

To check the relationship between our derivatives and antibiotics, we conducted further studies using the common checkerboard assay. Antibiotics such as ampicillin, gentamicin, streptomycin and vancomycin as well as *Enterococcus* spp. selected from both tested groups were used.

In the first stage, we checked the activity of selected antibiotics and determined the limit concentrations (MIC). In the next stage, we conducted research assessing the relationship between the tested derivatives and selected antibiotics, where we used MIC and lower concentrations of the tested compounds. The antibiotics taken into consideration in the study are important preparations in the treatment of infections caused by *Enterococcus* spp. The results are presented in Tables 5 and 6.

Table 5. Interactions of cinnamic acid derivatives with antibiotics on resistant strains of *Enterococcus* spp. HLAR.

Strains	Antibiotic	MIC Antibiotic (mg/mL)		Cinnamic Acid Derivative	MIC Cinnamic Acid Derivative (mg/mL)		FICI	Outcome
		Alone	Comb.		Alone	Comb.		
Enterococcus faecalis 12214	ampicillin	10	0.001	16a	0.004	0.0005	0.126	synergy
			0.001	16c	0.004	0.0005	0.126	synergy
			0.002	16d	0.001	0.001	1	additivity
			0.001	16f	0.004	0.0005	0.126	synergy
	gentamycin	2	0.001	16a	0.004	0.002	0.5	synergy
			0.001	16c	0.004	0.0005	0.125	synergy
			0.001	16d	0.0005	0.0005	1	additivity
			0.001	16f	0.002	0.0005	0.25	synergy
	streptomycin	10	0.001	16a	0.004	0.002	0.25	synergy
			0.001	16c	0.004	0.0005	0.126	synergy
			0.001	16d	0.002	0.001	0.5	synergy
			0.001	16f	0.002	0.0005	0.25	synergy
Enterococcus faecalis 12338	ampicillin	0.8	0.001	16a	0.004	0.0005	0.126	synergy
			0.001	16c	0.004	0.0005	0.126	synergy
			0.001	16d	0.002	0.0005	0.375	synergy
			0.001	16f	0.004	0.0005	0.126	synergy
	gentamycin	2	0.001	16a	0.008	0.002	0.25	synergy
			0.001	16c	0.008	0.0005	0.062	synergy
			0.001	16d	0.001	0.001	1	additivity
			0.001	16f	0.004	0.001	0.25	synergy
	streptomycin	10	0.001	16a	0.004	0.001	0.25	synergy
			0.001	16c	0.002	0.001	0.5	synergy
			0.001	16d	0.001	0.0005	0.5	synergy
			0.002	16f	0.002	0.0005	0.25	synergy

Comb.—combination: compound + antibiotic or antibiotic + compound.

Table 6. Interactions of cinnamic acid derivatives with antibiotics on resistant strains of *Enterococcus* spp. VRE.

Strains	Antibiotic	MIC Antibiotic (mg/mL)		Cinnamic Acid Derivative	MIC Cinnamic Acid Derivative (mg/mL)		FICI	Outcome
		Alone	Comb.		Alone	Comb.		
E. faecium 966351 VRE	Ampicillin	0.8	0.016	16a	0.008	0.0005	0.082	synergy
			0.008	16c	0.016	0.0005	0.041	synergy
			0.002	16d	0.002	0.0005	0.252	synergy
			0.016	17c	0.016	0.0005	0.082	synergy
	Gentamycin	2	0.001	16a	0.004	0.001	0.25	synergy
			0.001	16c	0.002	0.001	0.5	synergy
			0.001	16d	0.001	0.001	1	additivity
			0.032	17c	0.008	0.008	1.016	additivity
	Streptomycin	10	0.001	16a	0.004	0.002	0.5	synergy
			0.032	16c	0.008	0.008	1.003	additivity
			0.001	16d	0.001	0.0005	0.5	synergy
			0.032	17c	0.008	0.008	1.003	additivity
	Vancomycin	0.008	0.001	16a	0.004	0.0005	0.25	synergy
			0.001	16c	0.002	0.001	0.625	partial synergism
			0.001	16d	0.001	0.001	1.125	additivity
			0.001	17c	0.008	0.0005	0.188	synergy
E. faecium 830981 VRE	Ampicillin	0.5	0.016	16a	0.008	0.0005	0.082	synergy
			0.008	16c	0.016	0.0005	0.041	synergy
			0.002	16d	0.002	0.0005	0.252	synergy
			0.016	17c	0.016	0.0005	0.082	synergy
	Gentamycin	2	0.016	16a	0.002	0.0005	0.33	synergy
			0.016	16c	0.001	0.0005	0.58	partial synergism
			0.008	16d	0.001	0.001	1	additivity
			0.001	17c	0.008	0.0005	0.063	synergy
	Streptomycin	5	0.001	16a	0.002	0.002	1	additivity
			0.001	16c	0.002	0.001	0.5	synergy
			0.001	16d	0.001	0.0005	0.5	synergy
			0.002	17c	0.008	0.001	0.125	synergy
	Vancomycin	1	0.002	16a	0.004	0.0005	0.126	synergy
			0.002	16c	0.004	0.0005	0.126	synergy
			0.001	16d	0.001	0.0005	0.5	synergy
			0.001	17c	0.016	0.004	0.251	synergy

Comb.—combination: compound + antibiotic or antibiotic + compound.

The cinnamic acid derivatives used in the research show a synergistic effect with antibiotics against selected HLAR strains. The exception is compound **16d**, which presents additive properties with ampicillin and gentamicin. Compounds **16a**, **16c** and **16f** are synergistic compounds with the tested antibiotics. These compounds may become potential preparations for clinical use in combination with currently used antibiotics against HLAR strains. However, the results obtained for selected VRE strains are not as homogeneous as for HLAR strains. Most of the tested compounds in a mixture with antibiotics show synergism. However, some compounds (**16a, 16c, 16d** and **17c**), when combined with antibiotics (gentamicin, streptomycin and vancomycin), give additive effects. Compound **16a** exhibits synergistic properties with all the tested antibiotics against selected VRE strains. In turn, all the compounds show synergy with ampicillin. The remaining tested compounds (**16c, 16d** and **17c**) show differentiated interactions with antibiotics: synergism or additivity.

3. Discussion

In our previous study, we showed that cinnamic acid derivatives with 4-chloro-2-mercaptobenzenesulfonamide moiety were active against reference and clinical strains of *Enterococcus* spp. The tested enterococci strains were mostly HLAR and included both *E. faecalis* and *E. faecium* strains. Only two of the tested isolates were VRE strains. In this work, we decided to test the activity of cinnamic acid derivatives against *Enterococcus* characterized by VRE.

The results of our previous research conducted by Bułakowska et al. [18] showed that the most active derivatives against *Enterococcus* spp. HLAR were **16a, 16c, 16d** and **16f**. Compounds **16d** and **17c** were the most active against *Enterococcus* spp. VRE. Both derivatives contain a chlorine atom as the substituent R^1 and naphthyl or piperonyl as the R^2 substituent. Moreover, derivatives **16a** and **16c** turned out to be very active against *Enterococcus* spp. VRE as well as for HLAR strains. Derivative **16f** was less active against VRE than against HLAR strains.

Based on the obtained results, it can be concluded that the activity of the tested derivatives against *Enterococcus* spp. HLAR and VRE was mainly due to the presence of the substituent R^2—naphthyl, and the substituent R^1 = H, F, NO_2 was secondary. The high activity of compounds **16d** and **17c** against *Enterococcus* spp. of the VRE group could mean that the substituent R^1 = Cl determines the main activity of the compound with the substituent R^2 only in the second place. When comparing the MIC values, obtained by serial dilution, to the standard (co-trimoxazole), the tested compounds turned out to be significantly more active against the tested *Enterococcus* strains. This is most likely related to the structure of the compounds—the combination of sulfonamide with cinnamic acid in one molecule and a different mechanism of action on microorganisms than the composition of co-trimoxazole.

Mingoia et al. [10] investigated the antibacterial properties of several hydroxy- and phenyl-substituted *trans*-cinnamic acid derivatives conjugated with an antimicrobial pharmacophore such as carvacrol in order to select the best candidate for the treatment of cutaneous infections caused by pathogens. Among the list of derivatives, only DM2 and DM8 turned out to be active against the tested bacterial strains. Compound DM2 was more active against *E. faecium* (MIC_{50} 32 mg/L) than *E. faecalis* (MIC_{50} 256 mg/L). The authors [9] suggest that the presence of a hydroxyl group in the *ortho* position in the phenyl nucleus is important for the effect on the cell membrane of enterococci. Therefore, the DM8 compound turned out to be the most active against *E. faecium* (MIC_{50} = 32 mg/L). It needs to be highlighted that the authors themselves, in Table 2, presented the range of the antibacterial activity of selected derivatives, including MD8, which for *E. faecalis* was in the range of 32–512 mg/mL and for *E. faecium* was in the range of 16–512 mg/mL. Hence, the authors' suggestion as to the mechanism is not that clear.

Guzman et al. [15] reported that cinnamic acid was active against *E. faecalis* and its minimum inhibitor concentration was 6.75 mM. In turn, the MICs of ferulic acid and its 4-*O*-acetyl derivative for *E. faecalis* ATCC 29212 were determined as 659 μM and 540 μM, respectively. Among natural and synthetic cinnamic esters, activity was demonstrated by 5-*O*-caffeoylquinic acid (MIC 181 μM) against *E. faecalis* OGRF1, rosmarinic acid (MIC 833 μM) and methyl rosmarinate (MIC 801 μM) against *E. faecalis* C159-6, and finally caffeic acid phenethyl ester (MIC 400 μM) against *E. faecalis* ATCC 29212. 4-*tert*-butylphenyl ferulate and 4-isopropylphenyl ferulate were active against *E. faecalis* ATCC 29212 at the concentrations of 391 μM and 51 μM, respectively. In turn, the MIC of 4-chloro-3-methylphenyl ferulate was 50 μM. Among cinnamic aldehydes, alcohols and their derivatives, the most active against *E. faecalis* turned out to be cinnamaldehyde at a concentration of 1.89 mM.

Many research groups are engaged in the construction of hybrid compounds using cinnamic acid. Cephem hybrid with cinnamic aldehyde gave results of activity against *E. faecalis* A20688 as 1.6 μM, 1.5 μM, 1.4 mM and 364 nM. Oxazolidinone hybrids are active against *E. faecium* ATTC 700221 (VRE; MIC 388 nM) and *E. faecalis* ATCC 29212 (MIC 194 nM) [15].

Gómez et al. [21] examined the antimicrobial properties of natural essential oil components, including cinnamaldehyde, against three species of bacteria: *Enterococcus* spp., *Staphylococcus* spp., and *Pseudomonas* spp. (10 clinical strains of each). Cinnamaldehyde (CIN) presented the highest activity for all tested bacterial strains—the MICs within the range of 10–50 mg/mL. The research was conducted in Mueller Hinton (MH) broth or cation-adjusted Mueller Hinton II broth (MH II).

Teethaisong et al. [22] investigated the effect of *Stephania suberosa* extract (SSE) against *E. faecium* strains and obtained MIC values of 0.5 mg/mL.

Biofilm consists of organized spaces, a multi-layer cluster of cells of one or several species of microorganisms, formed on biotic and abiotic surfaces. Microorganisms concentrated in biofilm are characterized by diverse metabolic activity. There are also antibiotic-resistant bacteria that "protect" the susceptible bacteria. Biofilm-forming bacteria are surrounded by a special extracellular polymeric substance (EPS) matrix. It is already known that Enterococcal surface protein (ESP) significantly enhanced *E. faecalis* biofilm formation in a glucose-dependent manner [22]. Biofilm is the cause of many life-threatening infections of humans and animals. Due to its complex structure, it is very difficult to remove; EPS is difficult for disinfectants and antibiotics to penetrate.

The compounds **16a**, **16c**, **16d**, **16f** and **17c** were tested at concentrations of 0.5 MIC, 2 × MIC and 4 × MIC and inhibited the formation of biofilm by both groups of enterococci, but the inhibition of the VRE strains was more efficient than that of the HLAR strains. However, the activity of the tested compounds against the already formed biofilm was low in both groups of bacteria; only compound **16f** was active against *Enterococcus* spp. HLAR and inhibited the formation of the biofilm to about 90% in comparison to the control. In our studies, we determined the amount of biofilm with crystal violet, as was previously described in [18].

Ali et al. [19], using BHI medium, examined the effect of *trans*-cinnamaldehyde (0.5%, 0.75% and 1%) on the biofilm formed by *E. faecalis* (clinical isolate) for 72 h. The authors treated the biofilm with the compounds for 5 and 15 min or 24 h and demonstrated, using 2,3-bis-(2-methoxy-4-nitro-5-sulfophenyl)-2*H*-tetrazolium-5-carboxanilide (XTT), that a 15-min action of cinnamaldehyde kills bacterial cells. Derivatives studied in our work had a bacteriostatic effect on planktonic bacterial cells in the tested concentration range. Due to the higher resistance of biofilm cells to chemicals than free-living cells, we chose crystal violet for biofilm determination in our studies. Crystal violet shows the size (biomass) of the biofilm presence or its absence rather than the presence of living cells, as was described in Ali et al. [19].

Akshaya et al. [23] examined the effect of cinnamaldehyde in the concentration range of 62.5–1000 μM on the biofilm formed by the *E. faecalis* strain (MTCC 2729) using BHI medium with 2% glucose for 72 h. The researchers used crystal violet and XTT [2,3-bis-(2-methoxy-4-nitro-5-sulfophenyl)-2*H*-tetrazolium-5-carboxanilide] as markers. Cinnamaldehyde prevented the growth of *E. faecalis* biofilm from a concentration of 62.5 μM, according to the crystal violet-staining technique. It was found that cinnamaldehyde at a concentration of 1000 μM inhibited the production of *E. faecalis* biofilm by 85%.

Akshaya et al. [23] studied the effect of cinnamaldehyde on the expansion and gelatinase activity of *E. faecalis* strains, which is important in the biofilm formation process. Gelatinase activity has been reported also to be involved in the initial steps of the generation of biofilm. In our studies, we detected phenotypically the presence of gelatinase produced by the tested strains. Unfortunately, we do not notice a correlation between the ability to form a biofilm and the presence of enzymes. The gelatinase activity was demonstrated by the following strains: *E. faecalis* 12245, 12214, 12338, 3937152 and *E. faecium* 264281, 508171, 16247; these strains formed a strong or a weak biofilm, as shown in Figure 1.

Hashem et al. [24] showed, using *gelE(−)* mutants, that the lack of the enzyme did not result in the lack of biofilm formation, which is consistent with our results.

The literature states [23] that the biofilm-forming activity of *E. faecalis* in the presence of glucose varies. Based on our results (Figure 2) (e.g., in the case of *E. faecalis* 12214, 12245, 12338, 12961), the presence of 2% glucose in two different media did not result in biofilm formation at the same level. There must be other factors that influence biofilm formation, depending on the medium used.

Enterococci possess in their genome the *fsr* locus that shares significant homology with the *agr* locus of staphylococci, which acts as an accessory global regulator of virulence factors and metabolism, including biofilm formation. Pillai et al. [25] showed that biofilm formation by *E. faecalis* OG1RF was greater in TSB supplemented with 1% glucose, but the same effect was not evident in *fsr*, *gelE* or *sprE* mutants. This could suggest that a glucose-dependent transcriptional regulator controlled *fsr*, either directly or indirectly, and that *fsr* exerts catabolite control over biofilm formation through GelE and SprE downstream proteases.

Kim et al. [26] examined the effect of tryptone–yeast extract broth with 0% glucose + 0% sucrose, 0.5% glucose, 1% glucose, 0.5% sucrose or 1% sucrose on *Enterococcus faecalis* planktonic and biofilm In vitro. They showed that the virulence-associated gene expression was the highest in broth with 1% sucrose (biofilm growth conditions) and in broth with 1% glucose (planktonic growth conditions). A higher bacteria and exopolysaccharide (EPS) bio-volume in sucrose was observed than in 0% glucose + 0% sucrose or glucose.

Interestingly, many researchers study the impact of chemical compounds on the already formed biofilm but do not check the preventive effect. Certainly, destroying the formed biofilm is a very important issue in the search for compounds that act on bacteria, but the administration of preventive preparations or coating materials used for catheterization, drainage, etc., may also be an important element in the fight against infections with resistant strains.

Caballero Gómez et al. [21], using TSB medium, examined the effect of natural essential oil components (including cinnamaldehyde) at MIC and 0.5 MIC concentrations, and their combination with EDTA (12.5–25 mM in water) and HLE (disinfectant solution—composed of 3–6% H_2O_2; 2.2–4.4% lactic acid) on the biofilm formed by selected strains. Crystal violet was used to determine the presence of biofilm. Cinnamaldehyde inhibited the formation of *Enterococcus* sp. strain M28M12 biofilm by 80%; for the other two strains, the effect was not so spectacular. However, a synergistic effect between cinnamaldehyde with HLE and EDTA was visible. CA + HLE caused 2–6 $\log_{10}$ reductions in CFU (colony-forming units) of enterococci and CA + EDTA 2–3 $\log_{10}$ reductions in CFU of enterococci in biofilm.

The presence of whole peripheral blood (Method 4.5) with its antibacterial mechanisms and the presence of phagocytic cells may have resulted in a slight decrease in the number of bacteria in the control samples. It seems that a similar mechanism occurred in the case of the lowest concentrations (0.5 µg/mL) of the tested compounds. This may be due to the fact that *Enterococcus* spp. do not have many virulence factors, like staphylococci, that neutralize the defense mechanisms present in the blood of mammals. In tests with higher concentrations of compounds, the number of viable bacterial cells changes significantly. These changes are a combination of the mechanisms of the immune system present in the blood and the bacteriostatic effect of the concentrations of compounds. The results obtained may be due to the influence of the tested derivatives on delays in the division of bacterial cells, which, when transferred to a solid substrate without the tested agent, have an extended doubling time and did not produce visible colonies even after 48 h of incubation. We suggested that the tested compounds have constant, stable bacteriostatic activity in whole blood, and they do not inhibit the activity of the cells of the immune system. This could be a basis for further research into potential drugs against resistant!bacteria.

Doyle et al. [27] cite that *trans*-cinnamaldehyde has properties that limit its use: low solubility in water, sensitivity to light and air, and it is not very stable in the blood where it is converted into cinnamic acid. Present in cosmetics in concentrations above 0.005%, it causes allergies and adverse reactions. The authors emphasize the need to test aldehyde derivatives for toxicity. The derivatives we tested show toxic activity to the peripheral blood of domestic sheep at concentrations of 32 µg/mL, as we demonstrated in the publication by Bułakowska et al. [18]. These compounds present stable activity against MRSA and *Enterococcus* spp. strains (data above) in the tested concentration range, during 24 h of testing. However, it would be necessary to carry out tests on the stability of the antimicrobial activity of compounds in biological systems over an extended period of time and to transform the derivatives we studied into water-soluble forms.

Enterococcus spp. are bacteria that are naturally resistant to many antibiotics, and the treatment of infections is mainly based on combining several antibiotics in order to achieve a synergistic effect. This effect is intended to fight the infection caused by multidrug-resistant strains. We wanted to check whether our compounds have any interactions with conventional antibiotics.

The cinnamic acid derivatives used in the research show a synergistic effect with antibiotics against selected HLAR strains. The exception is compound **16d**, which presents additive properties with ampicillin and gentamicin. It should be emphasized here that the tested compounds reduce the MIC for antibiotics by 800 to 10,000 times. However, the MIC of the tested compounds in combination with antibiotics is reduced by 2 to 16 times. Compounds **16a**, **16c** and **16f** are compounds that act synergistically with the tested antibiotics. These compounds may become potential preparations for clinical use in combination with currently used antibiotics against HLAR-resistant strains. However, the results obtained for selected VRE strains are not as homogeneous as for HLAR strains. Most of the tested compounds in a mixture with antibiotics show synergism. However, some compounds (**16a**, **16c**, **16d** and **17c**), when combined with antibiotics (gentamicin, streptomycin and vancomycin), give additive effects. The tested compounds reduce the MIC of antibiotics by 8 to 10,000 times. However, the combination of the tested derivatives with antibiotics causes a decrease in the MIC values of the compound by 2 to 32 times. Compound **16a** exhibits synergistic properties with all the tested antibiotics against selected VRE strains. In turn, all the compounds show synergy with ampicillin. The next stage of further research would be to check the activity of concentrations showing synergism, how they act on bacteria over time, how they affect biofilm and whether their activity is stable in the blood.

Essential oil (from *C. zeylanicum*) exhibits synergistic activity with amikacin, gentamicin, imipenem and meropenem against *Acinetobacter baumannii* and has a positive interaction with colistin [26]. Essential oil obtained from *Cinnamomum burmannii* interacts with gentamicin against *S. epidermidis*, and *Cinnamomum verum* essential oil showed the ability to restore the sensitivity of *Escherichia coli* to piperacillin (the bacterium had the TEM-1 beta-lactamase gene) [26]. *Trans*-cinnamaldehyde from *C. zeylanicum* decreased the MIC of clindamycin for *Clostridium difficile* by 16-fold [26].

Doyle et al. [27] presented a report on the synergism of cinnamaldehyde in combination with ampicillin, bacitracin, clindamycin, erythromycin, novobiocin, penicillin, streptomycin, sulfamethoxazole and tetracycline against *Salmonella* Typhimurium SGI1 (*tet A*), *Escherichia coli* N00-666, *Staphylococcus aureus blaZ*, which was resistant to penicillin, and erythromycin-resistant *Streptococcus pyogenes ermB*.

Cinnamic acid showed synergism with amikacin, ampicillin, ciprofloxacin, erythromycin, or vancomycin against *E. coli* and *S. aureus* and a combination of cinnamic acid with ciprofloxacin against *P. aeruginosa*. Cinnamic acid displays synergistic effects with amikacin, clofazimine, isoniazid and rifampin against *Mycobacterium tuberculosis* and *M. avium* [27].

Teethaisong et al. [22], using the checkerboard method, determined that SSE plus ampicillin and SSE plus vancomycin combinations exhibited synergistic interactions against *E. faecium* isolates.

4. Materials and Methods

4.1. Materials

Sterile sheep blood was defibrinated (GrasoBiotech, Starogard Gdański, Poland). Co-trimoxazole (composition sulfamethoxazole 400 mg: trimethoprim 80 mg; WZF Polfa, Warszawa, Poland), ampicillin-Na-salt (Serva, Heidelberg, Germany), streptomycin sulfate salt (Pol-Aura, Dywity, Poland), gentamycin (40 mg/mL, solution for injection and infusion; (KRKA d.d., Novo mesto, Slovenia), amikacin disulfate salt (Pol-Aura, Dywity, Poland), norfloxacin (Pol-Aura, Dywity, Poland), levofloxacin (5 mg/mL, solution for infusion, (Pharmathen S.A, Pallini, Greece), vancomycin hydrochloride (Pol-Aura, Dywity, Poland), ciprofloxacin (10 mg/mL, solution for infusion, (KRKA d.d., Novo mesto, Slovenia), vancomycin hydrochloride (Pol-Aura, Dywity, Poland), doxycycline (20 mg/mL, solution for infusion (Polfa Tarchomin S.A., Warszawa, Poland). Brain–heart infusion broth (BHI, Becton Dickinson, Franklin Lakes, NJ, USA) was used for MIC and FICI determination, while BHI and tryptic soy broth (TSB, Becton Dickinson, Franklin Lakes, NJ, USA) medium supplemented with 2% glucose were used to culture the biofilm bacteria. Muller–Hinton agar (MH, Becton Dickinson, Franklin Lakes, NJ, USA) was used alongside the disc diffusion method. Bacterial strains and culture conditions: lists of strains tested in the publication are presented in Table 7a, b. *Enterococcus faecalis* ATCC 51299 and clinical strain *Enterococcus* spp. were cultured in an aerobic atmosphere at 37 °C for 48 h. To determine the bacterial viability, BHI blood agar plates were used.

Table 7. (**a**) List of full names of strains tested in our previous study [18] and in the present study. (**b**) List of full names of strains tested in this publication only.

(a)

List of Strains Listed in the Publication [18]	Full Strain Name and Specific Resistance Mechanism
Enterococcus hirae ATCC 10541	
Enterococcus faecalis ATCC 51299	*Enterococcus faecalis* ATCC 51299 VRE
Enterococcus sp. 12835	*Enterococcus faecium* 12835 HLAR
Enterococcus sp. 12848	*Enterococcus faecium* 12848 HLAR
Enterococcus sp. 12214	*Enterococcus faecalis* 12214 HLAR
Enterococcus sp. 12245	*Enterococcus faecalis* 12245 HLAR
Enterococcus sp.12961	*Enterococccus faecium* 12961HLAR
Enterococcus sp. 12338	*Enterococcus faecalis* 12338 HLAR
Enterococcus sp. 16247	*Enterococcus faecium* 16247 HLAR
Enterococcus faecalis 3937152	*Enterococcus faecalis* 3937152 HLAR, VRE
Enterococcus faecium 3934825	*Enterococcus faecium* 3934825 HLAR, VRE

(b)

List of Strains Listed Only in This Publication	Full Strain Name, and Specific Resistance Mechanism
Enterococcus sp. 773081	*Enterococcus faecium* 773081 HLAR, VRE
Enterococcus sp. 508171	*Enterococcus faecium* 508171 HLAR, VRE
Enterococcus sp. 830981	*Enterococcus faecium* 830981 HLAR, VRE
Enterococcus sp. 264281	*Enterococcus faecium* 264281 HLAR, VRE
Enterococcus sp. 967321	*Enterococcus faecium* 967321 HLAR, VRE
Enterococcus sp. 966351	*Enterococcus faecium* 966351 HLAR, VRE
Enterococcus sp. 576181	*Enterococcus faecium* 576181 HLAR, VRE
Enterococcus sp. 885041	*Enterococcus faecium* 885041 HLAR, VRE

HLAR (high-level aminoglycoside resistance), VRE (vancomycin-resistant *Enterococcus*).

4.2. Determination of Susceptibility to Antibiotics by the Agar Disc Diffusion Method

Disc diffusion methods for antibiotics [28] and antibiotic susceptibility were interpreted according to EUCAST clinical breakpoints (version 11.0) [29]. In our research, Muller–Hinton medium (Beckton-Dicinson, Franklin Lakes, NJ, USA) and antibiotic paper discs (BioMaxima S.A., Lublin, Poland, Country) like ampicillin 2 µg/mL, imipenem 10 µg/mL, norfloxacin 10 µg/mL, vancomycin 5 µg/mL, teicoplanin 30 µg/mL, co-trimoxazole 25 µg/mL, doxycycline 30 µg/mL, linezolid 10 µg/mL, gentamicin 120 µg/mL, and streptomycin 300 µg/mL were used.

4.3. Minimum Inhibitory Concentration Determination

The MIC determination for the reference and clinical strains was performed based on the methodology described by Bułakowska et al. [18]. The dry test samples were dissolved in dimethyl sulfoxide (DMSO) and diluted in water, resulting in a final concentration of about 500 µg/mL. Antibiotics were weighed and dissolved in water, resulting in a final concentration of ampicillin (200 mg/mL), streptomycin (200 mg/mL), amikacin (80 mg/mL), norfloxacin (40 mg/mL) and vancomycin (80 mg/mL). The other antibiotics were in concentrations: co-trimoxazole (composition sulfamethoxazole 400 mg: trimethoprim 80 mg), gentamycin (40 mg/mL), levofloxacin (5 mg/mL), ciprofloxacin (10 mg/mL), and doxycycline (20 mg/mL). These solutions were diluted and added to the first well of each microtiter line. Dilution in geometric progression was completed by transferring the mixture/dilution (100 µL) from the first to the twelfth well. An aliquot (100 µL) was discarded from the twelfth well. Then, 100 µL of bacterial suspension was added to each well. The final concentration of the synthetic compound used in the antimicrobial activity assay ranged from 125 to 0.006 µg/mL. The final concentration of the antibiotics was: ampicillin (from 10 to 0.05 mg/mL), streptomycin (from 10 to 0.05 mg/mL), gentamycin (from 2 to 0.001 mg/mL), amikacin (from 4 to 0.002 mg/mL), norfloxacin (from 2 to 0.001 mg/mL), levofloxacin (from 0.25 to 0.000125 mg/mL), ciprofloxacin (from 0.5 to 0.00025), vancomycin (from 4 to 0.002 mg/mL) and doxycycline (from 1 to 0.0005 mg/mL). Tests were incubated in adequate conditions described by Bułakowska et al. [18]. The MIC was considered the lowest concentration at which no visible growth was observed. Diluent concentration had no effect on the activity of the tested compounds. All experiments were carried out three times.

4.4. Inhibition of Biofilm (Prior to Biofilm and Post-Biofilm) Formation by the Cinnamic Acid Derivatives

Determination of the biofilm inhibitory concentration (before and after biofilm formation) was carried out according to the method described by Bułakowska et al. [18] with modification. For the determination of biofilm, we used TSB (tryptic soy broth) supplemented with 2% glucose, BHI (brain–heart infusion broth) medium supplemented with 2% glucose, and BHI medium supplemented with 5% bovine serum. We also increased the range of concentrations of the tested compounds of 0.5 × MIC, MIC, 2 × MIC and 4 × MIC. The final volume of the mixture was 200 µL. In the post-biofilm formation, biofilms were formed for 24 h at 37 °C, non-adherent cells were removed, and compounds at the concentrations of 0.5 × MIC, MIC, 2 × MIC and 4 × MIC were added into each well. After 24 h incubation at 37 °C, the contents of each well were discarded and washed 3 times with sterile deionized water in order to remove non-adherent cells. The biofilm was fixed with 2% formaldehyde (0.5 h) and then stained with 0.1% crystal violet solution for 1 h at 37 °C. Next, plates were rinsed with water until clean drops were obtained. The stained biofilm was dissolved by 96% ethanol, and growth of bacteria was quantified by measuring the OD at 560 nm using a microplate reader (Infinite® 200 PRO, Tecan, Männedorf, Switzerland). Positive control were bacteria without compounds. All experiments were carried out in three repetitions.

4.5. Blood Bacteriostatic Activity Tests

The assay was performed as previously described by Bułakowska [18] with a modification. Pure sheep blood was used for the research. Two strains of bacteria *E. faecalis* 12245 and *E. faecium* 264281 were used with an inoculum density of approximately 10^8 CFU/mL at time 0 (t_0). The final concentration of the compounds were 0.5, 1, 2, 4, 8 and 16 µg/mL, and the final volume of the assay tube was 1 mL. Bacterial survivors were determined on BHI agar plates (CFU/mL) at 24 h after exposure. All experiments were carried out in three repetitions.

4.6. Checkerboard Arrays for Planktonic Bacteria (Fractional Inhibitory Concentration Index)

The checkerboard arrays method was described in [22]. The BHI broth was used in the studies. Antibiotics (ampicillin, gentamicin, streptomycin, vancomycin) in the range of 16 to 1 µg/mL and tested compounds in the range of 8 to 0.5 µg/mL were tested. Bacteria were cultured 48 h in aerobic conditions. After incubation, the turbidity of the samples was visually determined and the results were read. The MICs of the antibiotic and the test compound were determined and substituted into the formula to calculate the Fractional Inhibitory Concentration Index (FICI):

$$\mathrm{FICI} = \mathrm{FIC_A} + \mathrm{FIC_B} = \mathrm{A/MIC_A} + \mathrm{B/MIC_B}$$

$\mathrm{MIC_A}$ and $\mathrm{MIC_B}$ are the MICs of drugs A and B alone, respectively. A and B are the concentrations of the drugs in combinations, respectively. FIC (index) values were interpreted as follows [30]: FIC index ≤ 0.5 indicates synergism, FIC index > 0.5 to < 1.0 shows partial synergism, FICI = 1.0 indicates addition, FIC index > 1.0 to 4.0 denotes indifference, and FIC index > 4.0 denotes antagonism [22].

4.7. Statistical Analysis

All experiments were performed at least three times. The intergroup differences were estimated by one- or two-way analysis of variance by statistical package Microsoft Excel 2010. The data are presented as mean and standard deviation (SD). A *p*-value was considered as statistically significant when it was less than 0.05.

5. Conclusions

In the current study, we continued the studies on cinnamic acid derivatives with 4-chloro-2-mercaptobenzenesulfonamide moiety on Gram-positive cocci—*Enterococcus* spp. We expanded the number of research objects; in addition to clinical strains with HLAR (MIC **16d**, **17c**, **16a** and **16c** values are published by Bułakowska et al. [18]), we added the strains with the VRE mechanism of resistance and determined the active concentrations of the tested compounds against these bacteria. The most active compounds for the group of VRE strains were **16c**, **17c**, **16a** and **16d**. Whereas, for the HLAR group, the most active turned out to be **16a**, **16c**, **16d** and **16f**. Compounds **16d** and **17c** contain two or three chlorine atoms per molecule, and a strong effect may result from HLAR and VRE bacterial cells. Compounds **16f**, **16a**, **16c** and **16d** were the most active and inhibited biofilm formation by the tested *Enterococcus* spp. HLAR strains. The biofilm formation of VRE strains was inhibited by **16a**, **16c**, **16d** and **17a**. Compounds **16a**, **16c** and **16d** showed a low effect on the already formed biofilm of the tested strains; only compound **16f** appeared to be the most effective and inhibited the biofilm. We have shown that the tested derivatives maintain stable activity, inhibiting the growth of bacteria in the peripheral blood of domestic sheep. The interactions between antibiotics and compounds **16a**, **16c** and **16f** presented a synergistic effect with ampicillin, gentamicin, streptomycin and vancomycin against HLAR strains. The compounds **16a**, **16c**, **16d** and **17c** exhibit synergism, partial synergism or additivity against VRE strains. It should be noticed that the tested compounds reduce the MIC for antibiotics by 8 to 10,000 times. The MIC of the tested compounds in combination with antibiotics is reduced by 2 to 32 times. In summary, our results indicate that the tested cinnamic acid derivatives may be promising in the treatment of bacterial infections.

Author Contributions: Conceptualization, R.H. and A.B.; methodology, R.H.; software, R.H. and M.S.; validation, R.H. and M.S.; formal analysis, R.H.; investigation, R.H.; resources, R.H. and A.B.; data curation, R.H.; writing—original draft preparation, R.H. and M.S.; writing—review and editing, A.B., U.M., A.R.-Z. and J.S.; visualization, R.H.; supervision, A.B., U.M., A.R.-Z. and J.S.; project administration, R.H.; funding acquisition, A.R.-Z. and J.S. All authors have read and agreed to the published version of the manuscript.

Funding: This research received no external funding.

Institutional Review Board Statement: Not applicable.

Informed Consent Statement: Not applicable.

Data Availability Statement: Data are contained within the article.

Acknowledgments: The authors would like to many thanks to dr Katarzyna Turecka or her assistance, support and uplifting spirit.

Conflicts of Interest: The authors declare no conflict of interest.

References

1. Ali, I.A.A.; Neelakantan, P. Antibiofilm activity of phytochemicals against *Enterococcus faecalis*: A literature review. *Phytother. Res.* **2022**, *36*, 2824–2838. [CrossRef] [PubMed]
2. Liu, F.; Suna, Z.; Wang, F.; Liu, Y.; Zhu, Y.; Duc, L.; Wanga, D.; Xu, W. Inhibition of biofilm formation and exopolysaccharide synthesis of Enterococcus faecalis by phenyllactic acid. *Food Microbiol.* **2020**, *86*, 103344. [CrossRef] [PubMed]
3. Krawczyk, B.; Wityk, P.; Gałecka, M.; Michalik, M. The Many Faces of Enterococcus spp.—Commensal, Probiotic and Opportunistic Pathogen. *Microorganisms* **2021**, *9*, 1900. [CrossRef] [PubMed]
4. Woitschach, F.; Kloss, M.; Schlodder, K.; Borck, A.; Grabow, N.; Reisinger, E.C.; Sombetzki, M. Bacterial Adhesion and Biofilm Formation of *Enterococcus faecalis* on Zwitterionic Methylmethacrylat and Polysulfones. *Front. Cell. Infect. Microbiol.* **2022**, *12*, 868338. [CrossRef] [PubMed]
5. De Oliveira, D.M.P.; Forde, B.M.; Kidd, T.J.; Harris, P.N.A.; Schembri, M.A.; Beatson, S.A.; Paterson, D.L.; Walkera, M.J. Antimicrobial Resistance in ESKAPE Pathogens. *Clin. Microbiol. Rev.* **2020**, *33*, e00181-19. [CrossRef] [PubMed]
6. Cetinkaya, Y.; Falk, P.; Mayhall, C.G. Vancomycin-resistant enterococci. *Clin. Microbiol. Rev.* **2000**, *13*, 686–707. [CrossRef] [PubMed]
7. Codelia-Anjum, A.; Lerner, L.B.; Elterman, D.; Zorn, K.C.; Bhojani, N.; Chughtai, B. Enterococcal Urinary Tract Infections: A Review of the Pathogenicity, Epidemiology, and Treatment. *Antibiotics* **2023**, *12*, 778. [CrossRef]
8. Bag, M.A.S.; Arif, M.; Riaz, S.; Khan, M.S.R.; Islam, M.S.; Punom, S.A.; Ali, M.W.; Begum, F.; Islam, M.S.; Rahman, M.T.; et al. Antimicrobial Resistance, Virulence Profiles, and Public Health Significance of *Enterococcus faecalis* Isolated from Clinical Mastitis of Cattle in Bangladesh. *Hindawi BioMed Res.* **2022**, *2022*, 8101866. [CrossRef]
9. WHO (World Health Organization). Available online: https://www.who.int/health-topics/antimicrobial-resistance (accessed on 20 May 2021).
10. Mingoia, M.; Conte, C.; Di Rienzo, A.; Dimmito, M.P.; Marinucci, L.; Magi, G.; Turkez, H.; Cufaro, M.C.; Del Boccio, P.; Di Stefano, A.; et al. Synthesis and Biological Evaluation of Novel Cinnamic Acid-Based Antimicrobials. *Pharmaceuticals* **2022**, *15*, 228. [CrossRef]
11. Meesters, K.; Alemayehu, T.; Benou, S.; Buonsenso, D.; Decloedt, E.H.; Pillay-Fuentes Lorente, V.; Downes, K.J.; Allegaert, K. Pharmacokinetics of Antimicrobials in Children with Emphasis on Challenges Faced by Low and Middle Income Countries, a Clinical Review. *Antibiotics* **2023**, *12*, 17. [CrossRef]
12. Lagatolla, C.; Mehat, J.W.; La Ragione, R.M.; Luzzati, R.; Di Bella, S. In Vitro and In Vivo Studies of Oritavancin and Fosfomycin Synergism against Vancomycin-Resistant. *Enterococcus faecium*. *Antibiotics* **2022**, *11*, 1334. [CrossRef]
13. Babiker, A.; Clarke, L.; Doi, Y.; Shields, R.K. Fosfomycin for Treatment of Multidrug Resistant Pathogens Causing Urinary Tract Infection: A Real-World Perspective and Review of the Literature. *Diagn. Microbiol. Infect. Dis.* **2019**, *95*, 114856. [CrossRef] [PubMed]
14. Malheiro, J.F.; Maillard, J.-Y.; Borges, F.; Simões, M. Evaluation of cinnamaldehyde and cinnamic acid derivatives in microbial growth control. *Inter. Biodeter. Biodegrad.* **2019**, *141*, 71–78. [CrossRef]
15. Guzman, J.D. Natural cinnamic acids, synthetic derivatives, and hybrids with antimicrobial activity. *Molecules* **2014**, *19*, 19292–19349. [CrossRef] [PubMed]
16. Sova, M. Antioxidant and antimicrobial activities of cinnamic acid derivatives. *Mini-Rev. Med. Chem.* **2012**, *12*, 749–767. [CrossRef] [PubMed]
17. Ruwizhi, N.; Aderibigbe, B.A. Cinnamic acid derivatives and their biological efficacy. *Int. J. Mol. Sci.* **2020**, *21*, 5712. [CrossRef]

18. Bułakowska, A.; Sławiński, J.; Hałasa, R.; Hering, A.; Gucwa, M.; Ochocka, J.R.; Stefanowicz-Hajduk, J. An In Vitro Antimicrobial, Anticancerand Antioxidant Activity of *N*–[(2–Arylmethylthio)phenylsulfonyl]cinnamamide Derivatives. *Molecules* **2023**, *28*, 3087. [CrossRef]
19. Ali, I.A.A.; Cheung, B.P.K.; Matinlinna, J.P.; L'evesque, C.M.; Neelakanta, P. *Trans*-cinnamaldehyde potently kills *Enterococcus faecalis* biofilm cells and prevents biofilm recovery. *Microb. Pathog.* **2020**, *149*, 104482. [CrossRef]
20. Awakawa, T.; Barra, L.; Abe, I. Biosynthesis of sulfonamide and sulfamate antibiotics in actinomycete. *J. Ind. Microbiol. Biotechnol.* **2021**, *48*, kuab001. [CrossRef]
21. Gómez, C.N.; Manetsberger, J.; Benomar, N.; Castillo Gutiérrez, S.; Abriouel, H. Antibacterial and antibiofilm effects of essential oil components, EDTA and HLE disinfectant solution on Enterococcus, Pseudomonas and Staphylococcus sp. multiresistant strains isolated along the meat production chain. *Front. Microbiol.* **2022**, *13*, 1014169. [CrossRef]
22. Teethaisong, Y.; Chueakwon, P.; Poolpol, K.; Ayamuang, I.; Suknasang, S.; Apinundecha, C.; Eumkeb, G. *Stephania suberosa* Forman extract synergistically inhibits ampicillin- and vancomycin-resistant *Enterococcus faecium*. *Saudi J. Biol. Sci.* **2023**, *30*, 103557. [CrossRef] [PubMed]
23. Akshaya, B.S.; Premraj, K.; Iswarya, C.; Muthusamy, S.; Ibrahim, H.-I.M.; Khalil, H.E.; Ashokkumar, V.; Vickram, S.; Kumar, V.S.; Palanisamy, S.; et al. Cinnamaldehyde inhibits *Enterococcus faecalis* biofilm formation and promotes clearance of its colonization by modulation of phagocytes in vitro. *Microb. Pathog.* **2023**, *181*, 106157. [CrossRef] [PubMed]
24. Hashem, Y.A.; Abdelrahman, K.A.; Aziz, R. K Phenotype–Genotype Correlations and Distribution of Key Virulence Factors in *Enterococcus faecalis* Isolated from Patients with Urinary Tract Infections. *Infect. Drug Resist.* **2021**, *14*, 1713–1723. [CrossRef] [PubMed]
25. Pillai, S.K.; Sakoulas, G.; Eliopoulos, G.M.; Moellering, R.C., Jr.; Murray, B.E.; Inouye, R. T Effects of Glucose on *fsr*-Mediated Biofilm Formation in *Enterococcus faecalis*. *J. Infect. Dis.* **2004**, *190*, 967–970. [CrossRef]
26. Kim, M.-A.; Rosa, V.; Min, K.-S. Characterization of *Enterococcus faecalis* in different culture conditions. *Nat. Res. Sci. Rep.* **2020**, *10*, 21867. [CrossRef]
27. Doyle, A.A.; Stephens, J.C. A review of cinnamaldehyde and its derivatives as antibacterial agents. *Fitoterapia* **2018**, *139*, 104405. [CrossRef]
28. EUCAST Disk Diffusion Test Methodology, Available online:. Available online: https://www.eucast.org/ast_of_bacteria/disk_diffusion_methodology; (accessed on 2 January 2020).
29. Clinical Breakpoints - Breakpoints and Guidance. Available online: https://www.eucast.org/clinical_breakpoints (accessed on 2 January 2020).
30. Turecka, K.; Chylewska, A.; Kawiak, A.; Waleron, K.F. Antifungal Activity and Mechanism of Action of the Co(III) Coordination Complexes With Diamine Chelate Ligands Against Reference and Clinical Strains of *Candida* spp. *Front. Microbiol.* **2018**, *9*, 1594. [CrossRef]

antibiotics

MDPI

Article

Saponin-Derived Silver Nanoparticles from *Phoenix dactylifera* (Ajwa Dates) Exhibit Broad-Spectrum Bioactivities Combating Bacterial Infections

Mohd Adnan [1,2], Arif Jamal Siddiqui [1,2], Syed Amir Ashraf [2,3], Mohammad Saquib Ashraf [4], Sarah Owdah Alomrani [5], Mousa Alreshidi [1,2], Bektas Tepe [6], Manojkumar Sachidanandan [2,7], Corina Danciu [8,*] and Mitesh Patel [9,*]

1 Department of Biology, College of Science, University of Ha'il, Ha'il 55473, Saudi Arabia; drmohdadnan@gmail.com (M.A.)
2 Medical and Diagnostic Research Centre, University of Ha'il, Ha'il 55473, Saudi Arabia
3 Department of Clinical Nutrition, College of Applied Medial Sciences, University of Ha'il, Ha'il 55473, Saudi Arabia
4 Department of Medical Laboratory Science, College of Applied Medical Sciences, Riyadh ELM University, Riyadh 12734, Saudi Arabia
5 Department of Biology, College of Science and Arts, Najran University, Najran 66252, Saudi Arabia
6 Department of Molecular Biology and Genetics, Faculty of Science and Literature, Kilis 7 Aralik University, TR-79000 Kilis, Turkey
7 Department of Oral Radiology, College of Dentistry, University of Ha'il, Ha'il 55473, Saudi Arabia
8 Department of Pharmacognosy, Faculty of Pharmacy, "Victor Babes" University of Medicine and Pharmacy, 2 Eftimie Murgu Square, 300041 Timisoara, Romania
9 Research and Development Cell, Department of Biotechnology, Parul Institute of Applied Sciences, Parul University, Vadodara 391760, India
* Correspondence: corina.danciu@umft.ro (C.D.); patelmeet15@gmail.com (M.P.)

Abstract: The emergence of antibiotic resistance poses a serious threat to humankind, emphasizing the need for alternative antimicrobial agents. This study focuses on investigating the antibacterial, antibiofilm, and anti-quorum-sensing (anti-QS) activities of saponin-derived silver nanoparticles (AgNPs-S) obtained from Ajwa dates (*Phoenix dactylifera* L.). The design and synthesis of these novel nanoparticles were explored in the context of developing alternative strategies to combat bacterial infections. The Ajwa date saponin extract was used as a reducing and stabilizing agent to synthesize AgNPs-S, which was characterized using various analytical techniques, including UV–Vis spectroscopy, Fourier transform infrared (FTIR) spectroscopy, and transmission electron microscopy (TEM). The biosynthesized AgNPs-S exhibited potent antibacterial activity against both Gram-positive and Gram-negative bacteria due to their capability to disrupt bacterial cell membranes and the leakage of nucleic acid and protein contents. The AgNPs-S effectively inhibited biofilm formation and quorum-sensing (QS) activity by interfering with QS signaling molecules, which play a pivotal role in bacterial virulence and pathogenicity. Furthermore, the AgNPs-S demonstrated significant antioxidant activity against 2,2 diphenyl 1 picrylhydrazyl (DPPH) free radicals and cytotoxicity against small lung cancer cells (A549 cells). Overall, the findings of the present study provide valuable insights into the potential use of these nanoparticles as alternative therapeutic agents for the design and development of novel antibiotics. Further investigations are warranted to elucidate the possible mechanism involved and safety concerns when it is used in vivo, paving the way for future therapeutic applications in combating bacterial infections and overcoming antibiotic resistance.

Keywords: antibiofilm; anti-quorum sensing; cytotoxicity; antibacterial; antibiotic resistance; saponins; *Phoenix dactylifera*; Ajwa date

1. Introduction

Nanotechnology is a rapidly advancing area that deals with the manipulation and control of matter at the nanoscale level, typically involving structures with dimensions ranging from 1 to 100 nanometers [1]. At this scale, materials frequently display distinctive qualities and behaviors that are different from those of their bulk counterparts [2]. Nanotechnology has attracted significant attention due to its potential to revolutionize various industries and offer solutions to numerous challenges in many disciplines, such as pharmaceutical industries, electronics, energy, and environmental science [3–5]. One particular area of interest within nanotechnology is the utilization of nanoparticles, which are tiny particles with dimensions on the nanoscale [6,7]. Among the several kinds of nanoparticles, silver nanoparticles (AgNPs) have attracted a great deal of interest and have emerged as a prominent nanomaterial with diverse applications [8]. AgNPs have unique chemical, physical, and biological characteristics that make them highly versatile for a variety of applications [9,10]. The unique properties of AgNPs, such as their high surface-area-to-volume ratio, high electrical and thermal conductivity, and antimicrobial properties, contribute to their extensive applications in many disciplines such as the pharmaceutical industries, electronics, environmental science, and consumer products [11–13]. These characteristics make AgNPs versatile and attractive for use in relation to diverse technological advancements, paving the way for exciting developments in the nanotechnology arena [14].

The drugs previously used to inhibit or kill viruses, bacteria, and fungi have become less effective over time [15]. It has been found that the improper use and misuse of antimicrobials can lead to resistance in bacteria. This is particularly problematic in developing nations where patients can obtain antibiotics without a medical prescription [16]. Several antibiotics that are designed to inhibit the growth of bacteria and fungi are being phased out due to the fact that the target microorganisms are becoming resistant to them. Thus, antibiofilm effects and QS inhibition are currently regarded as two new methods that can be employed to tackle microbial resistance, thereby alleviating the ferocity of infections associated with them [17]. There are many kinds of bacteria that produce an extracellular polymeric protective coating, referred to as a biofilm, on abiotic or biotic surfaces. These coatings are most commonly found on surfaces with adequate nutrients or on food sources, and they protect bacteria against antibiotics, disinfectants, detergents, and defense systems that occur in the host body [18]. The process of QS involves the synthesis, diffusion, detection, and reaction of small signaling molecules known as autoinducers that signal to other cells. In fact, biofilm formation is a result of QS, which increases the resistance of bacteria to antibiotics 10–1000 times more than in their planktonic stage [19]. By disrupting the biofilm formation and QS in bacteria, it is possible to limit the expression of virulence factors in pathogenic bacteria, as well as the infection and contamination of such microorganisms.

It is widely recognized that natural foodstuffs such as fruits can provide human bodies with nutrients and a range of bioactive molecules that contribute to a healthy body. As strategic antimicrobials, these natural products are being looked into as potential food additives or nutraceuticals, which can serve as nutritional supplements for the good health of consumers. The inhibition of the production of signal molecules aided by synthesized signal molecules is a process called QS inhibition, which can be used to target cell-to-cell communication. When the production of the signal molecules is blocked, the bacteria are not able to form biofilms [20]. As a result, most scientists are currently working on the development of new therapeutic antibiotics by investigating plant products in order to find new antibiotics, which prevent the development of resistant bacteria strains by inhibiting QS mechanisms and controlling infections [21].

There is enormous interest in plants being used to synthesize different types of metal nanoparticles. Using plant metabolites in the synthesis of AgNPs is advantageous due to their natural origins and low toxicity [22]. In recent years, several reports have been published on the process by which plant-mediated AgNPs are synthesized. The results of these studies have shown that plant metabolites can be used to synthesize bioactive AgNPs with high efficiency. There are different types of secondary metabolites that can be found in plants, such as flavonoids, phenolic compounds, terpenoids, and saponins, which have been reported to play a role in reducing silver ions to their elemental state [23]. Due to the fact that plant species vary in terms of their composition and the quantity of secondary metabolites, it is important for us to examine a broad range of plant species to determine their ability and efficiency in biosynthesizing metal nanoparticles [24]. In this way, biomedical constraints and other production-related issues can be overcome. By using phyto-molecules to synthesize AgNPs, we may be able to avoid the problems associated with toxic chemical reagents in the production of AgNPs [25].

Ajwa dates (*Phoenix dactylifera* L.) are an expensive and popular fruit limited to Saudi Arabia's holy city of Madinah Al Munawara and its surrounding areas [26]. There is an abundance of dietary fiber in Ajwa dates, which may help to solve digestion problems. By providing natural roughage to the body and stimulating bowel movements, Ajwa dates effectively relieve constipation [27]. Furthermore, these dates contain large amounts of potassium, which is necessary for muscle contractions. Ajwa dates enrich breast milk with many nutrients that are beneficial for lactating women. Ajwa dates have also been shown to reduce disease and infection susceptibility in the children of mothers who eat them regularly [28]. Additionally, Ajwa dates are high in iron, which is another significant advantage. Besides assisting in the production of red blood cells, iron may also assist in treating and preventing anemia. As a result of their nutritional and health properties, Ajwa dates can be thought of as a potential bioactive component for the development of food products with nutraceutical significance for various health purposes [29]. Ajwa dates usually accumulate polyphenols, triterpenoids, saponins, and flavonoids, which confer some medicinal properties, including protection against cardiovascular disorders, diabetes, and cancer. Furthermore, their antimicrobial, anti-inflammatory, and antioxidant properties suggest their potential benefits in supporting immune function and reducing the risk of various infections [30].

The aim of this study was therefore to extract and synthesize saponin-derived AgNPs from Ajwa dates (AgNPs-S). Different biophysical methods were used to characterize the formation of AgNPs-S. Furthermore, the synthesized AgNPs-S were also tested against several bacterial pathogens to determine their antibacterial, nucleic acid, and protein leakage and their anti-QS and antibiofilm properties. The production of violacein, pyocyanin, and prodigiosin, which is considered a QS phenomenon, was examined in the presence of AgNPs-S. Additionally, the antioxidant activity of AgNPs-S against DPPH free radicals and their cytotoxic potential against human small lung cancer cells (A549s) were further assessed.

2. Materials and Methods

2.1. Collection of Ajwa Dates

The Ajwa dates used in the present study were purchased fresh from Al-Madina Al Munawwarah, the Kingdom of Saudi Arabia. After manual separation, the pulpy part of the date fruits was washed with double-distilled water, dried in an oven, and coarsely powdered using an electrical grinder. After the coarse powder was prepared for experimentation, it was kept in an airtight jar.

2.2. Extraction of Crude Saponins

In order to extract crude saponins from the Ajwa dates, powdered samples (20 g) were heated at 55 °C for 4 h with 100 mL of ethanol (20%). After the extract was filtered, residues were re-extracted using 200 mL of ethanol (20%). The extract was concentrated to 40 mL in a water bath and then combined with 20 mL of diethyl ether in a separating funnel. The mixture was vigorously agitated to separate the diethyl and aqueous layers. The aqueous phase was collected, and the diethyl ether fraction was discarded. N-butanol (60 mL) was added and thoroughly mixed in the aqueous layer. In the next step, 10 mL of 5% NaCl solution was added to the n-butanol extract. A water bath was used to concentrate the solution, and the saponin residues were dried in an oven [31].

2.3. Foam Test for Saponins

Saponins were diluted with 20 mL deionized water; then, samples were shaken for 15 min. The presence of saponins was suggested by the development of a stable foam.

2.4. Spectrophotometric Analysis of Saponins

A spectrophotometric method was used, with minor modifications, to quantitate the saponin-enriched fractions [32]. Quil-A (QA) was used as a standard. A solution of p-anisaldehyde (Sigma Aldrich®, Bengaluru, India) in ethyl acetate (0.5:99.5) and a solution of H_2SO_4 were mixed in equal amounts. QA and saponins were mixed with 2 mL of ethyl acetate. In the next step, reagents A and B were added (1 mL) to the reaction mixture. An incubation at 60 °C was performed in a water bath for 10 min on the mixture. After cooling the solutions for 10 min, they were measured at 430 nm for absorbance. The absorbance was measured using ethyl acetate as a control. To obtain a calibration curve, 75–175 µg of standard saponin was mixed in 2 mL of ethyl acetate. The overall saponins in the extract were calculated using a calibration curve for standard saponin.

2.5. High-Performance Thin-Layer Chromatography (HPTLC)

The HPTLC technique was used to analyze saponin-rich fractions obtained from Ajwa dates. After pre-washing with methanol and activating at 100 °C for 30 min, a silica gel 60 F_{254} plate (20 × 10 cm) was utilized for the chromatographic analysis. Separation was performed with chloroform, methanol, and water (6.4:3.2:1.2:0.8 $v/v/v$). Using an HPTLC autosampler (ATS4, CAMAG AG, Muttenz, Switzerland), a 10 µL sample was injected in 8 mm bands under a nitrogen flow (ATS4, CAMAG AG, Muttenz, Switzerland). HPTLC chambers were developed and presaturated with solvent systems and were used for separation until the migration of the solvent front reached 70 mm. In the following step, a vacuum-drying process was performed on the plates for 10 min [33].

2.6. Derivatization with p-Anisaldehyde Sulphuric Acid after Chromatography

The developed chromatographic plate was post-chromatographically derivatized by dipping it using a p-anisaldehyde sulphuric acid coloring solution (for 5 s). After drying for 10 min, a temperature of 70 °C was further applied to the plate for 5 min until bands appeared. A photo documentation system was used for the detection (TLC visualizer, CAMAG AG, Muttenz, Switzerland) of visible and ultraviolet light wavelengths. With a slit length of 5.00 × 0.45 mm and a wavelength of 545 nm, a densitometric measurement was performed (CAMAG AG, Muttenz, Switzerland). A densitogram was evaluated via winCats (CAMAG AG, Muttenz, Switzerland) [34].

2.7. Biosynthesis of Silver Nanoparticles Using Extracted Saponins (AgNPs-S)

The development of saponin-derived AgNPs was carried out by adding 4 mL of the extracted saponins drop by drop into 16 mL of 0.003 M aqueous silver nitrate and stirring it at 60 °C for 2 h [35]. The solution started to form silver nanoparticles as it changed color from yellow to brown. To further characterize the AgNPs-S, they were centrifuged, washed with ethanol, dried, and subsequently utilized for various biological assays.

2.8. Characterization of AgNPs-S

The first step in characterizing the AgNPs-S was the spectrophotometric analysis. A range of 300 to 700 nm was scanned with a resolution of 1 nm for AgNPs-S [36]. Fourier transform infrared spectroscopy (FT-IR) was further used to investigate the potential interaction between saponins and $AgNO_3$ (Bruker®, Billerica, MA, USA). The spectra were recorded in the range of 500 to 4000 cm^{-1} with 32 scans and a resolution of 4 cm^{-1} [37]. To estimate the shape and size of AgNPs-S, TEM measurements were also performed. The TEM analysis was carried out using a JEM-1400 Plus, Jeol, India. A TEM analysis was performed after smearing the AgNPs-S sample in a grid of carbon-coated copper and allowing it to evaporate for 1 h under a vacuum dryer [38].

2.9. Antibacterial Activity of AgNPs-S

An agar well diffusion technique was used to test the antibacterial activity of AgNPs-S against various Gram-positive and Gram-negative pathogenic bacteria, such as *Chromobacterium violaceum* MTCC-2656 (*C. violaceum*), *Pseudomonas aeruginosa* MTCC-741 (*P. aeruginosa*), *Escherichia coli* MTCC-9537 (*E. coli*), *Bacillus subtilis* MTCC-121 (*B. subtilis*), *Proteus vulgaris* MTCC-426 (*P. vulgaris*), *Serratia marcescens* MTCC-97 (*S. marcescens*), *Enterococcus faecalis* MTCC-439 (*E. faecalis*), and *Staphylococcus aureus* MTCC-96 (*S. aureus*) [39]. Using a sterile swab, the cultures of each bacterial strain, which had been developed overnight, were streaked onto an MHB agar plate. In the following step, using a sterile cork borer, wells were punctured, and AgNPs-S were transferred into each well. The plates were incubated at 37 °C for 24 h. Furthermore, the incubated samples were determined by measuring the inhibition zone.

2.10. Determination of Minimum Inhibitory Concentration (MIC)

The standard broth dilution assay was used to evaluate the MIC values of AgNPs-S against different bacterial pathogens [40]. The AgNPs-S were used in a series of double dilutions in MHB with an active bacterial culture (108 CFU/mL, 0.5 McFarland standard) to determine the MIC. The concentrations of the sample ranged from 1698.7 µg/mL to 1.65 µg/mL. A control was prepared using only inoculated broth, which was incubated at 37 °C for 24 h. The smallest concentration of AgNPs-S that prevents any growth on the tubes is known as the MIC. To verify the MIC value, the turbidity of the tubes was measured before and after incubation.

2.11. Determination of Nucleic Acid Leakage

Cell membrane integrity can be observed via the liberation of the cytoplasmic components of a cell that are indicative of the integrity of its membrane [41]. The incubation of *P. aeruginosa* bacteria was achieved using an LB medium at 37 °C for 12 h. Except for the control, the log-phase culture was treated with AgNPs-S (1 × MIC, 2 × MIC). After that, the incubation of samples was carried out at 37 °C for 6 and 24 h. The samples were filtered as soon as they were collected using an organic membrane with a 0.2 µm filter. The optical density of the supernatant was measured at 260 nm to estimate the amount of DNA and RNA released from the cytoplasm.

2.12. Determination of Protein Leakage

The effect of AgNPs-S on cell integrity was further determined by checking the release of proteins after the treatment of the AgNPs-S. Bradford's method was used to determine the protein concentrations in the supernatants [42]. The log-phase cultures of *P. aeruginosa* were treated with AgNPs-S (1 × MIC, 2 × MIC), except the control, and incubated at 37 °C for 6 h and 24 h. Centrifugation at 6000 rpm for 10 min at 4 °C was performed after incubation. The protein concentration was determined by adding 200 µL of the supernatant to 800 µL of the Bradford reagent at 595 nm via a UV spectrophotometer (UV-2600, Shimadzu, Japan). Bovine serum albumin (BSA) was used as a standard protein.

2.13. Determination of Antibiofilm Activity

Test tubes made of glass were used to investigate the antibiofilm effects of AgNPs-S as a hydrophilic surface [43]. Briefly, tubes containing 1 mL of an active bacterial culture and 500 µL of AgNPs-S (sub-MICs) received 3 mL of sterilized LB medium. After thorough mixing, the tubes were incubated in a shaker for 72 h at room temperature. After the tubes had been incubated, planktonic cells were taken out and washed with PBS. Inside the tubes, the biofilm that had grown was stained with crystal violet. By washing the stained biofilm with PBS and eliminating the excess dye, the developed biofilm was dissolved in acetic acid and its absorbance was measured at 595 nm using the UV spectrophotometer (UV-2600,

Shimadzu, Japan). Controls for the growth of biofilms were made using an LB medium containing individual bacterial strains. Biofilm inhibition was estimated as follows:

$$O.D._{control} - O.D._{test}/O.D._{control} \times 100$$

2.14. Determination of the Anti-QS Activity of AgNPs-S

The AgNPs-S were evaluated for their anti-QS properties against *C. violaceum*, *P. aeruginosa*, and *S. marcescens* via a well-diffusion assay. Bacterial cultures grown overnight were spread over Petri plates, and a gel puncture was used to make wells. The wells were punctured, 50 μL of AgNPs-S was added, and the plates were then incubated at 37 °C for 24 h. The anti-QS effects were seen the next day as a zone of clearance [44].

2.15. Assessment of Violacein Pigment Production in C. violaceum

In order to quantify violacein production, the standard procedure was followed [45]. A culture of *C. violaceum* was grown for 18 h at 30 °C without and with sub-MIC concentrations of AgNPs-S. Violacein pigment and bacterial cells were separated using centrifugation at 10,000 rpm for five minutes. To dissolve the pigment, the pellet was violently vortexed in 1 mL of DMSO for 5 min. The suspension was centrifuged again to spin down the bacterial debris. For the measurement of supernatant absorbance, a UV spectrophotometer was used (UV-2600, Shimadzu, Japan). The inhibition of violacein pigment production was estimated as follows:

$$O.D._{control} - O.D._{test}/O.D._{control} \times 100$$

2.16. Assessment of Pyocyanin Pigment Production in P. aeruginosa

Following the established standard protocols, the impact of AgNPs-S on the synthesis of pyocyanin in *P. aeruginosa* was examined in both the presence and the absence of AgNPs-S. [46]. The growth of *P. aeruginosa* in the LB medium in the presence and absence of sub-MICs of AgNPs-S took place overnight at 37 °C. Afterwards, 5 mL of the grown culture was centrifuged at 10,000 rpm for 10 min to collect the supernatant. The pyocyanin pigment production was then extracted from the supernatant of culture via extraction with 3 mL of chloroform. In the following step, the organic phase was collected and re-extracted with 1.2 mL of 0.2 N HCl. As a final step, the aqueous phase was taken, and absorbance was determined using a UV spectrophotometer (UV-2600, Shimadzu, Japan). The inhibition of pyocyanin pigment production was estimated as described above.

2.17. Assessment of Prodigiosin Pigment Production in S. marcescens

The effect of AgNPs-S on the production of prodigiosin synthesis in *S. marcescens* was investigated in both the presence and the absence of AgNPs-S by following standard procedures [47]. A test culture of *S. marcescens* was grown overnight at 30 °C in a sterile LB medium with and without AgNPs-S. After incubation, bacterial cells were collected using centrifugation for 10 min at 10,000 rpm. The resulting cell pellet was thoroughly stirred at room temperature into acidified ethanol (96 mL ethanol + 4 mL 1 M HCl). To eliminate cell debris, the mixture was centrifuged once more. The absorbance of the supernatant at 534 nm was then calculated using a spectrophotometer (UV-2600, Shimadzu, Japan). The inhibition of prodigiosin pigment production was estimated as described above.

2.18. Determination of DPPH Free-Radical-Scavenging Activity

The antioxidant activity of AgNPs-S was assessed against DPPH free radicals [48]. A freshly prepared DPPH solution in methanol (1 mM) was combined with equal volumes of different concentrations of AgNPs-S (1–1000 μg/mL) and mixed thoroughly. Following that, the solution was incubated for 30 min at room temperature in the dark. After incubation, a UV spectrophotometer (UV-2600, Shimadzu, Japan) was used to measure absorbance at 517 nm. Methanol served as a blank, and DPPH served as the control. The percentage of inhibition was used to calculate the free-radical-scavenging activity according to the following formula:

$$\% \text{ Scavenging activity} = \text{Pc} - \text{Ps}/\text{Pc} \times 100$$

where Pc is the absorbance of the control and Ps is the absorption of the AgNPs-S.

2.19. Determination of the Cytotoxic Potential of AgNPs-S

A549 (human non-small-cell lung cancer) and HEK293 (human embryonic kidney cells) were used to investigate the cytotoxic activity of the biosynthesized AgNps-S. Cells were raised in Dulbecco's Modified Eagle's Medium (DMEM) (MP Biomedicals, Eschwege, Germany) with 10,000 units/mL penicillin, 5 milligrams/mL streptomycin antibiotic solution, and 10% fetal bovine serum (Hi-Media, Mumbai, India) in T-25 flasks (25 cm^2) at 37 °C in humidified atmospheres with 5% CO_2. Cells were seeded in 96-well plates at a density of 10^4 cells per well after achieving 80% confluency. A hemocytometer was used to determine the viability of the cells after staining with Trypan Blue (0.4%) (Hi-Media®, Mumbai, India). In the following step, the cells were treated with different concentrations of AgNPs-S (1–1000 µg/mL) for 48 h. Following the removal of the plate from the incubator, the AgNPs-S-containing medium was aspirated. Each well was then incubated at 37 °C for 3 h under a humidified atmosphere (5% CO_2) with 200 µL of the medium containing 10% MTT reagent (MP Biomedicals, Eschwege, Germany). The formazan crystals were dissolved in 100 L of DMSO (Merck, Darmstadt, Germany) after the medium had been removed. With the help of an ELISA reader (EL10A, Biobase, China), the absorbance at 570 and 630 nm was measured in order to calculate the concentration of formazan crystals in the sample. To calculate the percentage of growth inhibition, a calculation was carried out by subtracting the values of the background and blank. Cisplatin was used as a positive control in this assay.

2.20. Statistical Analysis

Results are presented as the mean ± SD of the number of experiments performed. The significance of the results was determined for the treatments using an ordinary one-way ANOVA followed by Bonferroni's multiple comparisons test at $p < 0.05$. The analyses were carried out using the Graph Pad Prism software 8.0.

3. Results

3.1. Extraction and Confirmation of Saponins

The solvent-extraction method was used to extract crude saponins from the Ajwa dates. An initial qualitative test for saponins was conducted using the froth test, which was found to be successful in demonstrating the presence of saponins. In the HPTLC analysis, different compounds were detected with retention factors (Rf) of 0.021, 0.131, 0.187, 0.274, 0.610, and 0.769 for the extracted saponins from the extraction process (Figure 1A–D). Based on the spectrophotometric analysis, it was confirmed that the total crude saponin-enriched fraction yield was 415.89 µg/mL of crude saponins.

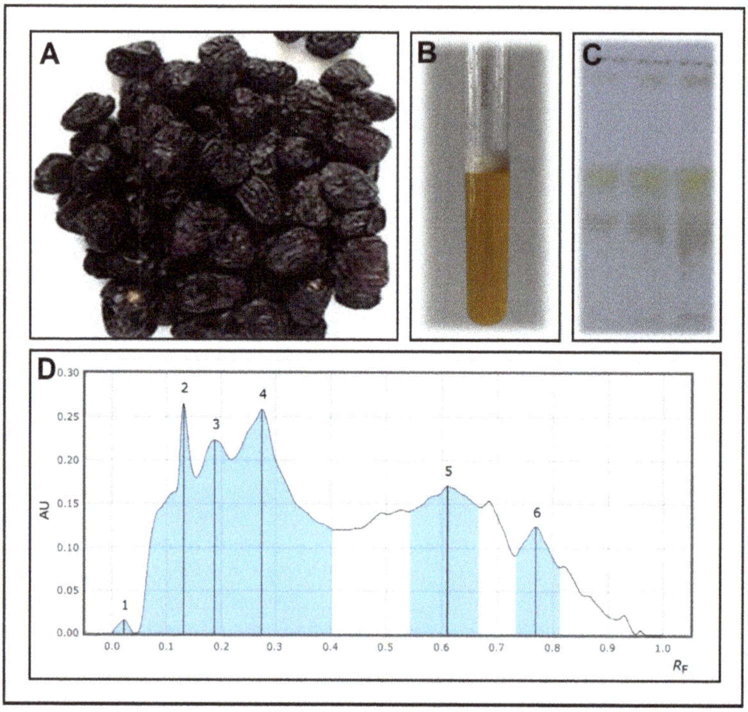

Figure 1. (**A**) Ajwa date fruits, (**B**) foam test of the saponin-enriched fractions of the Ajwa dates, (**C**) an HPTLC image of Ajwa dates with saponin-enriched fractions, (**D**) analyses of saponin-enriched fractions of Ajwa dates showing the separation of different compounds using HPTLC.

3.2. Synthesis and Characterization of AgNPs-S

AgNPs-S biosynthesis was achieved after extracting saponins from Ajwa dates and mixing them with a silver nitrate solution. During the incubation period, the sample color changed from yellow to dark brown. UV–visible spectroscopy is an important tool that is employed to detect AgNPs. UV–Vis spectroscopy was used as the primary method of checking the formation and constancy of synthesized AgNPs-S. A spectroscopy measurement after 24 h expressed an absorption spectrum with a peak maximum of 440 nm for the synthesized AgNPs-S (Figure 2A). Additionally, spectroscopy measurements were performed on the synthesized AgNPs-S after a period of one week, and the spectroscopic results showed no noticeable variation in the spectra of the nanoparticles, providing further evidence of their stability.

The FTIR spectra of crude saponins and AgNPs-S are shown in Figure 2. The FTIR spectra of AgNPs-S showed absorption bands at 1021.17 cm^{-1}, 1708.19 cm^{-1}, 2947.38 cm^{-1}, and 3293.53 cm^{-1}, corresponding to C–O stretching vibration of ethers or glycosides, C=O stretching vibration of carbonyls, C–H stretching vibration of alkanes, and O–H stretching vibration of hydroxyl groups. The FTIR spectra of crude saponins showed intense bands at 1019.36 cm^{-1}, 1720.87 cm^{-1}, 2947.49 cm^{-1}, and 3339.57 cm^{-1}, and a slight shift in the peak positions of IR bands in crude saponins and AgNPs-S was observed that indicates the functional groups and interactions involved in the synthesis and capping process. The size and morphology of the AgNPs-S were examined using TEM analysis. The resultant TEM images obtained at 120,000× magnifications and 80 KV are shown in Figure 2C,D. The TEM analysis revealed that the particles are spherical in nature and polydisperse. The sizes of the AgNPs-S, calculated via TEM analysis, were 2–10 nm.

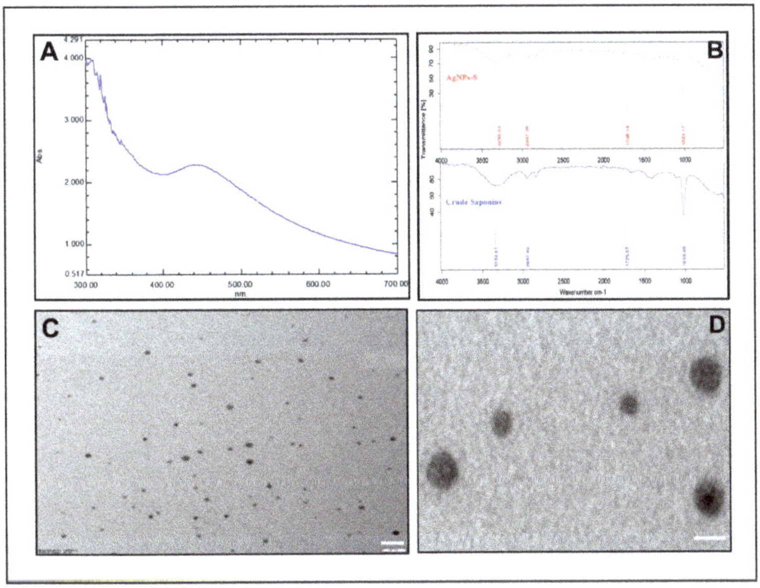

Figure 2. Characterization of AgNPs-S. (**A**) UV–visible absorption spectra of AgNPs-S. (**B**) FT-IR analysis of AgNPs-S. (**C**,**D**) Morphological analysis of AgNPs-S via TEM analysis, scale bar = 20 nm. (**D**) Enlargement of AgNPs-S, scale bar = 10 nm.

3.3. Antibacterial Potential of AgNPs-S

A well diffusion assay demonstrating the antibacterial properties of the biosynthesized AgNPs-S against Gram-positive and Gram-negative bacteria shows that they possess antibacterial properties. Zones of inhibition were used as a measure of antibacterial activity when assessing the results. The zone of inhibition was 14.00 mm against *C. violaceum*, 11.50 mm against *P. aeruginosa*, 11.48 mm against *B. subtilis*, 10.24 mm against *P. vulgaris*, 10.00 mm against *S. aureus*, 8.60 mm against *E. faecalis*, 8.46 mm against *S. marcescens*, and 8.24 mm against *E. coli* (Figure 3). A broth microdilution method was used to estimate the MIC of AgNPs-S against the selected pathogens. Furthermore, in order to determine the MIC of AgNPs-S against the tested pathogens, a broth microdilution method was used. The AgNPs-S had MIC values of 13.27 µg/mL for *C. violaceum*, 53.08 µg/mL for *P. aeruginosa*, *B. subtilis*, *P. vulgaris*, and *S. aureus*, and 106.16 µg/mL for *E. faecalis*, *S. marcescens*, and *E. coli* (Figure 4).

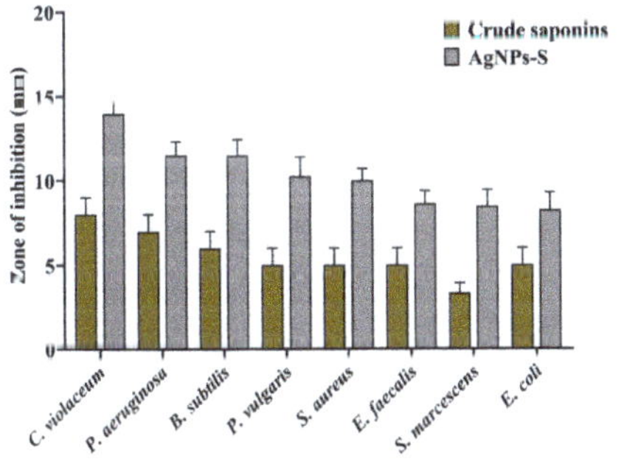

Figure 3. Antibacterial activity of crude saponins and AgNPs-S against different Gram-positive and Gram-negative bacterial pathogens. Values are represented as the mean ± SD of three independent experiments.

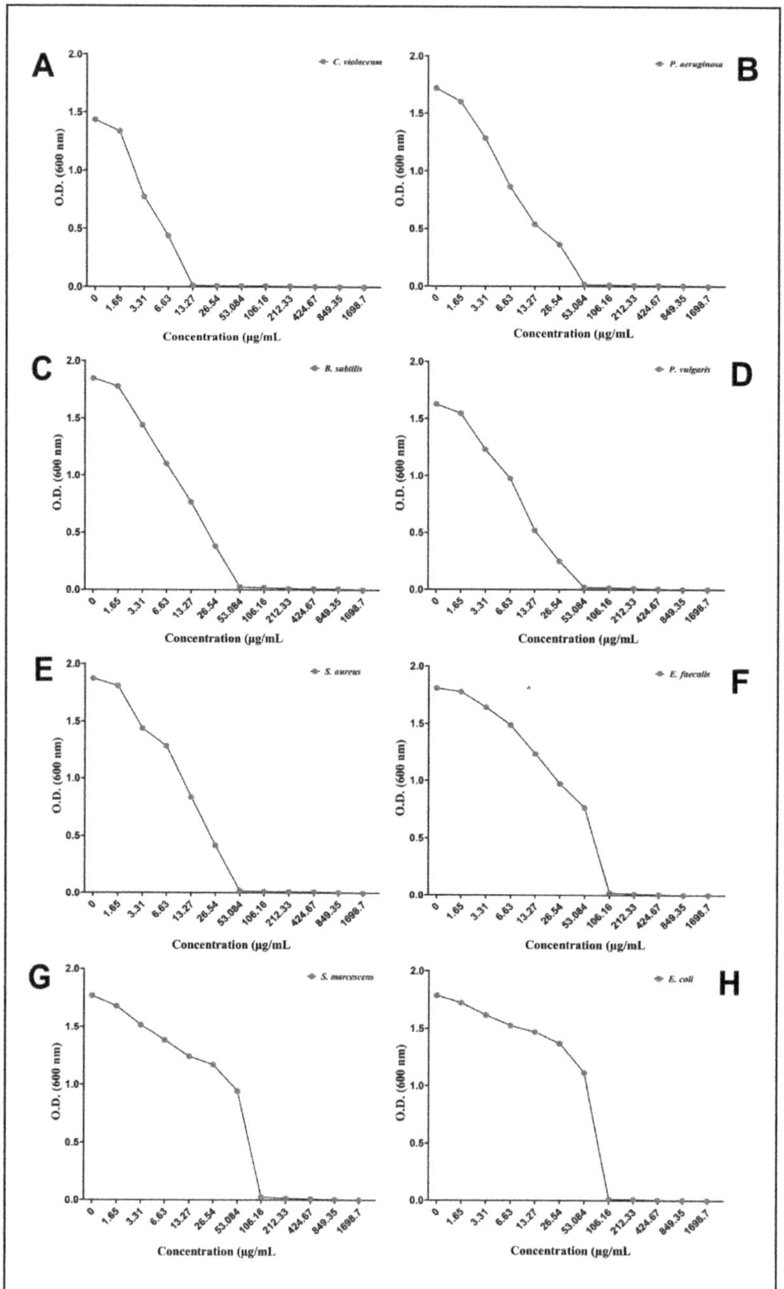

Figure 4. Determination of MIC after taking the optical density at 600 nm: (**A**) *C. violaceum*, (**B**) *P. aeruginosa*, (**C**) *B. subtilis*, (**D**) *P. vulgaris*, (**E**) *S. aureus*, (**F**) *E. faecalis*, (**G**) *S. marcescens*, and (**H**) *E. coli*.

3.4. Determination of the Effect of AgNPs-S on Nucleic Acids and Protein Leakage

As a possible mechanism of antibacterial action, the AgNPs-S were tested in order to determine whether they could suppress *P. aeruginosa* by leaking DNA and RNA via the membranes of the bacteria. When AgNPs-S were added to the bacterial culture, the results showed that the nucleic acids of the bacterial cell content were released into the medium, and these nucleic acid contents were released at an increasing rate with increasing doses of AgNPs-S. As a result of the *P. aeruginosa* treatment with supernatants of AgNPs-S (1 × MIC, 2 × MIC) for 6 and 24 h, the optical density (OD260) of the tested aliquot was much higher than that of the untreated controls. It is also worth noting that the optical density readings were observed to increase following the incubation intervals for 6 and 24 h (Figure 5A). There is an indication that AgNPs-S caused damage to the cell membrane of *P. aeruginosa*, which led to the disruption to the cell membrane and caused a leaking of macromolecules, including DNA and RNA.

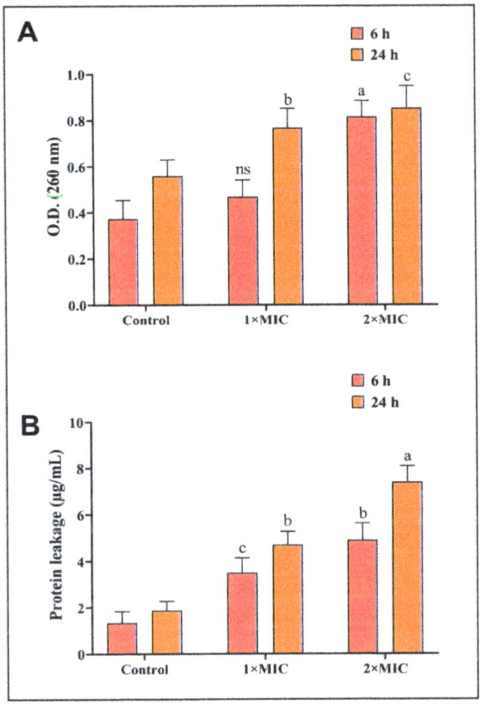

Figure 5. (**A**) AgNPs-S led to DNA and RNA leakage from *P. aeruginosa* bacteria. (**B**) AgNPs-S led to essential protein leakage from *P. aeruginosa* bacteria. Values are represented as the mean ± SD of three independent experiments. Different superscript letters indicate significant differences at $p \leq 0.05$ with respect to the control.

A further effect of AgNPs-S was observed via the disruption of proteins in the cell membranes of bacterial cells. According to the results shown in Figure 5B, AgNPs-S caused damage to the bacterial cell membrane of *P. aeruginosa*, which caused essential proteins to leak into the environment. In the untreated control, the leakage of proteins at the start of the experiment was much lower than the drip of proteins in the AgNPs-S-treated group. There was an increase in protein leakage not only with an increase in AgNPs-S concentrations, but also with an upsurge in the duration of the treatment. AgNPs-S caused a reduction in the content of cellular proteins due to their ability to penetrate and disrupt the membranes of cells.

3.5. Antibiofilm Potential of AgNPs-S

In the presence of AgNPs-S, *C. violaceum*, *P. aeruginosa*, and *S. marcescens* were observed to produce less biofilm in a concentration-dependent manner. At concentrations below the MIC, AgNPs-S reduced biofilm formation by 74.79%, 45.40%, and 29.32% in *C. violaceum*; 68.63%, 44.52%, and 40.55% in *P. aeruginosa*, and 55.87%, 53.34%; and 45.81% in *S. marcescens* (Figure 6A).

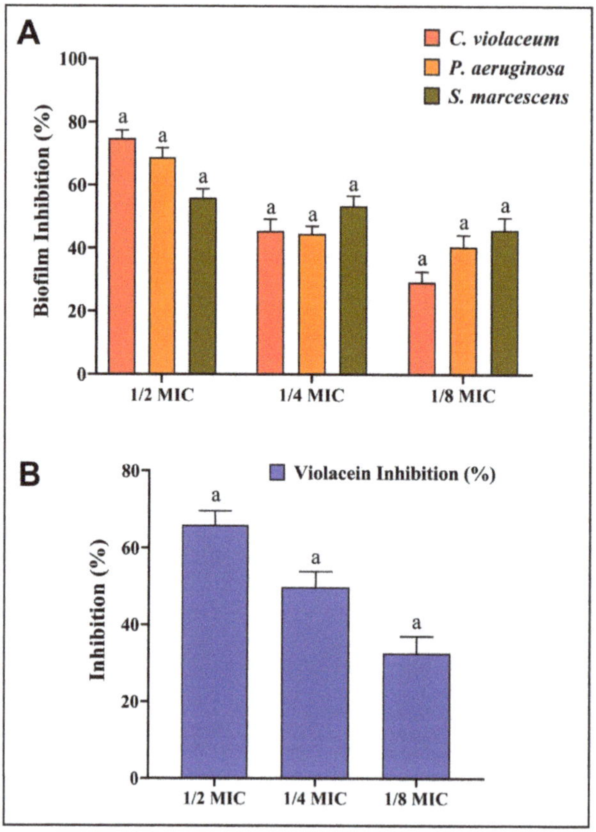

Figure 6. (**A**) Analysis of the quantitative inhibition of biofilm production using AgNPs-S. (**B**). Analysis of the quantitative inhibition of violacein in *C. violaceum* using AgNPs-S. Values are presented as the mean ± SD of three independent experiments. Different superscript letters indicate significant differences at $p \leq 0.05$ with respect to the control.

3.6. Anti-QS Potential of AgNPs-S

AgNPs-S were initially examined for their impact on *C. violaceum* QS activity. AgNPs-S prevented *C. violaceum* from producing violacein pigment at sub-MIC concentrations, which would indicate an inhibition of QS activity. Violacein production decreased by 65.89%, 49.69%, and 32.63% after treatment with 1/2, 1/4, and 1/8 MIC, respectively (Figure 6B). Furthermore, no inhibition was observed for the growth of *C. violaceum* when it was given treatments with AgNPs-S at sub-MIC levels.

The AgNPs-S were further studied for the inhibition of pyocyanin pigment to find out whether they could be effective in inhibiting the QS system of *P. aeruginosa*. Furthermore, pyocyanin is considered a powerful virulent factor that contributes to *P. aeruginosa* pathogenesis, virulence, and growth. A concentration-dependent reduction in pyocyanin formation at sub-MIC concentrations was achieved with AgNPs-S, and this reduction was measured at 74.83%, 68.21%, and 60.59%, respectively (Figure 7A).

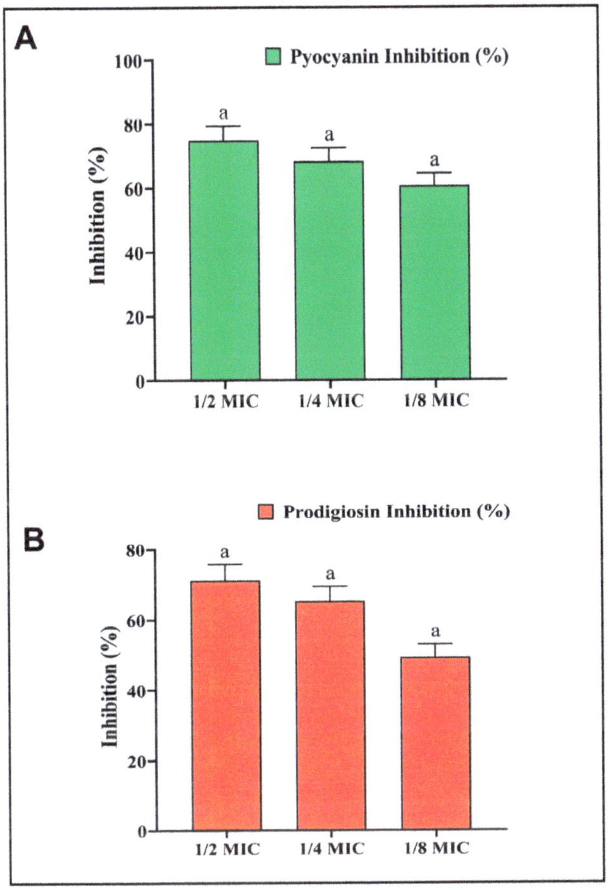

Figure 7. (**A**) Analysis of the quantitative inhibition of pyocyanin production in *P. aeruginosa* using AgNPs-S. (**B**) Analysis of the quantitative inhibition of prodigiosin in *S. marcescens* using AgNPs-S. Values are presented as the mean ± SD of three independent experiments. Different superscript letters indicate significant differences at $p \leq 0.05$ with respect to the control.

Moreover, the anti-QS activity of AgNPs-S was also studied in relation to the inhibition of prodigiosin activity in *S. marcescens*. Bacteria produce a pigment called prodigiosin, which is believed to play an essential role in promoting the growth, pathogenesis, and virulence of the organism. Prodigiosin production was reduced at sub-MIC doses by 71.10%, 65.22%, and 49.28% in a dose-dependent manner (Figure 7B).

3.7. In Vitro Antioxidant and Cytotoxic Potential of AgNPs-S

As part of the assessment of newly synthesized AgNPs-S and their antioxidant potential, they was tested against DPPH free radicals. Our novel synthesized AgNPs-S was observed to have good radical-scavenging abilities when exposed to DPPH free radicals. The antioxidant action of AgNPs-S was obtained in a dose-dependent manner, meaning that the antioxidant potency tended to rise with the increase in the sample concentration (Figure 8A). An MTT assay was used to assess the potential cytotoxic properties of AgNPs-S in contrast to non-small-cell lung cancer cells (A549) and normal human embryonic kidney cells (HEK-293). The obtained results indicated that the A549 cancer cells were inhibited in a dose-dependent manner after the treatment with AgNPs-S, whereas a low cytotoxicity of AgNPs-S was observed against HEK-293 cells at higher concentrations (Figure 8B).

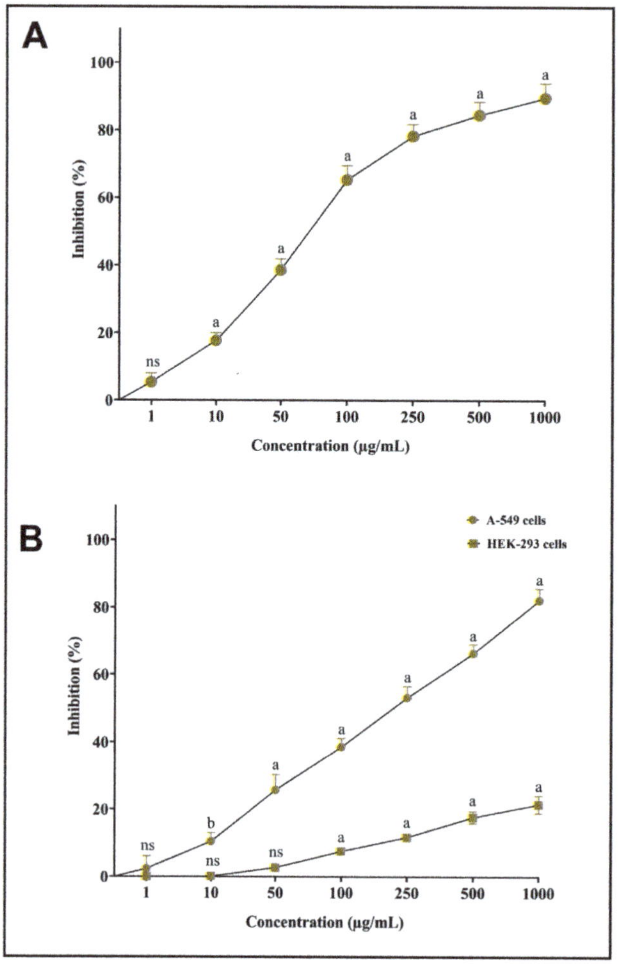

Figure 8. (**A**) Antioxidant potential of AgNPs-S against DPPH free radicals. (**B**) Cytotoxic activity of AgNPs-S against A549 human non-small-cell lung-cancer cells and normal human embryonic kidney cells (HEK-293). Values are presented as the mean ± SD of three independent experiments. Different superscript letters indicate significant differences at $p \leq 0.05$ with respect to the control.

4. Discussion

Natural compounds known as saponins can be found in a variety of plants, especially in legume seeds and roots, herbs, vegetables, and fruits [49]. Their name is derived from their ability to form soapy lathers when mixed with water. An important characteristic of saponins is that they are glycosides, meaning that they are a mixture of sugar molecules and non-sugar molecules. The non-sugar molecule in saponins is usually a steroid or triterpenoid, while saponins contain a variety of sugar molecules that give rise to a range of biological activities [50]. Saponins are known for forming stable foams or froths when they are shaken with water, one of their most well-known properties. Due to their natural foaming properties, they are often used in applications such as detergents, shampoos, and soaps, where they can act as natural foaming agents [51]. As well as being capable of providing surfactant properties, saponins have also been shown to possess a variety of biological properties that include antimicrobial, antifungal, anti-inflammatory, and anticancer properties [52–55].

In this study, we investigated the antibiofilm, antibacterial, and anti-QS activities of novel AgNPs synthesized from saponins derived from Ajwa dates. Recently, interest in the potential effectiveness of AgNPs as antibacterial agents has experienced an uptick due to their distinctive properties, including their improved surface area, improved reactivity, and potential to overcome antibiotic resistance [11–13]. Ajwa dates, known for their rich saponin content, proved to be an intriguing natural source for the development of AgNPs by means of potential antimicrobial activity [56]. As a result of the characterization studies, it was confirmed that AgNPs can be successfully synthesized using the saponins derived from Ajwa dates. The UV–Vis spectroscopy results revealed characteristic absorption peaks in the range associated with the formation of AgNPs, indicating that nanoparticles were formed during the synthesis process. The Fourier-transform infrared spectroscopy (FTIR) investigation revealed various functional groups from Ajwa date saponins that contribute to the stability and capping of AgNPs. The C-H stretching vibration of alkanes is usually seen around 2900 cm^{-1} and indicates the presence of aliphatic hydrocarbon chains in saponins. This peak may not change significantly after the synthesis of AgNPs, as the hydrocarbon chains are not involved in the reduction or capping process [57]. The C=O stretching vibration of carbonyls is usually seen around 1700 cm^{-1} and indicates the presence of carbonyl groups (C=O) in saponins. These groups can be part of ketones, esters, or carboxylic acids. This peak may shift or change in intensity after the synthesis of AgNPs, as the carbonyl groups can be involved in the reduction or capping process. For example, carboxylic acids can donate electrons to silver ions and form carboxylate groups that bind to the surface of AgNPs [58]. The O-H stretching vibration of alcohols or phenols is usually seen around 3400 cm^{-1} and indicates the presence of hydroxyl groups (O-H) in saponins. These groups can be part of sugars, glycosides, or phenolic compounds. This peak may shift or change in intensity after the synthesis of AgNPs, as the hydroxyl groups can be involved in the reduction or capping process. For example, phenols can donate electrons to silver ions and form phenolate groups that bind to the surface of AgNPs [59]. The C-O stretching vibration is found in ethers and glycosides. This peak is usually seen around 1100 cm^{-1} and indicates the presence of ether or glycosidic linkages (C-O-C) in saponins. These linkages connect different sugar units or aglycones in saponins. This peak may not change significantly after the synthesis of AgNPs, as the ether or glycosidic linkages are not involved in the reduction or capping process [59]. In the present study, a similar pattern of FTIR spectra was observed for crude saponins and AgNPs-S, which confirms the synthesis and capping process of AgNPs using crude saponins. Further confirmation of the successful synthesis of AgNPs was provided by transmission electron microscopy (TEM) images that showed polydispersed AgNPs 2–10 nm in size and with spherical shapes. As reported earlier [57], saponin-capped silver nanotriangles were prepared in an aqueous system using a *Trigonella foenum-graecum* seed extract. The synthesized nanoparticles were crystalline and triangular in shape, with an edge length of approximately 80 nm. Using UV/Vis spectroscopy, it was observed that the synthesized saponin-capped silver nanotriangles showed three absorption peaks at 360 nm, 432 nm, and 702 nm. For more than six months, these peaks remained in almost the same position, which confirms that the silver nanotriangles have a high level of stability. The FTIR spectra confirmed the presence of saponin on the surface of the silver nanotriangles, which acted as a capping agent and prevented their aggregation. In one study, AgNPs were synthesized using saponin-rich/poor leaf extracts from *Ocimum tenuiflorum* and *Phyllanthus urinaria* [60]. The results of the study showed that leaf extracts rich in saponins (WE) produced AgNPs that were smaller, more uniform in size, and more stable than extracts that were low in saponins

(EE). The AgNPs synthesized from WE had an average size of 9.6 nm, and an average size of 18.8 nm was measured for those synthesized from EE. There was a zeta potential of −29.3 mV for the AgNPs synthesized from WE and −17.4 mV for the AgNPs synthesized from EE. As a result of the FTIR analysis, it was confirmed that saponin was present on the surface of the AgNPs synthesized from WE as a capping agent. It was evident from the TEM images that the AgNPs synthesized from WE exhibited a spherical shape, while those synthesized from EE displayed an irregular shape. Similarly, AgNPs were also synthesized and characterized by [61] using saponin extracts from *Simarouba glauca* oil seed meal. With an average size of 10 nm, the synthesized AgNPs were spherical in shape. There were intense bands in the FTIR spectrum of saponin at 3350 cm^{-1}, 2827 cm^{-1}, 1704 cm^{-1}, and 1024 cm^{-1}, whereas the AgNPs showed absorption bands at 3375 cm^{-1}, 2928 cm^{-1}, 1707 cm^{-1}, and 1024 cm^{-1}, corresponding to O–H stretching vibrations, C–H stretching vibrations, and symmetric and asymmetric C–O–C stretching vibrations of carboxyl groups, respectively. In saponin and the synthesized AgNPs, there was a slight shift in the peak positions of the IR bands caused by the reduction process. The results of this study confirm that saponin can adsorb on the surfaces of AgNPs and that saponins can cap and stabilize nanoparticles.

In recent years, there has been rising concern about the formation of biofilms and the emergence of antibiotic resistance within various domains, such as pharmaceutical medicine, agriculture, and other industries [62]. A biofilm is composed of a variety of microbes, such as bacteria, fungi, and algae, which attach to surfaces and form an extracellular polymeric substance (EPS). Additionally, various reports suggest that biofilms could play a significant role in the development of numerous infections. Biofilm formation can occur on medical apparatuses, implants, and natural surfaces [63–65]. In the presence of a biofilm, bacteria exhibited significant levels of resistance to antibiotics, as well as being immune to the immune response of the host. [66]. A number of factors cause this resistance, including physical barriers, altered phenotypes, quorum sensing, and persistent cells [67]. In the healthcare setting, biofilms and antibiotic resistance pose significant challenges that need to be addressed. Infections associated with biofilms are often chronic and hard to treat and can result in the recurrence of infections even after the initial treatment has been completed. A second factor contributing to the spread of antibiotic resistance within a microbiome is the horizontal gene transfer of antibiotic resistance genes between bacteria and within their biofilm [68,69].

It is essential to take a multifaceted approach to addressing the issue of biofilms and antibiotic resistance in order to resolve this issue. A number of strategies are being explored, including the formulation of novel antimicrobial compounds that are specifically targeted in biofilms, the design of surface coatings that prevent biofilm formation, the use of combination therapies to treat multiple pathways, and the exploration of alternative treatments such as bacteriophages [70–74]. During the last few years, a tremendous amount of consideration has been paid to the inhibition of biofilm formation through targeting the QS mechanism. During the QS process, bacteria communicate with one another and coordinate their activities within a biofilm [75]. By interfering with the process of QS, the communication between bacterial cells is disrupted, causing the breakdown of the biofilm and the associated resistance mechanisms. As a consequence of this disruption, mature biofilms cannot be formed, resulting in the bacteria being more susceptible to antibiotics and other treatments [76]. Therefore, targeting the QS mechanism presents a promising avenue for inhibiting biofilm formation, reducing antibiotic resistance, and improving the effectiveness of antimicrobial treatment.

Saponins have long been recognized for their antimicrobial properties, which can be attributed to their amphiphilic nature and ability to disrupt bacterial cell membranes. The hydrophilic glycone portion and the lipophilic aglycone moiety of saponins contribute to their interactions with bacterial membranes. Saponins are inserted into the lipid bilayer, causing disruptions in the membrane's integrity. This disruption leads to increased permeability, the leakage of cellular contents, and eventual bacterial cell death. Moreover, saponins can also interfere with bacterial quorum sensing, a process critical for bacterial communication and virulence [77]. The combination of saponins with AgNPs has garnered interest as a means of enhancing antibacterial efficacy. Saponins can serve as stabilizing agents for AgNPs, preventing aggregation and maintaining their colloidal stability. This synergistic approach leverages the inherent antibacterial mechanisms of both compounds, leading to a cumulative effect on bacterial inhibition [78]. The newly synthesized AgNPs-S and their antibacterial activity were assessed against a variety of bacterial strains in order to determine their effectiveness. A pronounced inhibitory effect was observed in the zone of inhibition assays, indicating that AgNP-S can be effective in the fight against bacterial growth. Furthermore, the determination of the MIC values indicated that AgNPs-S can be effective against bacteria at low concentrations. In view of these findings, it is clear that AgNPs derived from the saponins of Ajwa dates possess potent antibacterial properties. However, the MIC values of AgNPs were found to be different against different Gram-positive and Gram-negative bacterial pathogens. This might be for several reasons; for instance, Gram-positive bacteria have a relatively thick peptidoglycan layer in their cell walls, which provides structural integrity and plays a crucial role in resisting the entry of foreign substances, including antibacterial agents [79]. This thicker peptidoglycan layer can act as a barrier, making it more difficult for antibacterial agents to penetrate and reach their target sites within the bacterial cell. As a result, Gram-positive bacteria may require higher concentrations of an antibacterial agent to achieve the same inhibitory effect, leading to a higher MIC value [80]. On the other hand, Gram-negative bacteria have an additional outer membrane composed of lipopolysaccharides (LPS) that surrounds their thin peptidoglycan layer. This outer membrane serves as an extra barrier and can restrict the entry of hydrophobic molecules, including some antibiotics, into the bacterial cell [81]. Therefore, Gram-negative bacteria might exhibit stronger resistance to certain antibacterial agents, resulting in higher MIC values. Moreover, Gram-negative bacteria possess efflux pumps that actively pump out various compounds, including antibiotics, from the bacterial cell. This efflux mechanism contributes to antibiotic resistance by quickly expelling the drug and reducing its effective concentration within the cell, which can lead to elevated MIC values. Therefore, the differences in cell wall structures, membrane properties, and resistance mechanisms between Gram-positive and Gram-negative bacteria can all contribute to variations in MIC values for antibacterial agents targeting these different types of bacteria [82].

AgNPs are well known to exert antibacterial effects against a variety of bacteria, including multi-drug-resistant strains. There are several ways in which AgNPs can interact with bacteria, depending on their size, shape, surface charge, and coating. Upon attachment to the bacterial cell wall, AgNPs can disrupt its integrity and leak cytoplasmic content and membrane potential [83,84]. DNA and RNA can be damaged by AgNPs that penetrate into the bacterial cytoplasm and bind to nucleic acids, preventing their replication, transcription, and translation [84]. Furthermore, AgNPs can also produce reactive oxygen species (ROS) and free radicals, which are capable of inducing DNA damage [83]. Bacterial proteins and enzymes can be denatured, aggregated, or inhibited by AgNPs [83,84]. Additionally, AgNPs can impact ribosomes and tRNAs, which are essential for protein synthesis [84]. The oxidative phosphorylation and ATP synthesis of bacteria can be interfered with by AgNPs [83,84]. It is possible for these mechanisms to lead to the death of bacteria through apoptosis or necrosis [83,84]. In the present study, synthesized AgNPs-S were able to leak nucleic acids and protein at concentrations of 1 × MIC and 2 × MIC after 6 h and 24 h in *P. aeruginosa*.

Furthermore, AgNPs-S also displayed remarkable antibiofilm activity. As AgNPs-S are capable of inhibiting biofilm formation, it indicates that they can be used for the prevention of bacterial infections and to fight against antibiotic resistance in the future. The disruption of biofilms by AgNPs-S indicates their potential to augment the effectiveness of conventional antibiotics to a considerable extent. This study shows that AgNPs-S have significant antibiofilm potential, which is consistent with the results from other studies that reported on the antibiofilm potential of AgNPs that were synthesized in different ways. For example, a study by [85] synthesized AgNPs from leaf extracts of *Allophylus cobbe* and tested their antibacterial and antibiofilm effects against *P. aeruginosa*, *E. coli*, and *S. aureus*. The results showed that AgNPs could disrupt the biofilm's integrity, penetrate into the biofilm matrix, interfere with the quorum-sensing system, and enhance the efficacy of antibiotics. The authors of [86] synthesized AgNPs from leaf extracts of *Semecarpus anacardium*, *Glochidion lanceolarium*, and *Bridelia retusa* and evaluated their antibacterial and antibiofilm activities against different bacterial pathogens. The results demonstrated that AgNPs could attach to the biofilm surface, disrupt its structure, cause the leakage of EPS, and induce oxidative stress, DNA damage, protein dysfunction, and cell death. A study by [87] chemically synthesized AgNPs and characterized their effect on the biofilm formation and EPS production of *P. aeruginosa* and *S. aureus*. The results revealed that AgNPs could inhibit biofilm formation, reduce EPS production, and alter the morphology of biofilm cells. A study by [88] synthesized AgNPs using sodium borohydride as a reducing agent and examined their antibiofilm activity against extended-spectrum β-lactamases-producing *E. coli* and *Klebsiella* spp. The results indicated that AgNPs could prevent biofilm formation, detach biofilm cells, and increase the susceptibility of biofilm cells to antibiotics. A study by [89] synthesized AgNPs–chitosan composites and assessed their antibiofilm activity against multi-drug-resistant *Acinetobacter baumannii*. The results suggested that the AgNPs–chitosan composites could inhibit biofilm formation, disrupt biofilm structure, reduce biofilm biomass, and enhance the activity of antibiotics.

The anti-QS activity of AgNPs-S was an intriguing aspect of this study. The QS mechanism is a means of communication among bacteria that produces and detects the signal molecules responsible for regulating virulence factors [19]. AgNPs-S derived from Ajwa date saponins were found to inhibit QS in bacteria, thereby inhibiting progress in bacterial communication and virulence by interfering with QS. As a consequence of this finding, AgNPs-S are not only considered to be potential antimicrobial agents but also factors that could influence bacterial behavior and bacteria's pathogenic capabilities.

An imbalance between the body's protective antioxidant mechanisms and the generation of reactive oxygen species (ROS) leads to oxidative stress [90]. ROS, including free radicals, result in damage to cells, proteins, and DNA, leading to oxidative stress and the development of various diseases [91]. Natural compounds possess powerful antioxidant activity that plays a pivotal role in countering oxidative stress and maintaining cellular health by combating oxidative damage [92]. The antioxidant activity of AgNPs makes them intriguing therapeutic candidates. There are several mechanisms through which AgNPs can exhibit antioxidant activity. They accomplish this by donating electrons or accepting free radicals, one of the most important mechanisms through which they scavenge and neutralize reactive oxygen species (ROS). Aside from this, AgNPs can actively stimulate the activity of endogenous antioxidant enzymes, such as catalase, glutathione peroxidase, and superoxide dismutase (SOD), which assist in the reduction of oxidative stress and the conservation of cellular homeostasis [93–95]. The strong antioxidant activity of AgNPs-S was also demonstrated in the present study by their capacity to scavenge DPPH free radicals.

Lung cancer is one of the most important health issues worldwide; it is caused by the uncontrolled growth of abnormal cells in the lungs. The disease has a high mortality rate and limited treatment options, causing high mortality among various cancer-related deaths [96]. Many conventional treatment options, such as surgery, chemotherapy, and radiation therapy, have limited efficacy and can cause a range of side effects [97]. Thus, it is essential that novel approaches for the management and treatment of cancers such as lung cancer should be explored. Regarding possible therapeutic options, AgNPs are an emerging research area. Several potential advantages can be gained from using AgNPs to treat lung cancer. In terms of their cytotoxicity, AgNPs have been shown to selectively target cancer cells while sparing healthy cells [98]. The potential benefits of this targeted strategy could include the possibility of minimizing damage to healthy lung tissue, as well as reducing the adverse effects associated with conventional treatment methods [99]. Second, AgNPs have demonstrated promising cytotoxic properties. The process of apoptosis (programmed cell death) or autophagy (the self-destruction of cancer cells) is thought to be the mechanism by which these compounds induce cell death [100,101]. As well as inhibiting tumor angiogenesis, AgNPs exert antiangiogenic effects by forming new blood vessels to support tumor growth [102]. Furthermore, nanoparticles synthesized from silver can be used as drug carriers or to enhance the effectiveness of existing chemotherapeutics. Anticancer drugs can be loaded or functionalized onto them, enabling targeted delivery to the tumor site and potentially improving bioavailability. By using this approach, drug resistance can be overcome and treatments enhanced [103]. The results of our study showed a significant inhibition of the viability of human non-small-cell lung cancer cells after the action of AgNPs-S. Therefore, AgNPs-S show great promise as a novel treatment for lung cancer.

Overall, saponin-derived AgNPs from Ajwa dates possess significant antibacterial, antibiofilm, anti-QS, antioxidant, and cytotoxic potential. These nanoparticles demonstrate broad-spectrum antimicrobial activity, inhibit biofilm formation, interfere with QS, and exhibit antioxidant and cytotoxic effects against lung cancer cells. The multifaceted activities of AgNPs-S open up new avenues for their application in combating bacterial infections, biofilm-related complications, and cancer.

5. Conclusions

The development of saponin-derived silver nanoparticles from Ajwa dates represents a novel and promising approach in nanotechnology and biomedical research. The findings discussed in this study highlight the successful synthesis of AgNPs utilizing bioactive saponins found in Ajwa dates and emphasize their potential in many fields. The antibacterial potential of the novel AgNPs-S was evident in preventing the growth of both Gram-positive and Gram-negative bacteria. Moreover, the novel AgNPs-S exhibited significant antibiofilm activity by impeding the formation and growth of bacterial biofilms. The observed anti-QS activity of AgNPs-S provides a novel avenue for mitigating bacterial pathogenicity by disrupting QS signaling and downregulating virulent gene expression. Additionally, AgNPs-S demonstrated noteworthy antioxidant and cytotoxic effects, exerting cytotoxicity against lung cancer cells. Overall, this investigation into the antibacterial, antibiofilm, anti-QS, antioxidant, and cytotoxicity potential of saponin-derived AgNPs from Ajwa dates offers valuable insights into their multifunctional properties. The outcomes of this study hold great promise for the advancement of innovative bio-therapeutic approaches against bacterial infections, biofilm-related complications, and cancer. Continued research in this area may be a promising approach to reforming the field of nanomedicine and addressing the pressing challenges associated with antimicrobial resistance and cancer therapy.

Author Contributions: Conceptualization, M.A. (Mohd Adnan), C.D. and M.P.; methodology, A.J.S., M.A. (Mousa Alreshidi), S.A.A., M.S.A., S.O.A., B.T. and M.S.; validation, A.J.S., M.A. (Mousa Alreshidi), S.A.A., M.S.A., S.O.A., B.T. and M.S.; formal analysis, C.D., M.P., M.A. (Mohd Adnan) and S.O.A.; investigation, A.J.S., M.A. (Mousa Alreshidi), S.A.A., M.S.A., S.O.A., B.T. and M.S.; data curation, A.J.S., M.A. (Mousa Alreshidi), S.A.A., M.S.A., S.O.A., B.T. and M.S.; writing—original draft preparation, M.P., C.D. and M.A. (Mohd Adnan); writing—review and editing, M.A. (Mohd Adnan), B.T. and M.S.; software, M.A. (Mohd Adnan) and M.P.; visualization, M.P. and A.J.S.; supervision, M.A. (Mohd Adnan) and C.D.; project administration, M.A. (Mohd Adnan). All authors have read and agreed to the published version of the manuscript.

Funding: This research has been funded by Scientific Research Deanship at the University of Ha'il-Saudi Arabia through project number MDR-22027.

Institutional Review Board Statement: Not applicable.

Informed Consent Statement: Not applicable.

Data Availability Statement: All data generated and analyzed during the course of this study are included in the article.

Acknowledgments: The authors are thankful to the Scientific Research Deanship at the University of Ha'il-Saudi Arabia for supporting this study through project number MDR-22027.

Conflicts of Interest: The authors declare no conflict of interest. The funders had no role in the design of the study; in the collection, analyses, or interpretation of data; in the writing of the manuscript; or in the decision to publish the results.

References

1. Bayda, S.; Adeel, M.; Tuccinardi, T.; Cordani, M.; Rizzolio, F. The history of nanoscience and nanotechnology: From chemical–physical applications to nanomedicine. *Molecules* **2019**, *25*, 112. [CrossRef] [PubMed]
2. Soliman, M.K.; Salem, S.S.; Abu-Elghait, M.; Azab, M.S. Biosynthesis of silver and gold nanoparticles and their efficacy towards antibacterial, antibiofilm, cytotoxicity, and antioxidant activities. *Appl. Biochem. Biotechnol.* **2023**, *195*, 1158–1183. [CrossRef] [PubMed]
3. Alsaba, M.T.; Al Dushaishi, M.F.; Abbas, A.K. A comprehensive review of nanoparticles applications in the oil and gas industry. *J. Pet. Explor. Prod. Technol.* **2020**, *10*, 1389–1399. [CrossRef]
4. Kumar, H.; Bhardwaj, K.; Kuča, K.; Kalia, A.; Nepovimova, E.; Verma, R.; Kumar, D. Flower-based green synthesis of metallic nanoparticles: Applications beyond fragrance. *Nanomaterials* **2020**, *10*, 766. [CrossRef] [PubMed]
5. Martínez, G.; Merinero, M.; Pérez-Aranda, M.; Pérez-Soriano, E.M.; Ortiz, T.; Villamor, E.; Begines, B.; Alcudia, A. Environmental impact of nanoparticles' application as an emerging technology: A review. *Materials* **2020**, *14*, 166. [CrossRef] [PubMed]
6. Lines, M. Nanomaterials for practical functional uses. *J. Alloys Compd.* **2008**, *449*, 242–245. [CrossRef]
7. Ozak, S.T.; Ozkan, P. Nanotechnology and dentistry. *Eur. J. Dent.* **2013**, *7*, 145–151.
8. Yaqoob, A.A.; Umar, K.; Ibrahim, M.N.M. Silver nanoparticles: Various methods of synthesis, size affecting factors and their potential applications–a review. *Appl. Nanosci.* **2020**, *10*, 1369–1378. [CrossRef]
9. Shanmuganathan, R.; Karuppusamy, I.; Saravanan, M.; Muthukumar, H.; Ponnuchamy, K.; Ramkumar, V.S.; Pugazhendhi, A. Synthesis of silver nanoparticles and their biomedical applications—A comprehensive review. *Curr. Pharm. Des.* **2019**, *25*, 2650–2660. [CrossRef]
10. Some, S.; Sen, I.K.; Mandal, A.; Aslan, T.; Ustun, Y.; Yilmaz, E.Ş.; Katı, A.; Demirbas, A.; Mandal, A.K.; Ocsoy, I. Biosynthesis of silver nanoparticles and their versatile antimicrobial properties. *Mater. Res. Express* **2018**, *6*, 012001. [CrossRef]
11. Keat, C.L.; Aziz, A.; Eid, A.M.; Elmarzugi, N.A. Biosynthesis of nanoparticles and silver nanoparticles. *Bioresour. Bioprocess.* **2015**, *2*, 47. [CrossRef]
12. Syafiuddin, A.; Salmiati; Salim, M.R.; Beng Hong Kueh, A.; Hadibarata, T.; Nur, H. A review of silver nanoparticles: Research trends, global consumption, synthesis, properties, and future challenges. *J. Chin. Chem. Soc.* **2017**, *64*, 732–756. [CrossRef]
13. Yusuf, M. Silver nanoparticles: Synthesis and applications. *Handb. Ecomater.* **2019**, 2343. [CrossRef]
14. Mohammadlou, M.; Maghsoudi, H.; Jafarizadeh-Malmiri, H. A review on green silver nanoparticles based on plants: Synthesis, potential applications and eco-friendly approach. *Int. Food Res. J.* **2016**, *23*, 446.
15. Walusansa, A.; Asiimwe, S.; Nakavuma, J.; Ssenku, J.; Katuura, E.; Kafeero, H.; Aruhomukama, D.; Nabatanzi, A.; Anywar, G.; Tugume, A.K.; et al. Antibiotic-resistance in medically important bacteria isolated from commercial herbal medicines in Africa from 2000 to 2021: A systematic review and meta-analysis. *Antimicrob. Resist. Infect. Control* **2022**, *11*, 11. [CrossRef]
16. Ayukekbong, J.A.; Ntemgwa, M.; Atabe, A.N. The threat of antimicrobial resistance in developing countries: Causes and control strategies. *Antimicrob. Resist. Infect. Control* **2017**, *6*, 47. [CrossRef]
17. Alfred Ngenge, T.; Kucukaydin, S.; Ceylan, O.; Duru, M.E. Evaluation of enzyme inhibition and anti-quorum sensing potentials of Melaleuca alternifolia and Citrus sinensis essential oils. *Nat. Prod. Commun.* **2021**, *16*, 1934578X211044565. [CrossRef]
18. Yum, S.-j.; Kwon, J.H.; Lee, K.-T.; Park, J.-T.; Jeong, H.-G. Efficacy of pristimerin against Staphylococcus aureus planktonic cultures and biofilms. *LWT* **2022**, *164*, 113627. [CrossRef]
19. Abebe, G.M. The role of bacterial biofilm in antibiotic resistance and food contamination. *Int. J. Microbiol.* **2020**, *2020*, 1705814. [CrossRef]
20. Skandamis, P.N.; Nychas, G.-J.E. Quorum sensing in the context of food microbiology. *Appl. Environ. Microbiol.* **2012**, *78*, 5473–5482. [CrossRef]
21. Tamfu, A.N.; Ceylan, O.; Cârâc, G.; Talla, E.; Dinica, R.M. Antibiofilm and anti-quorum sensing potential of cycloartane-type triterpene acids from cameroonian grassland propolis: Phenolic profile and antioxidant activity of crude extract. *Molecules* **2022**, *27*, 4872. [CrossRef] [PubMed]
22. Mittal, A.K.; Chisti, Y.; Banerjee, U.C. Synthesis of metallic nanoparticles using plant extracts. *Biotechnol. Adv.* **2013**, *31*, 346–356. [CrossRef] [PubMed]
23. Dauthal, P.; Mukhopadhyay, M. Noble metal nanoparticles: Plant-mediated synthesis, mechanistic aspects of synthesis, and applications. *Ind. Eng. Chem. Res.* **2016**, *55*, 9557–9577. [CrossRef]
24. Singh, P.; Kim, Y.-J.; Zhang, D.; Yang, D.-C. Biological synthesis of nanoparticles from plants and microorganisms. *Trends Biotechnol.* **2016**, *34*, 588–599. [CrossRef]
25. Ahmed, S.; Ahmad, M.; Swami, B.L.; Ikram, S. A review on plants extract mediated synthesis of silver nanoparticles for antimicrobial applications: A green expertise. *J. Adv. Res.* **2016**, *7*, 17–28. [CrossRef]

26. Zhang, C.-R.; Aldosari, S.A.; Vidyasagar, P.S.; Nair, K.M.; Nair, M.G. Antioxidant and anti-inflammatory assays confirm bioactive compounds in Ajwa date fruit. *J. Agric. Food Chem.* **2013**, *61*, 5834–5840. [CrossRef]
27. Al-Shahib, W.; Marshall, R.J. The fruit of the date palm: Its possible use as the best food for the future? *Int. J. Food Sci. Nutr.* **2003**, *54*, 247–259. [CrossRef]
28. Al-Farsi, M.A.; Lee, C.Y. Nutritional and functional properties of dates: A review. *Crit. Rev. Food Sci. Nutr.* **2008**, *48*, 877–887. [CrossRef]
29. Hasan, N.S.; Amom, Z.H.; Nor, A.; Norhafizah, M.; Norhaizan, M.E.; Azrina, A. Nutritional composition and in vitro evaluation of the antioxidant properties of various dates extracts (*Phoenix dactylifera* L.) from Libya. *Asian J. Clin. Nutr.* **2010**, *2*, 208–214. [CrossRef]
30. Khalid, S.; Khalid, N.; Khan, R.S.; Ahmed, H.; Ahmad, A. A review on chemistry and pharmacology of Ajwa date fruit and pit. *Trends Food Sci. Technol.* **2017**, *63*, 60–69. [CrossRef]
31. Edeoga, H.O.; Okwu, D.; Mbaebie, B. Phytochemical constituents of some Nigerian medicinal plants. *Afr. J. Biotechnol.* **2005**, *4*, 685–688. [CrossRef]
32. Uematsu, Y.; Hirata, K.; Saito, K.; Kudo, I. Spectrophotometric determination of saponin in Yucca extract used as food additive. *J. AOAC Int.* **2000**, *83*, 1451–1454. [CrossRef] [PubMed]
33. Bobby, M.N.; Wesely, E.; Johnson, M. High performance thin layer chromatography profile studies on the alkaloids of Albizia lebbeck. *Asian Pac. J. Trop. Biomed.* **2012**, *2*, S1–S6. [CrossRef]
34. Venkatesh, P.; Mukherjee, P.K.; Kumar, N.S.; Bandyopadhyay, A.; Fukui, H.; Mizuguchi, H.; Islam, N. Anti-allergic activity of standardized extract of Albizia lebbeck with reference to catechin as a phytomarker. *Immunopharmacol. Immunotoxicol.* **2010**, *32*, 272–276. [CrossRef]
35. Atarod, M.; Nasrollahzadeh, M.; Sajadi, S.M. Green synthesis of Pd/RGO/Fe3O4 nanocomposite using Withania coagulans leaf extract and its application as magnetically separable and reusable catalyst for the reduction of 4-nitrophenol. *J. Colloid Interface Sci.* **2016**, *465*, 249–258. [CrossRef]
36. Liu, C.; Xu, B.; McClements, D.J.; Xu, X.; Cui, S.; Gao, L.; Zhou, L.; Xiong, L.; Sun, Q.; Dai, L. Properties of curcumin-loaded zein-tea saponin nanoparticles prepared by antisolvent co-precipitation and precipitation. *Food Chem.* **2022**, *391*, 133224. [CrossRef]
37. Geethalakshmi, R.; Sarada, D. Characterization and antimicrobial activity of gold and silver nanoparticles synthesized using saponin isolated from *Trianthema decandra* L. *Ind. Crops Prod.* **2013**, *51*, 107–115.
38. Muniyan, A.; Ravi, K.; Mohan, U.; Panchamoorthy, R. Characterization and in vitro antibacterial activity of saponin-conjugated silver nanoparticles against bacteria that cause burn wound infection. *World J. Microbiol. Biotechnol.* **2017**, *33*, 147. [CrossRef]
39. Shameli, K.; Ahmad, M.B.; Yunus, W.M.Z.W.; Ibrahim, N.A.; Rahman, R.A.; Jokar, M.; Darroudi, M. Silver/poly (lactic acid) nanocomposites: Preparation, characterization, and antibacterial activity. *Int. J. Nanomed.* **2010**, *5*, 573–579. [CrossRef]
40. Biedenbach, D.; Lob, S.; Badal, R.; Sahm, D. Variability of Susceptibility and Multidrug Resistance among K. pneumoniae from IAI in Asia/Pacific Countries–SMART 2012–2013. *Int. J. Antimicrob. Agents PO BOX* **2015**, *211*, 1000.
41. Chen, C.Z.; Cooper, S.L. Interactions between dendrimer biocides and bacterial membranes. *Biomaterials* **2002**, *23*, 3359–3368. [CrossRef] [PubMed]
42. Bradford, M.M. A rapid and sensitive method for the quantitation of microgram quantities of protein utilizing the principle of protein-dye binding. *Anal. Biochem.* **1976**, *72*, 248–254. [CrossRef] [PubMed]
43. Ghaima, K.K.; Rasheed, S.F.; Ahmed, E.F. Antibiofilm, antibacterial and antioxidant activities of water extract of Calendula officinalis flowers. *Int. J. Biol. Pharm. Res.* **2013**, *4*, 465–470.
44. Zahin, M.; Hasan, S.; Aqil, F.; Khan, M.; Ahmad, S.; Husain, F.M.; Ahmad, I. Screening of certain medicinal plants from India for their anti-quorum sensing activity. *Indian J. Exp. Boil.* **2010**, *48*, 1219–1224.
45. Matz, C.; Deines, P.; Boenigk, J.; Arndt, H.; Eberl, L.; Kjelleberg, S.; Jürgens, K. Impact of violacein-producing bacteria on survival and feeding of bacterivorous nanoflagellates. *Appl. Environ. Microbiol.* **2004**, *70*, 1593–1599. [CrossRef]
46. Essar, D.W.; Eberly, L.; Hadero, A.; Crawford, I. Identification and characterization of genes for a second anthranilate synthase in Pseudomonas aeruginosa: Interchangeability of the two anthranilate synthases and evolutionary implications. *J. Bacteriol.* **1990**, *172*, 884–900. [CrossRef]
47. Slater, H.; Crow, M.; Everson, L.; Salmond, G.P. Phosphate availability regulates biosynthesis of two antibiotics, prodigiosin and carbapenem, in Serratia via both quorum-sensing-dependent and-independent pathways. *Mol. Microbiol.* **2003**, *47*, 303–320. [CrossRef]
48. Bhakya, S.; Muthukrishnan, S.; Sukumaran, M.; Muthukumar, M. Biogenic synthesis of silver nanoparticles and their antioxidant and antibacterial activity. *Appl. Nanosci.* **2016**, *6*, 755–766. [CrossRef]
49. Kareem, O.; Ali, T.; Dar, L.A.; Mir, S.A.; Rashid, R.; Nazli, N.; Gulzar, T.; Bader, G. Positive Health Benefits of Saponins from Edible Legumes: Phytochemistry and Pharmacology. In *Edible Plants in Health and Diseases: Volume II: Phytochemical and Pharmacological Properties*; Springer: Singapore, 2022; pp. 279–298.
50. Oleszek, M.; Oleszek, W. Saponins in Food. In *Handbook of Dietary Phytochemicals*; Springer: Singapore, 2020.
51. Kora, A.J. Plant saponin biosurfactants used as soap, hair cleanser, and detergent in India. *Appl. Next Gener. Biosurfactants Food Sect.* **2023**, 459–477. [CrossRef]
52. Desai, S.D.; Desai, D.G.; Kaur, H. Saponins and their biological activities. *Pharma Times* **2009**, *41*, 13–16.

53. Fleck, J.D.; Betti, A.H.; Da Silva, F.P.; Troian, E.A.; Olivaro, C.; Ferreira, F.; Verza, S.G. Saponins from Quillaja saponaria and Quillaja brasiliensis: Particular chemical characteristics and biological activities. *Molecules* **2019**, *24*, 171. [CrossRef] [PubMed]
54. Rai, S.; Acharya-Siwakoti, E.; Kafle, A.; Devkota, H.P.; Bhattarai, A. Plant-derived saponins: A review of their surfactant properties and applications. *Sci* **2021**, *3*, 44. [CrossRef]
55. Sparg, S.; Light, M.; Van Staden, J. Biological activities and distribution of plant saponins. *J. Ethnopharmacol.* **2004**, *94*, 219–243. [CrossRef] [PubMed]
56. Sani, I. Proximate Analysis, Phytochemical Screening And Antioxidant Potential Of Ajwa Date From Medina, Saudi Arabia. *Int. Res. J. Pharm. Biosci.* **2015**, *2*, 12–17.
57. Debnath, B.; Das, R. Controlled synthesis of saponin-capped silver nanotriangles and their optical properties. *Plasmonics* **2019**, *14*, 1365–1375. [CrossRef]
58. Srivastava, N.; Choudhary, M.; Singhal, G.; Bhagyawant, S.S. SEM studies of saponin silver nanoparticles isolated from leaves of Chenopodium album L. for in vitro anti-acne activity. *Proc. Natl. Acad. Sci. India Sect. B Biol. Sci.* **2020**, *90*, 333–341. [CrossRef]
59. Singh, J.; Bajaj, R.; Harpreet, K.; Harjot, K.; Navneet, K.; Sukhmeen, K.; Muhit, R. Chemo-bio synthesis of silver nanoparticles. *J. Nanomed. Res.* **2016**, *4*, 00092.
60. Nguyen, D.H.; Vo, T.N.N.; Le, N.T.T.; Thi, D.P.N.; Thi, T.T.H. Evaluation of saponin-rich/poor leaf extract-mediated silver nanoparticles and their antifungal capacity. *Green Process. Synth.* **2020**, *9*, 429–439. [CrossRef]
61. Paramesh, C.C.; Halligudra, G.; Gangaraju, V.; Sriramoju, J.B.; Shastri, M.; Rangappa, D.; Subbegowda, R.K.; Shivaramu, P.D. Silver nanoparticles synthesized using saponin extract of Simarouba glauca oil seed meal as effective, recoverable and reusable catalyst for reduction of organic dyes. *Results Surf. Interfaces* **2021**, *3*, 100005. [CrossRef]
62. Uddin, T.M.; Chakraborty, A.J.; Khusro, A.; Zidan, B.R.M.; Mitra, S.; Emran, T.B.; Dhama, K.; Ripon, M.K.H.; Gajdács, M.; Sahibzada, M.U.K.; et al. Antibiotic resistance in microbes: History, mechanisms, therapeutic strategies and future prospects. *J. Infect. Public Health* **2021**, *14*, 1750–1766. [CrossRef]
63. Adnan, M.; Patel, M.; Deshpande, S.; Alreshidi, M.; Siddiqui, A.J.; Reddy, M.N.; Emira, N.; De Feo, V. Effect of Adiantum philippense extract on biofilm formation, adhesion with its antibacterial activities against foodborne pathogens, and characterization of bioactive metabolites: An in vitro-in silico approach. *Front. Microbiol.* **2020**, *11*, 823. [CrossRef] [PubMed]
64. Awadelkareem, A.M.; Siddiqui, A.J.; Noumi, E.; Ashraf, S.A.; Hadi, S.; Snoussi, M.; Badraoui, R.; Bardakci, F.; Ashraf, M.S.; Danciu, C. Biosynthesized Silver Nanoparticles Derived from Probiotic Lactobacillus rhamnosus (AgNPs-LR) Targeting Biofilm Formation and Quorum Sensing-Mediated Virulence Factors. *Antibiotics* **2023**, *12*, 986. [CrossRef] [PubMed]
65. Patel, M.; Ashraf, M.S.; Siddiqui, A.J.; Ashraf, S.A.; Sachidanandan, M.; Snoussi, M.; Adnan, M.; Hadi, S. Profiling and role of bioactive molecules from puntius sophore (Freshwater/brackish fish) skin mucus with its potent antibacterial, antiadhesion, and antibiofilm activities. *Biomolecules* **2020**, *10*, 920. [CrossRef]
66. Dufour, D.; Leung, V.; Lévesque, C.M. Bacterial biofilm: Structure, function, and antimicrobial resistance. *Endod. Top.* **2010**, *22*, 2–16. [CrossRef]
67. Alam, A.; Kumar, A.; Tripathi, P.; Ehtesham, N.Z.; Hasnain, S.E. Biofilms: A phenotypic mechanism of bacteria conferring tolerance against stress and antibiotics. In *Mycobacterium Tuberculosis: Molecular Infection Biology, Pathogenesis, Diagnostics and New Interventions*; Springer: Singapore, 2019; pp. 315–333.
68. Nirwati, H.; Sinanjung, K.; Fahrunissa, F.; Wijaya, F.; Napitupulu, S.; Hati, V.P.; Hakim, M.S.; Meliala, A.; Aman, A.T.; Nuryastuti, T. Biofilm formation and antibiotic resistance of Klebsiella pneumoniae isolated from clinical samples in a tertiary care hospital, Klaten, Indonesia. *BMC Proc.* **2019**, *13*, 20. [CrossRef]
69. Vestby, L.K.; Grønseth, T.; Simm, R.; Nesse, L.L. Bacterial biofilm and its role in the pathogenesis of disease. *Antibiotics* **2020**, *9*, 59. [CrossRef]
70. Bhattacharya, M.; Wozniak, D.J.; Stoodley, P.; Hall-Stoodley, L. Prevention and treatment of Staphylococcus aureus biofilms. *Expert Rev. Anti-Infect. Ther.* **2015**, *13*, 1499–1516. [CrossRef]
71. Khatoon, Z.; McTiernan, C.D.; Suuronen, E.J.; Mah, T.-F.; Alarcon, E.I. Bacterial biofilm formation on implantable devices and approaches to its treatment and prevention. *Heliyon* **2018**, *4*, e01067. [CrossRef]
72. Koo, H.; Allan, R.N.; Howlin, R.P.; Stoodley, P.; Hall-Stoodley, L. Targeting microbial biofilms: Current and prospective therapeutic strategies. *Nat. Rev. Microbiol.* **2017**, *15*, 740–755. [CrossRef]
73. Markowska, K.; Grudniak, A.; Wolska, K. Silver nanoparticles as an alternative strategy against bacterial biofilms. *Acta Biochim. Pol.* **2013**, *60*, 523–530. [CrossRef]
74. Römling, U.; Balsalobre, C. Biofilm infections, their resilience to therapy and innovative treatment strategies. *J. Intern. Med.* **2012**, *272*, 541–561. [CrossRef] [PubMed]
75. Paluch, E.; Rewak-Soroczyńska, J.; Jędrusik, I.; Mazurkiewicz, E.; Jermakow, K. Prevention of biofilm formation by quorum quenching. *Appl. Microbiol. Biotechnol.* **2020**, *104*, 1871–1881. [CrossRef] [PubMed]
76. Preda, V.G.; Săndulescu, O. Communication is the key: Biofilms, quorum sensing, formation and prevention. *Discoveries* **2019**, *7*, e10. [CrossRef] [PubMed]
77. Tagousop, C.N.; Tamokou, J.-d.-D.; Kengne, I.C.; Ngnokam, D.; Voutquenne-Nazabadioko, L. Antimicrobial activities of saponins from Melanthera elliptica and their synergistic effects with antibiotics against pathogenic phenotypes. *Chem. Cent. J.* **2018**, *12*, 97. [CrossRef] [PubMed]

78. Zhong, J.; Tan, L.; Chen, M.; He, C. Pharmacological activities and molecular mechanisms of Pulsatilla saponins. *Chin. Med.* **2022**, *17*, 59. [CrossRef]
79. Parvekar, P.; Palaskar, J.; Metgud, S.; Maria, R.; Dutta, S. The minimum inhibitory concentration (MIC) and minimum bactericidal concentration (MBC) of silver nanoparticles against Staphylococcus aureus. *Biomater. Investig. Dent.* **2020**, *7*, 105–109. [CrossRef]
80. Van de Vel, E.; Sampers, I.; Raes, K. A review on influencing factors on the minimum inhibitory concentration of essential oils. *Crit. Rev. Food Sci. Nutr.* **2019**, *59*, 357–378. [CrossRef]
81. Kowalska-Krochmal, B.; Dudek-Wicher, R. The minimum inhibitory concentration of antibiotics: Methods, interpretation, clinical relevance. *Pathogens* **2021**, *10*, 165. [CrossRef]
82. Walsh, C. Molecular mechanisms that confer antibacterial drug resistance. *Nature* **2000**, *406*, 775–781. [CrossRef]
83. Mansoor, S.; Zahoor, I.; Baba, T.; Padder, S.; Bhat, Z.; Koul, A.; Jiang, L. Fabrication of silver nanoparticles against fungal pathogens. *Front. Nanotechnol.* **2021**, *3*, 679358. [CrossRef]
84. Alavi, M.; Hamblin, M.R. Antibacterial silver nanoparticles: Effects on bacterial nucleic acids. *Cell. Mol. Biomed. Rep.* **2023**, *3*, 35–40. [CrossRef]
85. Gurunathan, S.; Han, J.W.; Kwon, D.-N.; Kim, J.-H. Enhanced antibacterial and anti-biofilm activities of silver nanoparticles against Gram-negative and Gram-positive bacteria. *Nanoscale Res. Lett.* **2014**, *9*, 373. [CrossRef] [PubMed]
86. Mohanta, Y.K.; Biswas, K.; Jena, S.K.; Hashem, A.; Abd_Allah, E.F.; Mohanta, T.K. Anti-biofilm and antibacterial activities of silver nanoparticles synthesized by the reducing activity of phytoconstituents present in the Indian medicinal plants. *Front. Microbiol.* **2020**, *11*, 1143. [CrossRef] [PubMed]
87. Siddique, M.H.; Aslam, B.; Imran, M.; Ashraf, A.; Nadeem, H.; Hayat, S.; Khurshid, M.; Afzal, M.; Malik, I.R.; Shahzad, M. Effect of silver nanoparticles on biofilm formation and EPS production of multidrug-resistant Klebsiella pneumoniae. *Biomed Res. Int.* **2020**, *2020*, 6398165. [CrossRef]
88. Ansari, M.A.; Khan, H.M.; Khan, A.A.; Cameotra, S.S.; Pal, R. Antibiofilm efficacy of silver nanoparticles against biofilm of extended spectrum β-lactamase isolates of Escherichia coli and Klebsiella pneumoniae. *Appl. Nanosci.* **2014**, *4*, 859–868. [CrossRef]
89. Dos Santos, E.M.P.; Martins, C.C.B., de Oliveira Santos, J.V.; da Silva, W.R.C.; Silva, S.B.C.; Pelagio-Flores, M.A.; Galembeck, A.; Cavalcanti, I.M.F. Silver nanoparticles–chitosan composites activity against resistant bacteria: Tolerance and biofilm inhibition. *J. Nanoparticle Res.* **2021**, *23*, 196. [CrossRef] [PubMed]
90. Adwas, A.A.; Elsayed, A.; Azab, A.; Quwaydir, F. Oxidative stress and antioxidant mechanisms in human body. *J. Appl. Biotechnol. Bioeng.* **2019**, *6*, 43–47.
91. Sharma, N. Free radicals, antioxidants and disease. *Biol. Med.* **2014**, *6*, 1. [CrossRef]
92. López-Alarcón, C.; Denicola, A. Evaluating the antioxidant capacity of natural products: A review on chemical and cellular-based assays. *Anal. Chim. Acta* **2013**, *763*, 1–10. [CrossRef]
93. Bedlovičová, Z.; Strapáč, I.; Baláž, M.; Salayová, A. A brief overview on antioxidant activity determination of silver nanoparticles. *Molecules* **2020**, *25*, 3191. [CrossRef]
94. Keshari, A.K.; Srivastava, R.; Singh, P.; Yadav, V.B.; Nath, G. Antioxidant and antibacterial activity of silver nanoparticles synthesized by Cestrum nocturnum. *J. Ayurveda Integr. Med.* **2020**, *11*, 37–44. [CrossRef]
95. White, P.A.; Oliveira, R.C.; Oliveira, A.P.; Serafini, M.R.; Araújo, A.A.; Gelain, D.P.; Moreira, J.C.; Almeida, J.R.; Quintans, J.S.; Quintans-Junior, L.J.; et al. Antioxidant activity and mechanisms of action of natural compounds isolated from lichens: A systematic review. *Molecules* **2014**, *19*, 14496–14527. [CrossRef]
96. Bade, B.C.; Cruz, C.S.D. Lung cancer 2020: Epidemiology, etiology, and prevention. *Clin. Chest Med.* **2020**, *41*, 1–24. [CrossRef]
97. Huang, C.-Y.; Ju, D.-T.; Chang, C.-F.; Reddy, P.M.; Velmurugan, B.K. A review on the effects of current chemotherapy drugs and natural agents in treating non–small cell lung cancer. *Biomedicine* **2017**, *7*, 23. [CrossRef] [PubMed]
98. Huy, T.Q.; Huyen, P.; Le, A.-T.; Tonezzer, M. Recent advances of silver nanoparticles in cancer diagnosis and treatment. *Anticancer Agents Med. Chem.* **2020**, *20*, 1276–1287. [CrossRef] [PubMed]
99. Chen, J.; Ning, C.; Zhou, Z.; Yu, P.; Zhu, Y.; Tan, G.; Mao, C. Nanomaterials as photothermal therapeutic agents. *Prog. Mater. Sci.* **2019**, *99*, 1–26. [CrossRef] [PubMed]
100. Gopinath, P.; Gogoi, S.K.; Sanpui, P.; Paul, A.; Chattopadhyay, A.; Ghosh, S.S. Signaling gene cascade in silver nanoparticle induced apoptosis. *Colloids Surf. B Biointerfaces* **2010**, *77*, 240–245. [CrossRef]
101. Mao, B.-H.; Tsai, J.-C.; Chen, C.-W.; Yan, S.-J.; Wang, Y.-J. Mechanisms of silver nanoparticle-induced toxicity and important role of autophagy. *Nanotoxicology* **2016**, *10*, 1021–1040. [CrossRef]
102. Gurunathan, S.; Lee, K.-J.; Kalishwaralal, K.; Sheikpranbabu, S.; Vaidyanathan, R.; Eom, S.H. Antiangiogenic properties of silver nanoparticles. *Biomaterials* **2009**, *30*, 6341–6350. [CrossRef]
103. Ivanova, N.; Gugleva, V.; Dobreva, M.; Pehlivanov, I.; Stefanov, S.; Andonova, V. *Silver Nanoparticles as Multifunctional Drug Delivery Systems*; IntechOpen: London, UK, 2018

antibiotics

Article

Integration of Antimicrobials and Delivery Systems: Synergistic Antibiofilm Activity with Biodegradable Nanoemulsions Incorporating Pseudopyronine Analogs

Jungmi Park [1], Neel Mahida [1,†], Gabrielle Ho [1,†], Elizabeth Pena [1,†], Jessa Marie V. Makabenta [1], Stanley Aneke [1], Mingdi Jiang [1], Leah M. Bouthillette [2], Stephanie E. Holz [2], Muhammad Aamir Hassan [1], Amanda L. Wolfe [2] and Vincent M. Rotello [1,*]

[1] Department of Chemistry, University of Massachusetts Amherst, Amherst, MA 01003, USA; jungmipark@umass.edu (J.P.); nmahida@umass.edu (N.M.); gho@umass.edu (G.H.); epena@umass.edu (E.P.); jmakabenta@umass.edu (J.M.V.M.); saneke@umass.edu (S.A.) mingdijiang@umass.edu (M.J.); muhammadaami@umass.edu (M.A.H.)

[2] Department of Chemistry and Biochemistry, University of North Carolina Asheville, Asheville, NC 28804, USA; lbouthil@ucsc.edu (L.M.B.); sholz@unca.edu (S.E.H.); awolfe@unca.edu (A.L.W.)

* Correspondence: rotello@umass.edu

† These authors contributed equally to this work.

Abstract: Multi-drug-resistant (MDR) bacteria, including methicillin-resistant *Staphylococcus aureus* (MRSA), pose a significant challenge in healthcare settings. Small molecule antimicrobials (SMAs) such as α-pyrones have shown promise as alternative treatments for MDR infections. However, the hydrophobic nature of many SMAs limits their solubility and efficacy in complex biological environments. In this study, we encapsulated pseudopyronine analogs (PAs) in biodegradable polymer nanoemulsions (BNEs) for efficient eradication of biofilms. We evaluated a series of PAs with varied alkyl chain lengths and examined their antimicrobial activity against Gram-positive pathogens (*S. aureus*, MRSA, and *B. subtilis*). The selected PA with the most potent antibiofilm activity was incorporated into BNEs for enhanced solubility and penetration into the EPS matrix (PA-BNEs). The antimicrobial efficacy of PA-BNEs was assessed against biofilms of Gram-positive strains. The BNEs facilitated the solubilization and effective delivery of the PA deep into the biofilm matrix, addressing the limitations of hydrophobic SMAs. Our findings demonstrated that the PA2 exhibited synergistic antibiofilm activity when it was loaded into nanoemulsions. This study presents a promising platform for addressing MDR infections by combining pseudopyronine analogs with antimicrobial biodegradable nanoemulsions, overcoming challenges associated with treating biofilm infections.

Keywords: biofilm infections; nanoemulsions; pseudopyronine analogs; essential oils

1. Introduction

Multi-drug-resistant (MDR) bacteria annually cause at least 2 million infections, leading to 23,000 deaths and increased hospitalizations each year [1]. Some of the most concerning MDR bacteria include methicillin-resistant *Staphylococcus aureus* (MRSA) [2]. MDR bacteria are challenging to treat due to their adapted ability to tolerate high levels of therapeutics [3–5]. Not addressing MDR bacterial infections contributes to increased persistence of infection, even resulting in mortality [6]. Biofilms formed by MDR bacteria are particularly challenging, not only from the inherent ability of associated bacteria to tolerate high levels of therapeutics [7], but also the protective environment, resulting in antibiotic therapy being ineffective [8]. The extracellular polymeric substances (EPSs) matrix in a biofilm, in particular, is a barrier to most antibiotics, resulting in increased antimicrobial resistance and prolonged infection [9].

Small molecule antimicrobials (SMAs) provide effective therapeutics and can offer a large design space that can be explored for drug development as an alternative solution to MDR infections [10]. α-Pyrones are a class of natural products produced by a variety of microorganisms as both biosynthetic precursors and secondary metabolites that have been found to possess antibiotic, antifungal, cytotoxic, and anti-atherosclerotic activity [11–15]. Pseudopyronine A (Figure 1) and pseudopyronine B are α-pyrone natural products produced by multiple species of bacteria that have saturated alkyl chains on C3 and C6 [16–19]. The pseudopyronines act as antibiotics against both resistant and non-resistant Gram-positive bacteria via selective membrane disruption and inhibition of fatty-acid synthase (FAS) II [19–21]. Recently, we synthesized and evaluated a series of C3/C6 pseudopyronine analogs and found that alkyl chain length at these positions directly affects antibacterial activity with analogs with longer alkyl chains (up to 6/7 carbons) showing the highest potency against susceptible strains of *S. aureus* and *B. subtills* both Gram-positive pathogens [22].

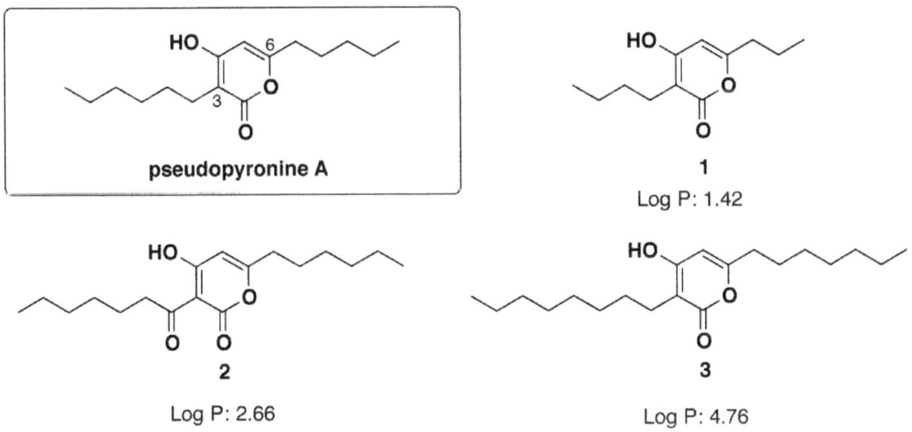

Figure 1. Chemical structures of pseudopyronine A and pseudopyronine analogs (PA) 1, 2, and 3.

Hydrophobic SMAs have limited aqueous solubility, making them challenging to use in complex biological environments like biofilms [23]. Combination strategies employing dual antimicrobials to combat biofilm infections have been studied; however, their efficacy toward mature biofilms is limited due to heterogeneous compositions deactivating many therapeutics [24].

Nanoemulsions involving essential oils have shown promising potential in treating bacterial infections with broad-spectrum activity, high biocompatibility, and a high barrier against resistance development [25,26]. Polymeric carriers based on poly(oxanorbornenimide) (PONI) backbones have been utilized for antimicrobial delivery [27]. In our previous studies, we introduced functionalized PONI-polymers incorporating guanidinium, maleimide, and tetramethylene glycol monoethyl ether (PONI-GMT) to create nanoemulsions with nature-derived essential oils including eugenol, carvacrol, linalool, and methyl eugenol [26]. We further explored this system to load hydrophobic antimicrobial therapeutics for the synergistic treatment of bacterial biofilms, leveraging the amphiphilic properties of nanoemulsions. Therefore, we hypothesized that polymer based biodegradable nanoemulsions (BNEs) can be utilized along with pseudopyronine analogs (PAs) to encapsulate and solubilize to reach deep into the EPS matrix and produce enhanced antibiofilm activity. For this study, we chose to examine three compounds with varied activity from the original series, PA1 (C = 3,4), PA2 (C = 6,7), and PA3 (C = 7,8) [28]. From these leads, PA2 had the best synergistic antibiofilm activity with the BNE. PA-BNE reduced bacterial viability against *S. aureus* and MRSA and *B. subtilis* biofilms compared with when

PA2 worked alone. Notably, PA-BNEs showed minimum cytotoxicity to fibroblast cells. Taken together, these studies demonstrated that careful choice of therapeutic and carrier presents a strategy to access a large design space of small molecules to address limitations of SMAs including solubility and biofilm penetration.

2. Results

2.1. Antimicrobial Activity of Analog Compounds against Gram-Positive Planktonic Bacteria

The intrinsic antimicrobial activity of analogs was evaluated against Gram-positive bacteria including MRSA by determining minimum inhibitor concentration (MIC) values (Table 1). PA1 was found to have MIC of 250 mg/L against *S. aureus* and *B. subtilis*, respectively. The most potent activity against *S. aureus* was observed for PA2 with MIC value of 0.5 mg/L. For longer alkyl chain analogs, PA2 and 3 showed more potent activity against *S. aureus* with 0.5 mg/L and 25 mg/L, respectively. We also tested the analogs against a drug-resistant strain of *S. aureus*, specifically MRSA, where the MIC values were higher than *S. aureus*.

Table 1. In vitro antimicrobial activity of PAs.

Compound	MIC (mg/L)		
	S. aureus	**MRSA**	***B. subtilis***
PA1	500	>500	500
PA2	0.5	12.5	50
PA3	25	177	50

S. aurues (CD-35), MRSA (IDRL-6169), and *B. subtilis* (FD6b).

2.2. Fabrication of PAs-Loaded Biodegradable Nanoemulsions (PA-BNEs)

2.2.1. Solubility of PAs in Eugenol

BNEs were fabricated by emulsifying essential oils (eugenol) with amphiphilic polymers using an oil–water interface and cross-linking [26]. The essential oil can be used to load hydrophobic components [29]. In this study, eugenol was chosen for its wide spectrum of antimicrobial activity and ability to disrupt biofilm when it was delivered with BNEs. PAs were dissolved in eugenol, and the solubility of each compound was recorded (Table 2). The solubility was high for PAs close to log P of eugenol (log P: 2.49). The PA2 have similar log P values of eugenol, affording the highest concentrations of around 100 mg/mL (PA2 log P: 2.66). However, PA1 and PA3 have higher or lower log P values (PA1 log P: 1.42, PA3 log P: 4.76), and show somewhat lower solubility compared with PA2. Taken together, PA2 was chosen for further studies due to its higher antimicrobial activity and better carrier solubility.

Table 2. Solubility test result of the PAs in eugenol.

	PA1	**PA2**	**PA3**
Drug concentrations in eugenol (mg/mL)	48	100	25

2.2.2. Generation and Characterization of PA-BNEs

Eugenol was used to dissolve PA2 (up to 24 mg/mL), and serial diluted to generate different formulations of PA2-loaded nanoemulsions (PA-BNE) (Figure 2a). In each fabrication, 500 μL of PA-BNE solution containing different PA2 levels was afforded and defined as 100% solution (*v/v*). The hydrodynamic size of PA-BNEs was measured by dynamic light scattering (DLS) and formed around 290 nm with narrow size distributions (polydispersity index: 0.08) (Figure 2b, Figure S1). The measured zeta potential of PA-BNEs was +10 mV, attributed to positively charged guanidinium groups on the polymers (Figure 2c).

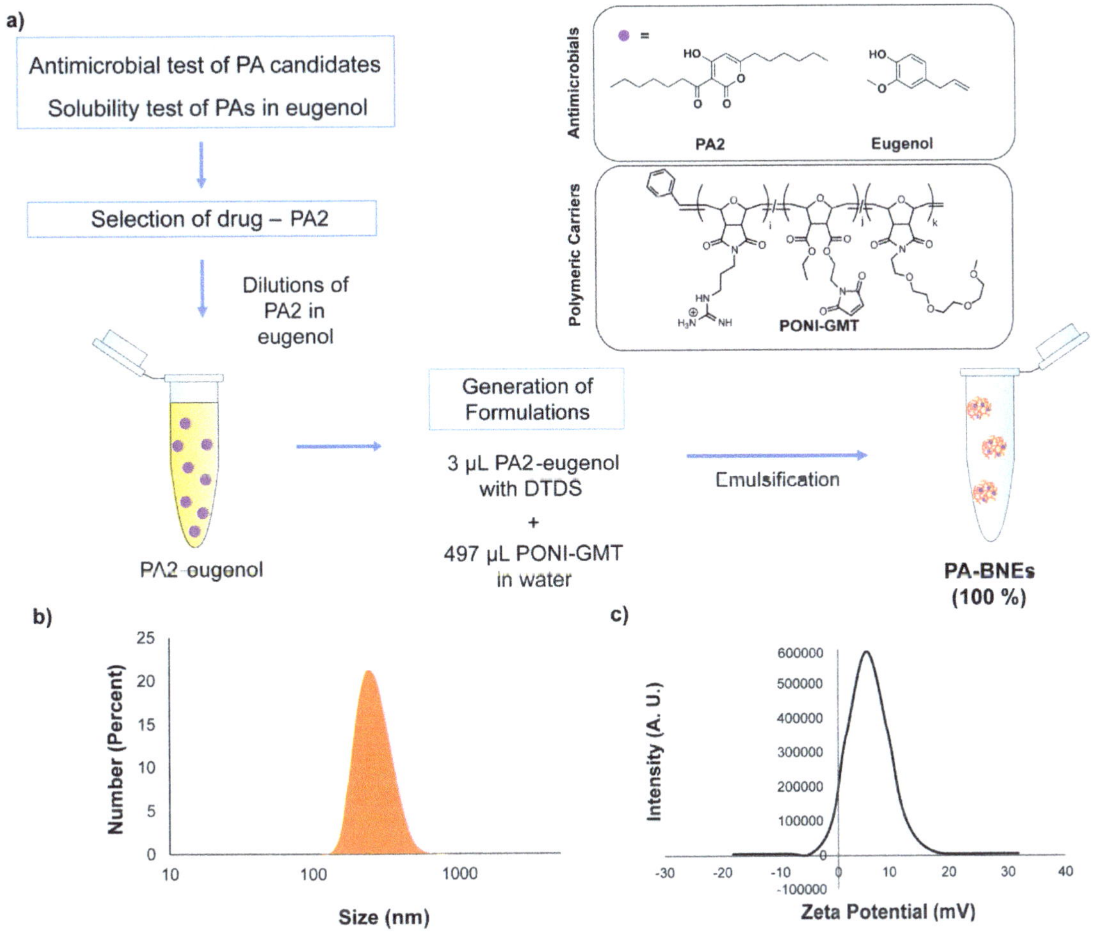

Figure 2. (**a**) Schematic representation of the workflow for preparation of PA-loaded nanoemulsions (PA-BNE) after solubility test and antimicrobial testing; (**b**) hydrodynamic size of PA-BNE measured by dynamic light scattering (DLS); (**c**) intensity graph of zeta-potential measurement.

2.3. Antimicrobial Activity of PA-BNE

2.3.1. Antimicrobial Activity of PA-BNEs

We next evaluated the antimicrobial activity of PA-BNE against MRSA (IDRL 6169). The minimum bactericidal concentrations (MBCs) were determined for each material PA2 and BNE. The PA2 alone was 12 mg/L and BNE was 16% (Table 3). Then, we varied PA2 loading to generate PA-BNEs and check the MBC. We observed 8% concentrations of BNE with 4 mg/L, showing eradication of MRSA the next day. The MBCs of PA2 were a third time less with BNE, and the MBC of BNE was half-fold than when treated alone, indicating a positive additive effect of those two systems.

Table 3. Minimal bactericidal concentrations (MBCs) of PA2, BNE and PA-BNE against MRSA.

Materials	MBC
	MRSA (IDRL-6169)
PA2	12 mg/L
BNE	16% (*v/v*)
PA-BNE	8% (*v/v*), 4 mg/L

2.3.2. Antibiofilm Activity of PA-BNEs

We next evaluated the antimicrobial activity of PA in the nanoemulsions against *S. aureus* (CD-35) and *B. subtilis* (FD6b) biofilm. The minimum biofilm bactericidal concentrations (MBBCs) were initially determined for each component using high-throughput screening. The PA2 alone was 4 mg/L where BNE was >16% (Figure 3a) against *S. aureus*. For *B. subtilis*, PA2 was presenting limited antibiofilm activity (>100 mg/L). Subsequently, we used PA-BNE with different levels of PA2 loading to assess their combined effects and best formulations for delivering PA to biofilm through checkerboard titrations. We observed that PA2 was active at 16% (*v/v*) concentrations of BNE, showing eradication at 32-fold lesser concentrations (0.125 mg/L) with BNE than PA2 alone (Figure 3b). For *B. subtilis*, a similar trend was observed, where PA-BNE (with 4 mg/L of PA2) showed eradication of biofilms after treatment (Figure S2). The additive effect was determined between PA2 and eugenol by fractional inhibitory concentration index (FICI = 0.531). Furthermore, we tested PA-BNE against MRSA biofilms with vancomycin as a control to evaluate the therapeutic potential of the system. Notably, the PA-BNE showed the most reduction in bacterial viability as comparable to the antibiotics.

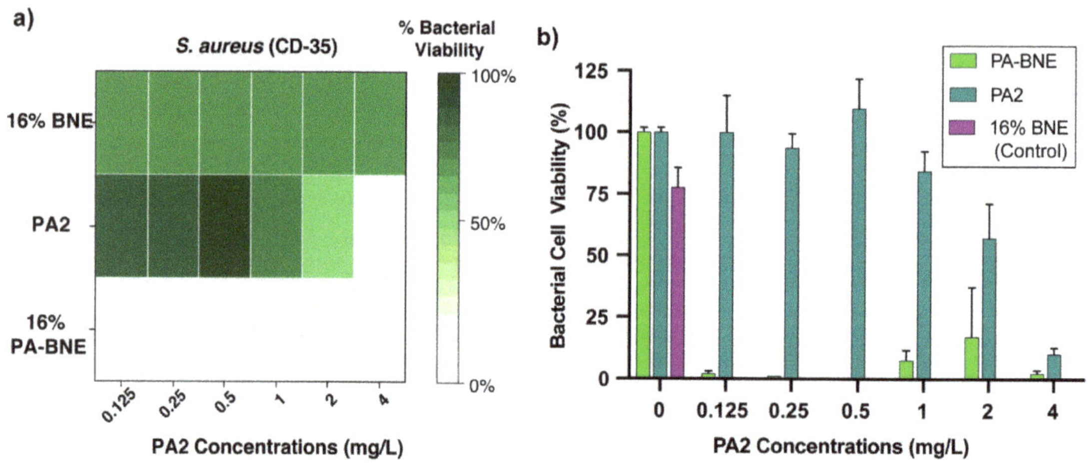

Figure 3. (**a**) Minimum biofilm bactericidal concentrations (MBBCs) of BNEs, PA2, and PA-BNE against *S. aureus* biofilm represented as a heatmap and (**b**) bacterial viability (%) of *S. aureus* biofilm at 16% of BNE varying PA2 concentrations after treatment. The data shown are averages of triplicates with the error bars indicating standard deviations.

2.4. Cytotoxicity of PA-BNE In Vitro Fibroblast Cell

Lack of toxicity to mammalian cells of combined PA-BNEs was demonstrated by mammalian cell viability test against 3T3 fibroblast cells, which is an epithelial cell line that is damaged during bacterial biofilm infections at the wound site. PA-BNEs showed safety towards mammalian cells, maintaining cell viability levels above 90% [30]. These results were comparable to those observed for the drug alone, indicating the safety of the combined system through nanoemulsions. Across the concentration range tested, PA-BNEs consistently demonstrated no significant adverse effects on cell viability, indicating its potential for safe implementation in various applications.

3. Discussion

Small molecule antimicrobials (SMAs) present a new and effective approach to developing therapeutics, offering a wide range of possibilities for drug design to combat drug-resistant infections [31,32]. Pseudopyronines (PAs) are a class of α-pyrone natural products, synthesized by multiple bacterial species [31,33]. In this study, we screened antimicrobial activity of synthesized derivatives of PAs, varying the number of carbons from 3,4 (PA1), 6,7 (PA2), and 7,8 (PA3) on C6 and C3 positions respectively. We confirmed the longer alkyl chains, but particularly PA2 with 6,7 carbons and a ketone on the C3 alkyl side chain, exhibited the highest potency against Gram-positive (*S. aureus*, MRSA and *B. subtilis*) strains of bacteria (Table 1). However, the application of SMAs is hindered by their low solubility in water, posing challenges in complex biological settings such as biofilms [31].

Polymers with poly(oxanorbornenimide) (PONI) backbones have been used as carriers to deliver antimicrobials [33]. We previously reported functionalized PONI-polymers with guanidinium, maleimide and tetramethylene glycol monoethyl ether (PONI-GMT) to form nanoemulsions with essential oils by using amphiphilic properties of polymers [26]. Essential oils are promising antimicrobials, but their activity against biofilm is reduced due to their hydrophobicity, which limits their penetration through the biofilm matrix [34]. Therefore, essential oils using nanoemulsions featured efficient penetration resulting in enhanced antimicrobial activity against biofilm [26]. BNEs were also used for the delivery of additional antimicrobials, such as hydrophobic triclosan [28]. In the current study, we employed nanoemulsions for the delivery of PAs to eradicate bacterial biofilms, using efficient loading of PAs to amphiphilic BNEs.

The BNEs used in our studies are composed of both hydrophobic and hydrophilic materials, enabling the incorporation of hydrophobic antimicrobials like PAs. Firstly, we tested the compatibility of PAs with essential oil by dissolving PAs into eugenol. Eugenol was chosen for its broad antimicrobial activity and ability to disrupt biofilms forming stable nanoemulsions with PONI-GMT polymers [26,35,36]. The solubility of PAs was tested and PA2 showed the highest solubility (100 mg/mL) among the PAs (Table 2). PA2 also demonstrated potent antimicrobial activity, suggesting that PA2 can be a promising candidate for co-delivery with eugenol in BNEs to enhance the accumulation of therapeutics and achieve synergistic bacterial killing against the biofilms.

Using the stock solution of PA2-eugenol, we generated formulations of PA-BNEs using emulsification (Figure 2a). We demonstrated the successful fabrication of nanoemulsions loaded with chosen analogs PA2, with size ~290 nm (Figure 2b, Figure S1) with positive surface charge +10 mV in an aqueous solution (Figure 2c). The formulated PA-BNEs were tested against MRSA to determine minimal bactericidal concentrations (MBCs) with PA2 and BNE controls. The result indicated PA-BNE featured an additive effect by lowering MBCs of PA2 and BNE when they were treated individually. Next, we screened formulations by varying PA2 concentrations to determine their synergistic effect between PA2 and eugenol using a checkerboard assay to determine MBBC. We demonstrated PA-BNEs showed a 32-fold reduction up to 0.125 mg/L relative to PA2 alone (4 mg/L). For *B. subtilis*, the MBBC of PA-BNE was determined at 4 mg/L with BNE while PA2 alone showed now significant antibiofilm activity (>100 mg/L). These results suggest the activity of PA2 was enhanced through the nanoemulsions system by enhanced delivery of PA2 across the mature biofilms (Figure 3a and Figure S2).

We assessed the antimicrobial activity of PA-loaded nanoemulsions against biofilms of *S. aureus* (CD-35), *B. subtilis* (FD6b), and MRSA (IDRL-6169). For *B. subtilis*, PA-BNE (containing 4 mg/L of PA2) effectively eliminated the biofilms. Furthermore, we tested the PA-BNE against MRSA biofilms, using vancomycin as a control to evaluate the therapeutic potential of the system (Figure S3). Notably, the PA-BNE exhibited a significant reduction in bacterial viability, comparable to the effects of the antibiotics.

Our findings demonstrate that PA-loaded nanoemulsions, specifically PA-BNE, effectively target and eradicate biofilms of *S. aureus*, *B. subtilis*, and MRSA. The combination of PA2 and eugenol within the nanoemulsion formulation shows enhanced antibiofilm activity, highlighting the therapeutic potential of this system.

Biofilm formation at infection sites can prolong the healing process regulated by fibroblast skin cells [37,38]. To evaluate the compatibility of PA-BNEs, we tested their cytotoxicity at concentrations used to eliminate established biofilms. In in vitro 3T3 fibroblast cells, PA-BNEs did not exhibit any significant toxicity towards fibroblast cells within the relevant concentration range (Figure 4). Overall, this result indicates that combination therapy of PA2 and BNEs has minimal toxicity towards mammalian cells.

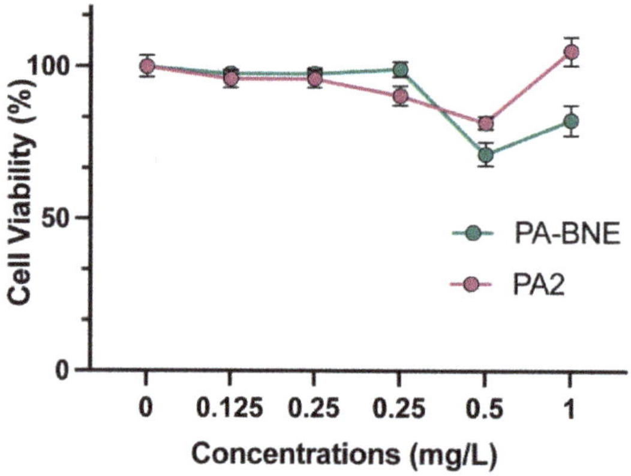

Figure 4. Cell viability of 3T3 fibroblast cells measured band quantified by Alamar blue assay. Treatment was performed for 3 h with materials. Values are expressed as mean ± standard deviation of ≥3 replicates.

4. Materials and Methods

The following bacteria strains were used for this study: *S. aureus* (CD-35), MRSA (IDRL-6169), and *B. subtilis* (FD6b). Overnight cultures of bacteria were prepared by transferring the isolated colony from the agar plate to culture tubes with sterile media broth. The bacterial cultures were then incubated overnight at 37 °C with aeration and agitation (275 rpm) until they reached the desired growth phase. Isolates with code IDRL were from the Infectious Diseases Research Laboratory at Mayo Clinic (Rochester, MN, USA). CD were from the Cooley Dickenson (Northampton, MA, USA). NIH-3T3 cells (ATCC CRL-1658) were purchased from ATCC. Dulbecco's Modified Eagle's Medium (DMEM) (DMEM; ATCC 30-2002) and fetal bovine serum (SH3007103) (Thermo Fisher Scientific, Waltham, MA, USA) were used for cell culture. Invitrogen™ alamarBlue™ Cell Viability Reagent (DAL 1100) was purchase from Thermo Fisher Scientific (Waltham, MA, USA) and used following the manufacturer's protocol.

4.1. Determination of Minimum Inhibitory Concentration (MIC) and Minimum Bactericidal Concentrations (MBCs)

The bacteria were grown in TSB medium under specific conditions. Once they reached the mid-log phase, the cultures were collected through centrifugation and washed with a sodium chloride solution. The concentration of the bacterial solution was determined by measuring the optical density at 600 nm. Dilutions of the bacterial solution were fabricated using M9 medium to achieve a concentration of 1×10^6 cfu/mL. In a 96-well plate, 50 µL of these diluted bacteria in M9 was mixed with 50 µL of testing materials in M9, resulting in a final bacterial concentration of 5×10^5 cfu/mL. The testing concentration was adjusted according to a standard protocol. Control groups, including a growth control with only a bacterial solution and a sterile control, were included in each experiment. The plate was then incubated for 16 h. The experiment was performed in triplicates, and at least two independent experiments were conducted on different days. The minimum inhibitory concentration (MIC) was determined as the lowest concentration of the testing chemical that prevented visible growth observed with the naked eye. Subsequently, the testing solutions (up to 4-fold MICs) exhibiting no visible growth were further diluted and enumerated on tryptic soy agar (TSA) plate. The MBC value was determined if it showed ~99% reduction in CFU/mL.

4.2. Preparation of PA-BNE

PA-BNEs were created by emulsifying eugenol loaded with PA2 and DTDS into an aqueous solution of PONI-GMT. Solid PA2 was dissolved in eugenol at different concentrations up to 33 mg/mL, along with DTDS at a concentration of 3 wt %. A total of 3 μL of the oil mixture and 497 μL of the aqueous PONI-GMT solution were combined and emulsified using an amalgamator for 50 s. The resulting emulsions were left to rest overnight before being utilized in the experiment.

4.3. Minimal Biofilm Bactericidal Concentration (MBBC) Determination

The minimum biofilm bactericidal concentrations (MBBCs) of the BNEs, PA2, and PA-BNEs were determined following established protocols. Bacterial solutions were prepared from overnight cultures and diluted 1/50th using tryptic soy broth (TSB) and incubated at 275 rpm and 37 °C until they reached the mid-log phase. Next, 150 μL of the bacterial culture was added to each well of a 96-well microtiter plate with pegged lids and incubated at 37 °C and 50 rpm for 6 h. Subsequently, the pegged lids were rinsed by submerging them in 200 μL of PBS for 30 s, followed by transfer to a separate 96-well plate containing two-fold serial dilutions of the therapeutic agents prepared in 5% TSB in M9 media. The plate was then incubated at 37 °C for 24 h. Afterward, the biofilms on the lids were treated with PBS as described earlier and transferred to a new plate containing fresh media. This plate was further incubated at 37 °C to determine the MBBC. The MBBC of the antibiofilm agents was determined through visual inspection and confirmed using spectrophotometry by measuring the optical density at 600 nm (OD600).

4.4. Antibiofilm Study

Bacterial seeding solutions were prepared in Tryptic Soy Broth (TSB) to achieve an optical density (OD) of 0.1. To a 96-well plate, 100 μL of the seeding solution was added. The plates were covered and incubated at room temperature under static conditions for 2 days to allow biofilm formation. After the incubation period, the biofilms were washed three times with phosphate-buffered saline (PBS) to remove any planktonic bacteria. PA-BNE fabricated in M9 media (5% *v/v* of TSB) were added to each well of the microplate. The microplate was then incubated at 37 °C under static conditions for 3 h. Following the incubation, the biofilms were washed with PBS three times, and the viability of the bacteria was assessed using an Alamar blue assay, following the manufacturer's protocol. This assay provides a measure of bacterial viability.

4.5. Mammalian Cell Viability Assay

The cytotoxicity of different components was evaluated using established protocols. To begin, 20,000 NIH 3T3 fibroblast cells (ATCC CRL-1658) were cultured in a 96-well plate using Dulbecco's modified Eagle medium (DMEM, ATCC 30-2002) supplemented with 1% antibiotics and 10% bovine calf serum. The cells were incubated in a humidified atmosphere with 5% CO_2 at 37 °C for 48 h. After incubation, the media was removed, and the cells were washed with phosphate-buffered saline (PBS) before incubation with the therapeutic agents. The PA2 or PA-BNE, solutions were prepared in media containing 10% serum and incubated with the cells in the 96-well plate for 3 h under humidified conditions at 37 °C.

Alamar blue assays were performed following the manufacturer's protocol from Invitrogen Bio-source to assess cell viability. The reduction in the Alamar blue agent resulted in red fluorescence, which was quantified using a Spectromax M5 microplate reader (Ex: 560 nm, Em: 590 nm). The percentage of cell viability was determined relative to the cells incubated with no materials, which were considered 100% viable controls. Each experiment was conducted in triplicate and repeated on two different days.

5. Conclusions

In summary, our study explored the use of small molecule antimicrobials (SMAs) and nanoemulsions for combating drug-resistant infections, particularly biofilms. Our studies found that longer alkyl chain derivatives of pseudopyronine analogs 2 (PA2) exhibited the highest potency against Gram-positive bacteria with MIC of 0.5 mg/L. By incorporating PAs into nanoemulsions, we enhanced their solubility and antimicrobial activity. The synergistic effect of PA2 and eugenol in the nanoemulsion system resulted in a significant reduction up to 32-fold less in biofilm eradication concentration. Importantly, our PA-loaded nanoemulsions demonstrated compatibility with mammalian cells. Overall, these findings indicate that SMA-carrier combinations offer a promising strategy to effectively target biofilms and combat multidrug-resistant infections.

Supplementary Materials: The following supporting information can be downloaded at: https://www.mdpi.com/article/10.3390/antibiotics12081240/s1, Figure S1: Dynamic Light Scattering Histogram of PA-BNE as of Intensity (percent); Figure S2: Minimum biofilm bactericidal concentrations (MBBC) of BNEs, PA2, and PA-BNE against B. subtilis biofilms represented as a heatmap after overnight treatment. Figure S3. Bacterial viability of MRSA (IDRL-6169) biofilms after the treatment with materials and vancomycin control.

Author Contributions: The manuscript was written through the contributions of all authors. J.P., J.M.V.M., A.L.W. and V.M.R. conceived the idea and designed the experiments. L.M.B. and S.E.H. synthesized pseudopyronine analogs. J.P. synthesized polymers and G.H. characterized materials. J.P., N.M. and S.A. performed solubility test of materials. G.H., N.M., S.A., J.M.V.M. and M.A.H. performed in vitro antimicrobial tests. J.P., N.M., G.H. and E.P. performed related analyses. M.J. cultured mammalian cells and performed in vitro cell studies and related analyses. J.P., A.L.W. and V.M.R. wrote the manuscript with significant contributions from E.P. All authors discussed results and provided suggestions for the manuscript. All authors have read and agreed to the published version of the manuscript.

Funding: This research was funded by Research Corporation for Science Advancement, North Carolina Biotechnology Center (2015-BRG-1201), Research Corporation for Science Advancement Cottrell Scholar Award (23975), and the National Institutes of Health under R01 AI134770. The content is solely the responsibility of the authors and does not necessarily represent the official views of the National Institutes of Health.

Institutional Review Board Statement: Not applicable.

Informed Consent Statement: Not applicable.

Data Availability Statement: Data are contained within the article.

Acknowledgments: Clinical isolates obtained from the Infectious Diseases Research Laboratory at Mayo Clinic, were kindly provided by Robin Patel. Clinical samples were obtained from the Cooley Dickinson Hospital Microbiology Laboratory (Northampton, MA, USA) and were kindly provided by Margaret Riley.

Conflicts of Interest: The authors declare no conflict of interest.

References

1. CDC. *Antibiotic Resistance Threats in The United States 2019*; U.S. Department of Human Health and Services, CDC: Atlanta, GA, USA, 2019; p. 10.
2. Richardson, L.A. Understanding and Overcoming Antibiotic Resistance. *PLoS Biol.* **2017**, *15*, e2003775. [CrossRef]
3. Ventola, C.L. The Antibiotic Resistance Crisis: Part 1: Causes and Threats. *Pharm. Ther.* **2015**, *40*, 277–283.

4. Jamal, M.; Ahmad, W.; Andleeb, S.; Jalil, F.; Imran, M.; Nawaz, M.A.; Hussain, T.; Ali, M.; Rafiq, M.; Kamil, M.A. Bacterial Biofilm and Associated Infections. *J. Chin. Med. Assoc.* **2018**, *81*, 7–11. [CrossRef]
5. Nikaido, H. Multidrug Resistance in Bacteria. *Annu. Rev. Biochem.* **2009**, *78*, 119–146. [CrossRef]
6. Hirsch, E.B.; Tam, V.H. Impact of Multidrug-Resistant *Pseudomonas aeruginosa* Infection on Patient Outcomes. *Expert. Rev. Pharmacoecon Outcomes Res.* **2010**, *10*, 441–451. [CrossRef]
7. Lebeaux, D.; Ghigo, J.-M.; Beloin, C. Biofilm-Related Infections: Bridging the Gap between Clinical Management and Fundamental Aspects of Recalcitrance toward Antibiotics. *Microbiol. Mol. Biol. Rev.* **2014**, *78*, 510–543. [CrossRef]
8. Vestby, L.K.; Grønseth, T.; Simm, R.; Nesse, L.L. Bacterial Biofilm and Its Role in the Pathogenesis of Disease. *Antibiotics* **2020**, *9*, 59. [CrossRef]
9. Flemming, H.C.; Wingender, J. The Biofilm Matrix. *Nat. Rev. Microbiol.* **2010**, *8*, 623–633. [CrossRef]
10. Makabenta, J.M.V.; Nabawy, A.; Li, C.H.; Schmidt-Malan, S.; Patel, R.; Rotello, V. Nanomaterial-based therapeutics for antibiotic-resistant bacterial infections. *Nat. Rev. Microbiol.* **2021**, *19*, 23–36. [CrossRef]
11. Suzuki, A.; Fukuda, T.; Kobayashi, K.; Ohshiro, T.; Tomoda, H. Pseudopyronine B, an Inhibitor of Sterol O-acyltransferase, Produced by *Pseudomonas* sp. *BYK11209*. *J. Antibiot.* **2017**, *70*, 96–97. [CrossRef]
12. McGlacken, G.P.; Fairlamb, I.J. 2-Pyrone Natural Products and Mimetics: Isolation, Characterization, and Biological Activity. *Nat. Prod. Rep.* **2005**, *22*, 369–385. [CrossRef] [PubMed]
13. Zhang, H.; Saurav, K.; Yu, Z.; Mándi, A.; Kurtán, T.; Li, J.; Tian, X.; Zhang, Q.; Zhang, W.; Zhang, C. α-Pyrones with Diverse Hydroxy Substitutions from Three Marine-Derived *Nocardiopsis* Strains. *J. Nat. Prod.* **2016**, *79*, 1610–1618. [CrossRef] [PubMed]
14. McMullin, D.R.; Nsiama, T.K.; Miller, J.D. Isochromans and α-Pyrones from *Penicillium corylophilum*. *J. Nat. Prod.* **2014**, *77*, 206–212. [CrossRef]
15. Lee, J.; Han, C.; Lee, T.G.; Chin, J.; Choi, H.; Lee, W.; Paik, M.J.; Won, D.H.; Jeong, G.; Ko, J.; et al. Marinopyrones A–D, α-Pyrones from Marine- Derived Actinomycetes of the Family Nocardiopsaceae. *Tet. Lett.* **2016**, *57*, 1997–2000. [CrossRef]
16. Grundmann, F.; Dill, V.; Dowling, A.; Thanwisai, A.; Bode, E.; Chantratita, N.; Bode, H.B. Identification and Isolation of Insecticidal Oxazoles from *Pseudomonas* spp. *Beilstein J. Org. Chem.* **2012**, *8*, 749–752. [CrossRef]
17. Chu, M.; Mierswa, R.; Xu, L.; He, J.; Terracciano, J.; Patel, M.; Zhao, W.; Black, T.A.; Chan, T.M. Structure of Sch 419560, a Novel α-Pyrone Antibiotic Produced by *Pseudomonas fluorescens*. *J. Antibiot.* **2002**, *55*, 215–218. [CrossRef] [PubMed]
18. Brachmann, A.O.; Brameyer, S.; Kresovic, D.; Hitkova, I.; Kopp, Y.; Manske, C.; Schubert, K.; Bode, H.B. Pyrones as Bacterial Signaling Molecules. *Nat. Chem. Biol.* **2013**, *9*, 573–578. [CrossRef] [PubMed]
19. Singh, M.P.; Kong, F.; Janso, J.E.; Arias, D.A.; Suarez, P.A.; Bernan, V.S.; Petersen, P.J.; Weiss, W.J.; Carter, G.; Greenstein, M. Novel α-Pyrones Produced by a Marine *Pseudomonas* sp. *F92S91: Taxonomy and Biological Activities*. *J. Antibiot.* **2003**, *56*, 1033–1044.
20. Bauer, S.J.; Ghequire, M.G.K.; Nett, M.; Josten, M.; Sahl, H.-G.; De Mot, R.; Gross, H. Biosynthetic Origin of the Antibiotic Pseudopyronines A and B in Pseudomonas putida BW11M1. *ChemBioChem* **2015**, *16*, 2491–2497. [CrossRef]
21. Giddens, A.C.; Nielsen, L.; Boshoff, H.I.; Tasdemir, D.; Perozzo, R.; Kaiser, M.; Wang, F.; Sacchettini, J.C.; Copp, B.R. Natural Product Inhibitors of Fatty Acid Biosynthesis: Synthesis of the Marine Microbial Metabolites Pseudopyronines A and B and Evaluation of Their Anti-infective Activities. *Tetrahedron* **2008**, *64*, 1242–1249. [CrossRef]
22. Bouthillette, L.M.; Darcey, C.A.; Handy, T.E.; Seaton, S.C.; Wolfe, A.L. Isolation of the Antibiotic Pseudopyronine B and SAR Evaluation of C3/C6 Alkyl Analogs. *Bioorg. Med. Chem. Lett.* **2017**, *27*, 2762–2765. [CrossRef]
23. Ishikawa, M.; Hashimoto, Y. Improvement in Aqueous Solubility in Small Molecule Drug Discovery Programs by Disruption of Molecular Planarity and Symmetry. *J. Med. Chem.* **2011**, *54*, 1539–1554. [CrossRef] [PubMed]
24. Gebreyohannes, G.; Nyerere, A.; Bii, C.; Sbhatu, D.B. Challenges of Intervention, Treatment, and Antibiotic Resistance of Biofilm-Forming Microorganisms. *Heliyon* **2019**, *5*, e02192. [CrossRef] [PubMed]
25. Simões, M.; Bennett, R.N.; Rosa, E.A.S. Understanding Antimicrobial Activities of Phytochemicals against Multidrug-Resistant Bacteria and Biofilms. *Nat. Prod. Rep.* **2009**, *26*, 746. [CrossRef]
26. Li, C.-H.; Chen, X.; Landis, R.F.; Geng, Y.; Makabenta, J.M.; Lemnios, W.; Gupta, A.; Rotello, V.M. Phytochemical-Based Nanocomposites for the Treatment of Bacterial Biofilms. *ACS Infect. Dis.* **2019**, *5*, 1590–1596. [CrossRef] [PubMed]
27. Gupta, A.; Makabenta, J.M.V.; Schlüter, F.; Landis, R.F.; Das, R.; Cuppels, M.; Rotello, V.M. Functionalized Polymers Enhance Permeability of Antibiotics in Gram-Negative MDR Bacteria and Biofilms for Synergistic Antimicrobial Therapy. *Adv. Ther.* **2020**, *3*, 2000005. [CrossRef]
28. Nabawy, A.; Makabenta, J.M.; Schmidt-Malan, S.; Park, J.; Li, C.-H.; Huang, R.; Fedeli, S.; Chattopadhyay, A.N.; Patel, R.; Rotello, V.M. Dual Antimicrobial-Loaded Biodegradable Nanoemulsions for Synergistic Treatment of Wound Biofilms. *J. Control. Release* **2022**, *347*, 379–388. [CrossRef]
29. Voytik-Harbin, S.L.; Brightman, A.O.; Waisner, B.; Lamar, C.H.; Badylak, S.F. Application and Evaluation of the Alamarblue Assay for Cell Growth and Survival of Fibroblasts. *In Vitr. Cell Dev. Biol. Anim.* **1998**, *34*, 239–246. [CrossRef]
30. Rampersad, S.N. Multiple Applications of Alamar Blue as an Indicator of Metabolic Function and Cellular Health in Cell Viability Bioassays. *Sensors* **2012**, *12*, 12347–12360. [CrossRef]
31. Breijyeh, Z.; Karaman, R. Design and Synthesis of Novel Antimicrobial Agents. *Antibiotics* **2023**, *12*, 628. [CrossRef]
32. Mantravadi, P.; Kalesh, K.; Dobson, R.; Hudson, A.; Parthasarathy, A. The Quest for Novel Antimicrobial Compounds: Emerging Trends in Research, Development, and Technologies. *Antibiotics* **2019**, *8*, 8. [CrossRef] [PubMed]

33. Liu, X.; Wang, Y.; Zaleta-Pinet, D.A.; Borris, R.P.; Clark, B.R. Antibacterial and Anti-Biofilm Activity of Pyrones from a Pseudomonas Mosselii Strain. *Antibiotics* **2022**, *11*, 1655. [CrossRef] [PubMed]
34. El-Tarabily, K.A.; El-Saadony, M.T.; Alagawany, M.; Arif, M.; Batiha, G.E.; Khafaga, A.F.; Elwan, H.A.M.; Elnesr, S.S.; Abd El-Hack, M.E. Using Essential Oils to Overcome Bacterial Biofilm Formation and Their Antimicrobial Resistance. *Saudi J. Biol. Sci.* **2021**, *28*, 5145–5156. [CrossRef]
35. Landis, R.F.; Li, C.-H.; Gupta, A.; Lee, Y.-W.; Yazdani, M.; Ngernyuang, N.; Altinbasak, I.; Mansoor, S.; Khichi, M.A.S.; Sanyal, A.; et al. Biodegradable Nanocomposite Antimicrobials for the Eradication of Multidrug-Resistant Bacterial Biofilms without Accumulated Resistance. *J. Am. Chem. Soc.* **2018**, *140*, 6176–6182. [CrossRef] [PubMed]
36. Ulanowska, M.; Olas, B. Biological Properties and Prospects for the Application of Eugenol—A Review. *Int. J. Mol. Sci.* **2021**, *22*, 3671. [CrossRef]
37. Madden, L.; Low, S.H.; Phillips, A.R.J.; Kline, K.A.; Becker, D.L. The Effects of *Staphylococcus Aureus* Biofilm Conditioned Media on 3T3 Fibroblasts. *FEMS Microbes* **2021**, *2*, xtab010. [CrossRef] [PubMed]
38. Kirker, K.R.; James, G.A. In Vitro Studies Evaluating the Effects of Biofilms on Wound-Healing Cells: A Review. *APMIS* **2017**, *125*, 344–352. [CrossRef]

antibiotics MDPI

Article

Discovery of Bactericidal Proteins from *Staphylococcus* Phage Stab21 Using a High-Throughput Screening Method

Ellisiv Nyhamar [1,2,†], Paige Webber [1,†], Olivia Liong [1], Özgenur Yilmaz [1,3], Maria Pajunen [1], Mikael Skurnik [1,*] and Xing Wan [1,2,*]

1 Department of Bacteriology and Immunology, Human Microbiome Research Program, Faculty of Medicine, University of Helsinki, 00290 Helsinki, Finland
2 Department of Microbiology, Faculty of Agriculture and Forestry, University of Helsinki, 00790 Helsinki, Finland
3 Faculty of Health Sciences, Kirklareli University, 39000 Kirklareli, Turkey
* Correspondence: mikael.skurnik@helsinki.fi (M.S.); xing.wan@helsinki.fi (X.W.)
† These authors contributed equally to this work.

Abstract: In the escalating battle against antimicrobial resistance, there is an urgent need to discover and investigate new antibiotic strategies. Bacteriophages are untapped reservoirs of such potential antimicrobials. This study focused on Hypothetical Proteins of Unknown Function (HPUFs) from a *Staphylococcus* phage Stab21. We examined its HPUFs for bactericidal activity against *E. coli* using a Next Generation Sequencing (NGS)-based approach. Among the 96 HPUFs examined, 5 demonstrated cross-species toxicity towards *E. coli*, suggesting the presence of shared molecular targets between *E. coli* and *S. aureus*. One toxic antibacterial HPUF (toxHPUF) was found to share homology with a homing endonuclease. The implications of these findings are profound, particularly given the potential broad applicability of these bactericidal agents. This study confirms the efficacy of NGS in streamlining the screening process of toxHPUFs, contributes significantly to the ongoing exploration of phage biology, and offers promises in the search for potent antimicrobial agents.

Keywords: bacteriophages; Hypothetical Proteins of Unknown Function (HPUFs); antimicrobial resistance; *Staphylococcus aureus*; cross-species toxicity

1. Introduction

Antimicrobial resistance is one of the most pressing challenges facing modern medicine. However, the rate of discovery and introduction of new classes of antibiotics has slowed drastically over the decades, with only two introduced to the market since 1962 [1]. The need for new antibiotic classes is only increasing as the potential for analogue development from existing classes is depleted. Pathogens that exhibit alarming resistance against current antimicrobial treatments are given the acronym of ESKAPE, including *Enterococcus faecium*, *Staphylococcus aureus*, *Klebsiella pneumoniae*, *Acinetobacter baumannii*, *Pseudomonas aeruginosa*, and *Enterobacter* species [2]. Among them, methicillin and vancomycin-resistant *Staphylococcus aureus* (MRSA/VRSA) are placed in the high-priority category by the World Health Organization to accelerate the development of new antimicrobial compounds for treating multi-drug-resistant *S. aureus* [3]. MRSA is usually acquired within a hospital environment and can cause various severe opportunistic infections and diseases [4]. Vancomycin has long been regarded as a drug of last resort for MRSA treatment. Unfortunately, the emerging VRSA jeopardises the efficiency of clinical treatments and leads to a significant increase in staphylococcal bacteraemia mortality [5].

Bacteriophages, especially lytic phages, are viruses that infect, propagate, and destroy bacteria. Throughout evolution, phages continuously adapt to confront their bacterial hosts for their own survival. This intertwined relationship endows the phages with highly specific mechanisms to reprogram bacterial cell metabolism. Phage-inspired antibacterial target discovery is another ascending approach to harnessing the antimicrobial activity of phages [6]. Identifying novel bacterial targets through phage research could help screen and design new small molecular compounds that replicate the growth-inhibitory effects of the antibacterial phage proteins. Intriguingly, a substantial proportion of phage gene products have completely unknown functions since they have not been characterized and have sequences that do not correspond with any proteins of known function. Screening hypothetical proteins of unknown function (HPUFs) from bacteriophages for toxic activity against bacteria may provide new and potentially life-saving approaches to combat bacterial infections [7,8]. An earlier extensive study on mining 26 *S. aureus* phage genomes revealed that 31 polypeptide families showed toxicity towards the bacterial host, including ORF104 from phage 77 [5]. The gene product of ORF104 interacted with bacterial essential protein DnaI, disrupting DNA synthesis and cell growth. The research team then used the protein pair to screen for small molecular inhibitors, and identified 36 of them interrupting the ORF104-DnaI interaction and 11 that were directly toxic against *S. aureus* [5].

Stab21 is a lytic *Staphylococcus* phage recently discovered by Oduor et al. [9]. The phage is taxonomically classified to the *Kayvirus* genus of the Twortvirinae subfamily in the Herelleviridae family (accession number LR215719, [9]). Stab21 has a wide host range and possesses no genes associated with antibiotic resistance or virulence [9]; therefore, it is a good candidate for therapeutical applications. Of all 238 predicted genes in the Stab21 genome, 203 were preliminarily annotated to encode HPUFs. Many lytic phages could possess genes encoding proteins that directly or indirectly mediate the destruction of their host bacterial cells [10]. Hence, among the HPUFs of Stab21, there is a great potential for the discovery of bactericidal proteins that alter bacterial pathways in an unprecedented manner.

The use of a next-generation sequencing (NGS)-based screening approach to screen for phage-encoded toxic proteins is shown to be as reliable as the alternative plating-based toxicity screening method. An earlier direct comparison was performed during the development of the NGS method, where it was concluded that the NGS-based assay not only provides similar screening results as the plating-based assays, but is also superior in efficiency, accuracy, and reliability [11,12].

In the study presented here, we investigated all hypothetical proteins and selected 96 true HPUFs for their bactericidal activity in *E. coli* using the NGS-based approach. We confirmed their bactericidal activities in *E. coli* and their potential anti-*S. aureus* abilities using various inducible expression systems. Five of the Stab21 gene products were shown to have cross-species toxicity towards *E. coli*. Through detailed in silico functional and structural analyses, we found that Gp024 shares high structural homology with a homing endonuclease. Our work not only underscores the potential of Stab21 HPUFs as antimicrobial agents, but also reinforces the efficacy of NGS in identifying these potential assets.

2. Results

The preliminary annotation of the Stab21 genome, based mainly on the Basic Local Alignment Search Tool (BlastP), identified 203 HPUFs [9]. This number was refined to 96 HPUFs after a more detailed examination through HHPred [13] searches and the identification of phage-particle-associated proteins by liquid chromatography–tandem mass spectrometry (LC-MS/MS) analysis [14].

2.1. *Potential Toxicity of Stab21 Gene Products*

The bactericidal potential of the 96 selected HPUF genes of Stab21 was investigated using the NGS approach [11]. The sum of four ligation joint sequences for each gene was calculated and used as its total read coverage. The relative number of joint sequence reads was calculated for all 96 genes by dividing the total read coverage of a single gene by the total number of joint sequence reads for all genes in the pool and expressed as a percentage (Table S1).

This method identified 16 gene products with toxic potential characterized by ratios under 0.5. Genes *g062c*, *g085*, and *g081c* exhibited the three lowest ratios. Additional 31 HPUF-encoded gene products with ratios between 1.0 and 0.5 were identified as potentially mildly toxic (Figure 1), while the remaining 42 genes with ratios above 1.0 were deemed non-toxic (Figure S1).

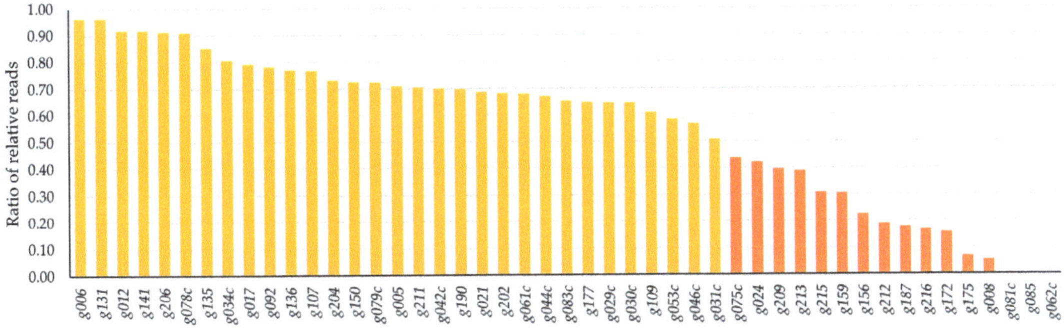

Figure 1. Results from the toxicity analysis using an NGS-approach of Stab21 phage HPUFs featuring ordered ratios of relative joint sequence reads for all 16 potentially toxic (orange bars) and 31 potentially mildly toxic genes (yellow bars). Non-toxic genes are elaborated in Figure S1.

Genes *g002* and *g018*, which had no detected ligation joint reads in the plasmid mixture, could not be conclusively evaluated. It is possible that the gene fragments were not successfully digested by restriction enzymes, leading to the absence of a suitable restriction site for ligation to the vector.

Ratios of relative reads for all the analysed HPUFs ranged between 0.0002 (for *g062c*) and 8.5133 (for *g196*). The complete results, including exact ratios and relative vector gene joint reads in both ligation mixtures and transformant plasmids, are listed in Table S1.

2.2. Five Stab21 Genes Products Inhibit the Growth of E. coli

A subsequent screening of the effect of toxHPUF candidates on *E. coli* DH5α was conducted via a drop test after cloning the candidate genes into the expression vector pBAD33. Arabinose-induced expression of the Stab21 HPUFs resulted in significant *E. coli* growth inhibition by 9 of the initially identified 16 genes, although with varying toxicity levels (Figure 2). Particularly, the gene products Gp081c, Gp159, Gp175, Gp209, Gp212, and Gp213 strongly suppressed the *E. coli* growth. Additionally, Gp172 seemed to diminish the overall viability of *E. coli*, as fewer colonies formed even in the presence of glucose compared to other nontoxic gene products. Gene products Gp024 and Gp187, on the other hand, only demonstrated mild toxicity to the host.

Employing a more stringent induction expression system with an anhydrotetracycline-inducible promoter [15], we followed the growth curves of the *E. coli* strains carrying these recombinant genes on the pRAB11N plasmids.

The drop test indicated that nearly all nine candidates displayed varying toxicity levels under inducing conditions of anhydrotetracycline (ATc) 0.4 μM (Figure S2). However, growth curve analysis offered a more reliable interpretation, ruling out false positives caused by mutagenesis from overnight incubation. As shown in Figure 3, after inducing the Stab21 HPUF genes with ATc, five genes significantly impeded the growth of *E. coli*, specifically genes *g024*, *g081c*, *g172*, *g187* and *g213*. Yet, after six hours, resistant mutants began to appear and resume the growth.

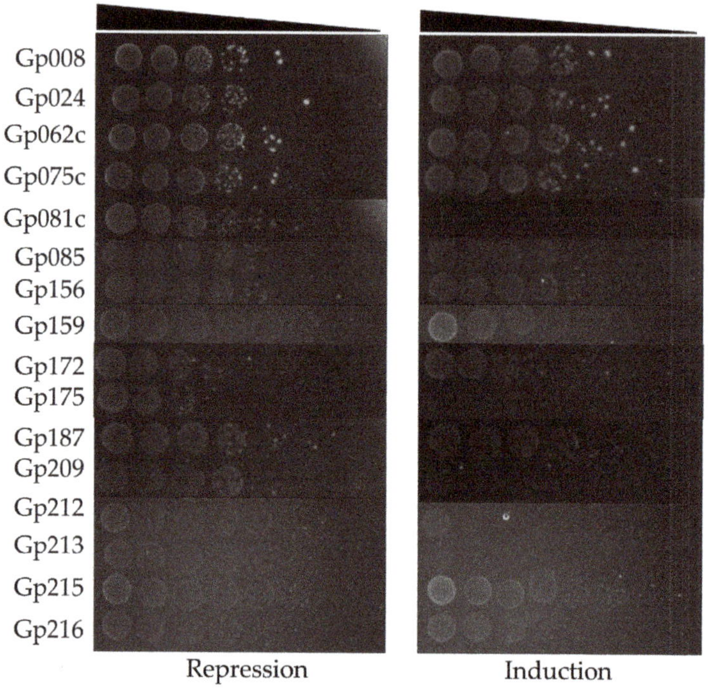

Figure 2. Initial drop test results of *E. coli* DH5α/pBAD33-HPUFs under repression (0.2% glucose) and induction (2% arabinose) conditions. Cell density from 10^{-1} to 10^{-8} dilutions is indicated with wedge.

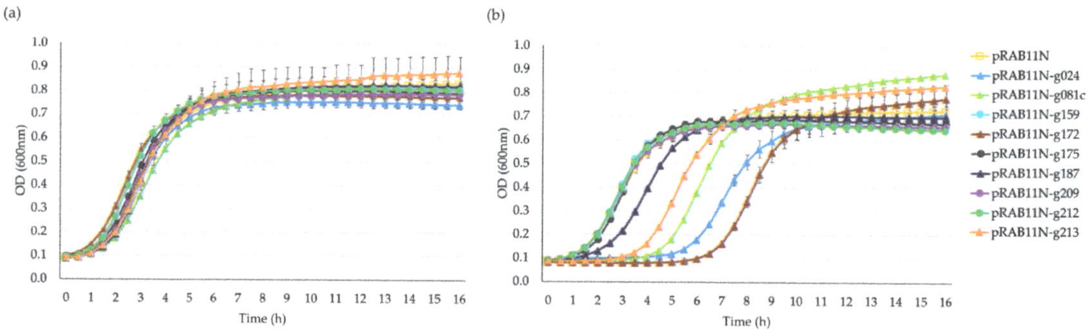

Figure 3. Growth curves of *E. coli* DH10B/pRAB11N-HPUFs for toxicity screening. (**a**) Toxicity screening without anhydrotetracycline (ATc) induction. (**b**) Toxicity screening with ATc 0.4 μM induction. Error bars show ± standard deviation calculated using triplicate results. OD, optical density.

2.3. *Stab21 Gp081c Might Also Inhibit the Growth of S. aureus*

The toxicity of Stab21 HPUFs on *S. aureus* was investigated via a drop test. Initially, chloramphenicol (Cm) was used to preserve the pRAB11N-HPUF plasmids in *S. aureus*. However, using both Cm and ATc seemed to be toxic to the host *S. aureus* strains, as the combination of Cm30 (30 μg/mL chloramphenicol) and ATc 0.4 μM inhibited even the growth of RN4220/pRAB11N. Similar inhibitory effect was also observed when using lower Cm concentration (Figure S3). Decreasing the ATc concentration, on the other hand, did not seem to be sufficient for the HPUF expression (Figure S4). Therefore, we decided to leave Cm out, and used only the ATc inducer. Under these conditions, upon induction, Gp024, Gp081c, Gp175, Gp187, Gp209, Gp212 and Gp213 showed toxicity (Figure 4).

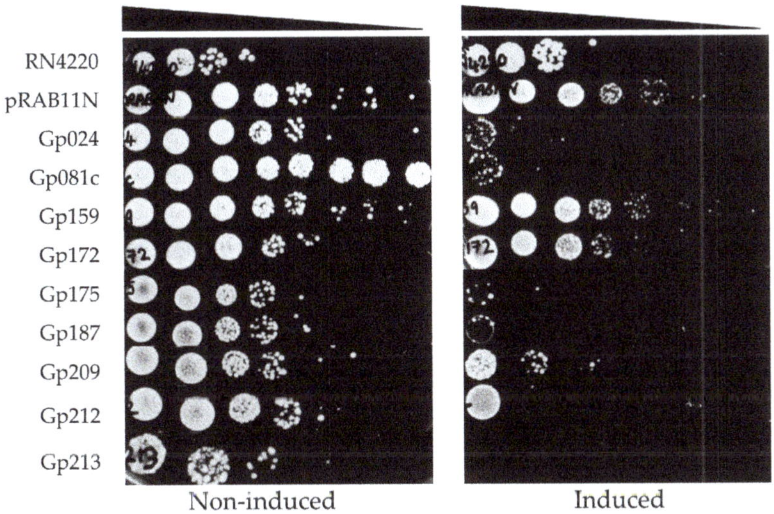

Figure 4. *S. aureus* RN4220/pRAB11N-HPUFs toxicity drop test under non-induced and induced conditions (ATc 0.4 μM). ATc, anhydrotetracycline. Cell density from 10^{-1} to 10^{-8} dilutions is indicated with wedge.

We also obtained growth curves for all strains under both ATc-induced and non-induced conditions in liquid cultures. In *S. aureus* RN4220, no HPUFs had a significant toxic effect when induced, but the known toxic gene product of ORF104 [7] did exhibit toxicity, even under the non-induced condition (Figure 5a). Gene products of *g081c* slightly delayed the *S. aureus* growth; however, the growth pace swiftly recovered due to the emergence of rescue mutants (Figure 5b).

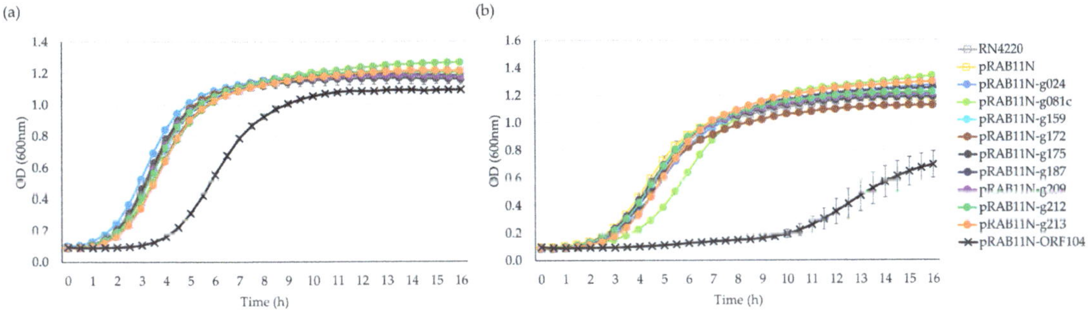

Figure 5. Growth curves of *S. aureus* RN4220 pRAB11N-HPUF. (**a**) Toxicity screening without ATc 0.4 μM induction. (**b**) Toxicity screening with ATc induction. Error bars show ± standard deviation calculated using triplicate results. OD, optical density.

2.4. Non-Inducing Mutation of g172 and g187 Tolerant Clones Located in tetR of pRAB11N

Upon induction, five gene products, Gp024, Gp081c, Gp172, Gp187, and Gp213, showed toxicity towards *E. coli*. However, after 6 h, the growth of toxin-tolerant mutants was observed from all recombinant strains. We suspected that the tolerant phenotype may have resulted from mutations in the plasmid DNA by inactivating the toxin, or in the *E.*

coli genomic DNA, potentially providing a clue of the identity of the target for the toxin. Therefore, to study this, we cultivated *E. coli* DH10B/pRAB11N-toxHPUFs in the presence of ATc for 16 h to allow the emergence of toxin-tolerant mutants. The presence of plasmids was examined by polymerase chain reaction (PCR). The plasmid was only detected in tolerant clones (denoted with '-T' suffix) recovered from DH10B/pRAB11N-*g172*-T and DH10B/pRAB11N-*g187*-T (Figure S5). Subsequent isolation and sequencing over the HPUF gene insertion of the plasmids pRAB11N-*g172*-T and pRAB11N-*g187*-T revealed that the inserts were 100% identical to the original toxic HPUF gene sequences. This indicated that no mutations in the toxHPUF genes could explain the tolerant phenotype.

Given this result, we re-evaluated the toxicity of Gp172 and Gp187 in the toxin-sensitive strains DH10B/pRAB11N-*g172* and DH10B/pRAB11N-*g187* and in the toxin-tolerant mutant strains DH10B/pRAB11N-*g172*-T and DH10B/pRAB11N-*g187*-T. Growth curves confirmed that upon ATc-induction the toxin-sensitive strains were inhibited up to 6 hr, and that the toxin-tolerant mutants remained non-toxic (Figure S6).

To identify the genomic mutation behind the toxin tolerance, the genomes of DH10B/pRAB11N-*g172*, -*g187*, -*g172*-T, and -*g187*-T were sequenced and subjected to de novo assembly. The obtained contigs were then compared to both the host genomic and the plasmid sequences. While the genomic sequence contigs of the four *E. coli* strains were 100% identical to the *E. coli* DH10B reference sequence (GenBank accession no. NC_010473), the plasmid sequences of DH10B/pRAB11N-*g172*-T and -*g187*-T carried both a single nucleotide mutation when aligned with the plasmid pRAB11N-*g172* and -*g187* sequences. Specifically, an A to C mutation was present at position 3654 in pRAB11N-g172-T, and a G to T mutation at position 3747 in pRAB11N-*g187*-T. Both mutations map into the *tetR* gene, causing Leu-113-Arg and Asp-82-Lys substitutions, respectively (Figure S7).

2.5. *Gp024 Is Homologous to a Homing Endonuclease*

The Phyre2 software (Version 2.0, http://www.sbg.bio.ic.ac.uk/~phyre2, accessed on 26 June 2023) was used to predict the functions of toxHPUFs Gp024, Gp081c, Gp172, Gp187, and Gp213. In Phyre2, a reliable model typically has an input and template sequence identity of over 30% and a confidence level of more than 90% [16]. Eighty residues (37% sequence coverage) of Gp024 were modelled with a 98.0% confidence to the C-terminus of *Bacillus* phage SPO1 homing endonuclease I-HmuI chain M (Protein Data Bank (PDB): c1u3eM). For *g081c*, a confidence of 85.5% was observed for 53 residues (a 48% sequence coverage), which matched to the *Saccharomyces cerevisiae* monopolin complex protein subunit CSM1. However, Gp172, Gp187, and Gp213 yielded models with low confidence scores, below 51%.

The HHpred [13] software was also used to predict functions of the same toxHPUFs by searching each toxHPUF against PDB mmcif70. In the HHpred analysis, a higher score value signifies a better sequence alignment quality and similarity. An expected value (E-value) close to zero indicates a strong identity by estimating the number of similar score hits that could occur randomly. Probability values further underscore the statistical significance of sequence and hit homology [17]. The best hit for Gp024 was also *Bacillus* phage SPO1 homing endonuclease I-HmuI (PDB: 1U3E) with a probability of 98.18%, a score of 42.4 and an *E*-value of 0.023. The Gp081c top model was *Enterobacter* phage 22 tail needle protein Gp26 with a probability of 95.31%, a score of 37.3 and an *E*-value of 0.21. The top model of Gp187 was *Homo sapiens* zinc finger protein SNA1 with a probability of 99.11%, a score of 75.52 and an *E*-value of 9.2^{-11}. The homologous models of Gp172 and Gp213 resulted in low probability and *E*-values.

Finally, we employed AlphaFold2 [18] to predict the structure of the five toxHPUFs (Figure S8). PyMOL was used to superimpose the functional models from Phyre2 and HHpred with the structural models of AlphaFold2. The root mean square deviation (RMSD) score measures the structural overlap between the two input models using the distance between aligned α-carbon atoms, with a score below 2.5 Å considered as an acceptable alignment [19]. When superimposing the truncated *Bacillus* phage SPO1 homing endonuclease I-HmuI (c1u3eM) obtained from the best Phyre2 model with the Gp024 AlphaFold2 model, the RMSD score was 1.581 Å between 138 atoms of the two proteins. Two C-terminal α-helixes from both proteins were found overlapping with each other (Figure 6a). When superimposing the best homologous model of I-HmuI (1U3E) from HHpred analyses with the predicted structure of Gp024, the RMSD score was 2.217 Å when aligning 181 atoms. The N-terminal DNA-binding surface of I-HmuI loosely overlapped with the N-terminus of Gp024 by two β-sheets and one α-helix (Figure 6b). Alignment of Gp081c with both Phyre2 and HHpred functional models resulted in RMSD scores of over 8 Å (Figure S9). The predicted structure obtained from AlphaFold2 for Gp187 was composed only of two β-sheets and so was omitted from further analysis.

(a)

(b)

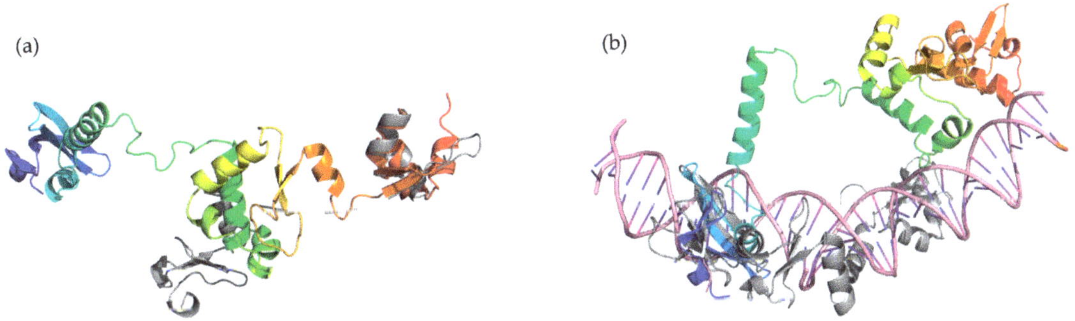

Figure 6. Structural and functional modelling of toxHPUFs Gp024 AlphaFold2 structural model (rainbow, N-terminus in blue, C-terminus in red) superimposed with *Bacillus* phage SPO1homing endonuclease I-HmuI (grey). (**a**) The model with the highest confidence from Phyre2. (**b**) The best model from HHpred, DNA structure is in pink.

3. Discussion

The escalating prevalence of antibiotic resistance in critical pathogens such as *S. aureus* demands the discovery of novel antimicrobial molecules [20]. Phages, with their unique genetic diversity, present a promising reservoir of potential antimicrobials, yet the majority of their genomes remain uncharacterized. Current phage research identifies a range of bacteriotoxic molecules such as endolysins and polysaccharide depolymerases that could potentially be harnessed against antibiotic resistant bacterial infections [21–23]. Given the wide genomic variation even among phages infecting the same host, there is significant potential for the discovery of new antimicrobial mechanisms and targets from the multitude of gene products currently deemed HPUF [24]. Such discoveries may yield innovative antibiotic treatments capable of countering the ever-increasing threat of antimicrobial resistance [6].

In this study, we employed an NGS-based screening assay to identify toxic proteins encoded by *Staphylococcal* phage Stab21. The HPUFs of Stab21 were screened for bacteriotoxic effects against *E. coli* and their bactericidal activities were confirmed in both *E. coli* and *S. aureus*. Our findings revealed that five gene products were toxic to *E. coli* DH10B using arabinose- and anhydrotetracycline-induced expression vectors. Crucially, this study verified that the application of this high-throughput NGS-based screening process in *E. coli* is not limited to examining HPUFs from only phages infecting Gram-negative bacteria.

Our study employed an already established protocol for NGS-based screening in *E. coli* [11,12], recognizing the value of this model organism in providing insights into cellular mechanisms that transcend species boundaries [25]. By adopting this protocol, we anticipate a rapid determination of any bacteriotoxic activity of HPUFs in both Gram-negative and Gram-positive strains.

In this context, we constructed the pCU1LK vector which contains the backbone of the *E. coli–S. aureus* shuttle vector pCU1 [26] that can accommodate up to 6 kb fragments cloned under the *lac* promoter. As the size of the inserted linker sequence was only 45 bp in pCU1LK, it should also allow cloning up to 6 kb fragments without problems to replicate freely in both hosts.

However, as the *lac* promoter is notoriously known as leaky, we selected another tighter expression vector pRAB11 with two *tet* operator *tetO* sites [27] to verify the toxicity of HPUFs. Nevertheless, we observed an unexpected growth inhibition of *S. aureus* strain RN4220/pRAB11N in the presence of ATc on solid media (Figures S3 and S4). This effect was not noticed in *E. coli* DH10B/pRAB11N. We do not have a clear explanation for this phenomenon. Despite the expectation that ATc should induce the gene expression at lower concentrations and with less toxicity than its parent antibiotic, tetracycline (Tc) [28], aged ATc has been found to generate toxic breakdown products that can interfere with *S. aureus* growth [29]. It is possible that these breakdown products are less effective on *E. coli* than on *S. aureus*, as observed in our study.

Though our study did not identify any toxHPUFs towards *S. aureus* among the nine *E. coli* -toxic candidates, further examination should be carried out for the remaining 87 HPUFs of Stab21, which were regarded as non-toxic to *E. coli.* That could involve pooling pCU1LK-HPUFs or pRAB11N-HPUFs ligation mixtures and subsequently screening successful transformants for toxicity-presenting an alternative to the NGS-based screening method. Alternatively, an arsenite-inducible plasmid, pT0021, which has been previously employed effectively to screen for toxHPUFs in *S. aureus* [7], could serve as another viable option for this investigation.

Furthermore, for future screening of HPUFs from various phages derived from different bacteria, the NGS screening technique presented in our study can be fine-tuned depending on the bacterial host by applying different inducible plasmid vectors such as the Tn7-based integration vector pTNS2 [30] for *Pseudomonas aeruginosa*, or vectors derived from the IncQ plasmid for *Acinetobacter baumannii* [31].

Among the structural studies of the top five identified toxic HPUFs, only Gp024 yielded a reliable protein model, aligning with the *Bacillus* phage SPO1 homing endonuclease I-HmuI. Although the predicted structure of Gp024 resembles different domains in HHpred and Phyre2, its function as a homing endonuclease cannot be completely ignored. Previous studies have identified phage HPUFs as homologs to homing endonucleases. A noteworthy example is found in the extensively researched *Escherichia* phage T4, which houses 15 homing endonuclease encoding genes, showing the evolutionary link between these proteins and phage biology [32]. Adding to the intrigue is the existence of colicins, DNases produced by *E. coli* that demonstrate toxicity against other *E. coli* strains. These colicins belong to the same H-N-H family of endonucleases [33] as the suspected homing endonuclease Gp024 of Stab21. The analogous functions and structural similarity of these proteins could suggest that Gp024 could exhibit characteristics of homing endonucleases like colicins. However, further experiments such as single-site mutations and DNA nicking assays are needed to confirm its role as a homing endonuclease.

Our findings that five HPUFs from Stab21 exhibit cross-species toxicity towards *E. coli* have profound implications. It is possible that these HPUFs share a conserved molecular target in both *E. coli* and *S. aureus*, significantly broadening the potential applicability of these bactericidal agents. In conclusion, our research opens a promising avenue for the discovery of novel, potent antimicrobial agents, providing hope in the fight against growing antimicrobial resistance.

4. Materials and Methods

4.1. Bacterial Strains, Plasmids, Phage and Culture Conditions

All bacterial strains and plasmids used for experimentation are listed in Table 1 and Table S2. Commercial electrocompetent *Escherichia coli* DH10B cells (Thermo Fischer Scientific, Waltham, MA, USA), in-house prepared electrocompetent *E. coli* DH5α and in-house prepared electrocompetent *Staphylococcus aureus* RN4220 were used as expression hosts.

Table 1. Bacterial strains, phage and plasmids used in this study.

Name	Usage	Source
Stab21	Bacteriophage; the genome was used as a template for HPUF amplification	[14]
E. coli DH10B	HPUF cloning and NGS-based screening	Themo Fischer Scientific. GenBank accession no. NC_010473
E. coli DH5α	HPUF cloning and screening with pBAD33	GenBank accession no. CP026085.1
S. aureus RN4220	HPUF cloning and screening with pRAB11N	GenBank accession no. CP076105.1
S. aureus Newman	ORF104 gene fragment isolation	GenBank accession no. NZ_CP087593.1
pCU1	Template for pCU1LK construction	[26] Kindly provided by Dr. Pentti Kuusela
pCU1LK	pCU1 containing multiple cloning sites between KpnI- PstI	This study
pBAD33	HPUF expression under arabinose-inducible promoter	[15]
pRMC2	Template for pRAB11 construction by insertion of second *tet* operator	[34]
pRAB11N	*E. coli/S. aureus* shuttle vector with tetracycline-inducible promoter for Stab21 HPUF expression	[27] Re-constructed in this study. GenBank accession no. JN635500

E. coli DH5α, DH10B and their derivatives were grown in Lysogeny broth (LB; 10 g/L Tryptone (Neogen, Lansing, MI, USA, Cat no. NCM02118A), 5 g/L Yeast Extract (Neogen, Cat no. NCM0218A), 10 g/L NaCl) or on agar (LA, LB supplemented with 1.5% Bacto agar). For toxicity tests, *E. coli* strains were grown in M9 minimal media (KH_2PO_4 3 g/L, 0.5 g/L NaCl, 6.78 g/L Na_2HPO_4, 1 g/L NH_4Cl, casamino acid 0.2% (*v*/*v*), $MgSO_4$ 2 mM, $CaCl_2$ 0.1 mM, thiamine 1 mg/L) supplemented with antibiotic to maintain the plasmid, and glucose for repression and arabinose for induction. *S. aureus* strains were grown in Tryptic Soy Broth (TSB; VWR Chemicals, Radnor, PA, USA, Cat. No. 470015-844) or on Tryptic Soy Agar (TSA, Vegitone, Sigma-Aldrich, St. Louis, MA, USA, Cat. No. 14432) or broth (Dehydrated TSB, VWR Chemicals). Liquid cultures were grown at 37 °C overnight with 200 RPM shaking unless stated otherwise. Solid cultures were incubated at 37 °C overnight. To maintain the plasmids, broth or agar was supplemented with either 100 µg/mL of ampicillin (Amp100) or 30 µg/mL of chloramphenicol (Cm30) unless stated otherwise.

4.2. DNA Manipulations

For plasmid isolations, individual colonies were obtained on a streak plate, and 1 colony was used for inoculation to obtain overnight cultures. Plasmids from *E. coli* strains were extracted, purified, and precipitated with either NucleoBond™ Xtra Midi kit and NucleoBond™ Finalizers (Machery-Nagel, Düren, Germany) from 200 mL overnight cultures or with the NuceloSpin Plasmid EasyPure Kit (Machery-Nagel) for 1 mL cultures, according to manufacturers' instructions. To isolate the plasmids from Gram-positive *S. aureus*, lysostaphin lyophilized powder from *Staphylococcus staphylolyticus* (Merck KGaA, Darmstadt, Germany) was added to the final concentration of 20 µg/mL and incubated for 1 h at 37 °C before using NucleoSpin Plasmid EasyPure Kit according to the manufacturer's manual. For the Illumina sequencing, plasmid pools were extracted with NucleoBond™ Xtra Midi kit, and eluted in a 200 µL Tris/HCl pH 8.5 elution buffer.

E. coli and *S. aureus* genomic DNA was isolated using the JetFlex Genomic DNA Purification Kit (Thermo Fischer Scientific) following the bacterial gDNA isolation protocol for Gram-negative and Gram-positive bacteria, the latter using a 20 µg/mL lysostaphin pre-treatment. The isolated DNA was rehydrated at 22 °C for 16 h.

DNA fragments were amplified by PCR using primers listed in Table S3. Stab21 phage DNA [14] was used as a template for amplification of HPUFs. *S. aureus* Newman gDNA was used to amplify the toxic control gene ORF104. Plasmid DNA and colonies were used as templates for confirmation of correct gene insertion. Phusion High-Fidelity DNA Polymerase (Thermo Fischer Scientific) was used for generating DNA fragments with the highest accuracy for cloning, while DreamTaq DNA Polymerase (Thermo Fisher Scientific) was used for screening the presence of a certain DNA fragment either from the colony or from the ligation mixture. The PCRs were run in a T100™ or iCycler Thermal Cycler (Bio-Rad Laboratories, Inc., Hercules, CA, USA) following standard manufacturer protocol for the polymerases.

All restriction enzymes used in this study were obtained from Thermo Fisher Scientific or New England Biolabs (MA, USA). Plasmid vectors were linearised with restriction enzymes as stated according to the manufacturer's instructions, and dephosphorylated with FastAP™ Thermosensitive Alkaline Phosphatase (Thermo Fisher Scientific) at 37 °C for 30 min followed by a 15 min heat inactivation at 65 °C.

Sticky-end ligation of double-digested individual HPUF-encoding gene fragments to linearised and dephosphorylated pCU1LK or pRAB11N vectors was carried out at a 1:3 vector to insert molar ratio, and the total DNA concentration was adjusted to 10 ng/μL. T4 DNA Ligase (5 U) (Thermo Fischer Scientific) was used for all the ligation reactions. The ligation reaction was incubated at room temperature overnight (15 h) before heat inactivation at 65 °C for 10 min.

NucleoSpin Gel and PCR Clean-up XS kit (Machery-Nagel) was used to purify and concentrate DNA after PCRs and enzymatic reactions.

For the NGS screening assay, the Stab21 HPUF-encoding genes and pCU1LK vector were first double digested with restriction enzymes NotI and NheI or KpnI FastDigest™ enzymes (Thermo Fisher Scientific) depending on the insertion fragments (Table S3) [11]. Every 16 ligation mixtures of the HPUF gene and vector pCU1LK were pooled before concentration by kit, and an elution volume of 20 μL in Baxter Sterile Water (Baxter Corporation, Deerfield, IL, USA) was used per pool. One microliter (ca. 200 ng) of each ligation pool was transferred to 50 μL of *E. coli* DH10B cells through electroporation. Plasmids from transformation reactions were isolated from a 3 h culture inoculated with all colonies formed on the transformation plates. DNA samples from both the ligation pool and the plasmid pool were sequenced with the 150 bp paired-end protocol in the Illumina HiSeq platform at NovoGene Company Ltd. (Cambridge, UK) as described by Kasurinen et al. [11].

4.3. Electroporation and Transformation

Electroporation was performed with a Gene Pulser™ apparatus (Bio-Rad Laboratories) using 0.2 mm cuvettes. For the transformation of *E. coli* strains, the parameters of 200 Ω resistance, 25 mF capacitance and 2.5 kV voltage resulted in a time constant between 4.5 and 5.0 ms. Transformed *E. coli* cells were recovered in a 1 mL super optimal broth (SOC; 2% Tryptone, 0.5% Yeast Extract, 10 mM NaCl, 2.5 mM KCl, 10 mM $MgCl_2$, 10 mM $MgSO_4$, 20 mM glucose) and incubated at 37 °C with a 200 rpm shaking for 45 min before being plated on LB Amp100 agar plates using 10 μL, 100 μL, and the remainder of cells collected through centrifugation. For NGS screening, every 50 μL of the recovered cells from each pool were spread onto LB Amp100 plates, resulting in 20 plates. The plates were incubated at 37 °C overnight.

For the transformation of *S. aureus* RN4220, the parameters of the Gene Pulser electroporator were set with a resistance of 100 Ω, a capacitance of 25 μF, and a voltage of 2.3 kV resulting in a time constant between 2.0 and 2.4 ms. Transformed *S. aureus* were recovered in a 850 μL TSB and a 150 μL 2 M sucrose and incubated at 37 °C with a 200 rpm shaking for 90 min. The same plating scheme and incubation conditions were used as those for *E. coli* electroporation.

4.4. Construction of Vectors pCU1LK and pRAB11N

To construct a vector suitable for screening the toxicity of all the 96 HPUFs in *E. coli*, we added a linker to the pCU1 plasmid. The KpnI-PstI linker containing restriction sites for BamHI, XbaI, NheI, NcoI, and NotI was constructed by annealing oligonucleotides NOTup and NOTdown (Table S3) with a final concentration of 50 μM in a 20 μL linker solution (50 mM Tris-HCl pH 8.0, 100 mM NaCl, 1 mM EDTA). The reaction mixture was incubated at 95 °C for 2 min, followed by 10 min at 52 °C. The annealed linker was phosphorylated with T4 polynucleotide kinase (T4 PNK, Thermo Fisher Scientific) before ligation to gel-purified pCU1 linearised with KpnI and PstI digestions. The resultant vector pCU1LK was used for the preliminary screening of the toxicity of all HPUFs in *E. coli*.

The *E. coli–S. aureus* shuttle vector pRAB11N was re-constructed to make an exact copy of the plasmid pRAB11, which could no longer be obtained from any source. The plasmid pRMC2 [34] was used as a template in plasmid-PCR using pRAB-fw and pRAB-rev as primers (Table S3). This PCR added a second *tet* operator to the *tetR* promoter region. A 30 µL aliquot of the obtained PCR product was digested with a 50 U DpnI (New England BioLabs, cat. no. R0176) in a reaction volume of 50 µL to eliminate the pRMC2 template before ligation. One of the confirmed transformants was named pRAB11N, and it was used as a shuttle expression vector in both *E. coli* and *S. aureus*.

The correctness of the obtained plasmid vectors was confirmed by Sanger sequencing at the Finnish Institute for Molecular Medicine (FIMM) Genomics Sequencing (Biomedicum, Tukholmankatu 8, Helsinki, Finland) using primers Puc19-F and Puc19-R for pCU1LK, and fR-346 for pRAB11N. Primers used in this study are listed in Table S3.

4.5. Bioinformatics

The NGS-based toxicity screening of HPUF encoding genes was carried out using the protocol described previously [11]. The DNA samples used for NGS are described in Section 2.3. For each pool of 16 HPUFs, the reads containing the four expected ligation joint sequences (VGF, GVF, VGR, and GVR, Figure 7, and Table S1) were identified and extracted from both the pooled ligation mixture DNA and the pooled plasmid DNA samples using the script and workflow described earlier [11]. The total number of the four ligation joint sequences for each HPUF-encoding gene was calculated and used to represent their total read coverage (N joint reads, Formula (1)). The relative number of joint sequence reads was calculated for all genes in the pools by dividing the total read coverage of a single gene by the total number of joint sequence reads for all genes in the pool and expressed as a percentage (relative gene percentage, Formula (1)). As described by Kasurinen et al., a low ratio (Formula (2)) between the relative joint sequence reads of individual genes from plasmid pools and those from the corresponding ligation mixture indicates the presence of toxHPUF gene, owing to the elimination of transformants carrying a toxic gene [11].

$$\text{Relative gene percentage} = \frac{\text{N joint-reads of single gene}}{\text{N joint-reads of all genes in pool}} \times 100\%, \tag{1}$$

$$\text{Ratio} = \frac{\text{Relative gene percentage from pooled plasmid DNA}}{\text{Relative gene percentage from ligation mixtures}}. \tag{2}$$

On the contrary, a ratio close to 1 or above indicates a non-toxic gene, reflecting the successful replication of the recombinant plasmid. In theory, a HPUF could be considered as bactericidal if this ratio is less than 1. In our study presented here, gene products exhibiting ratios between 0.5 and 1.0 were considered potentially mildly toxic, while those with a ratio under 0.5 were potentially bactericidal.

4.6. Toxicity Confirmation

The toxicity of the potentially toxic HPUFs towards host bacteria was primarily tested using a drop test on agar plates. Potentially toxic HPUFs genes were cloned either into the pBAD33 vector under an arabinose-inducible promoter (using the KpnI-XbaI restriction sites) or pRAB11N under an ATc-inducible promoter (using the BglII-KpnI sites). The correct gene insertions were confirmed by colony PCR using primers pBADF and pBADRev for pBAD33 constructions and pRAB11-F and fR-346 for pRAB11N constructions. The resultant PCR products were further analysed and identified by Sanger sequencing.

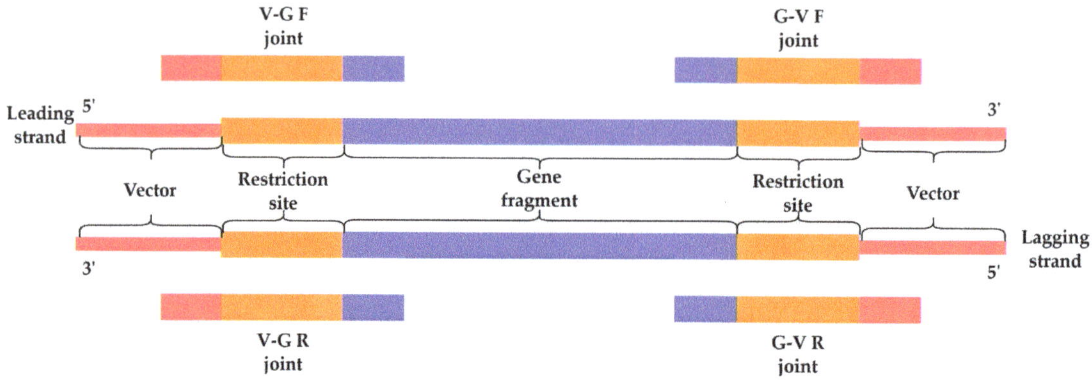

Figure 7. Illustration of the four ligation joint sequences used in the determination of sequence read coverage for each of the screened HPUFs (V, vector; G, gene fragment; F, forward; R, reverse). Adapted with permission from Nyhamar 2022 [12], University of Helsinki.

Subsequently, *E. coli* or *S. aureus* transformants carrying the desired recombinant plasmids (Table S2) were grown on suitable agar plates to obtain single colonies. Three isolated colonies containing the recombinant vector and positive-control colonies were resuspended and diluted to optical density at 600 nm (OD_{600}) 0.2 with sterile phosphate-buffered saline (PBS) pH 7.4. Five microliters of the serial dilutions from 10^{-1} to 10^{-8} of each culture were spotted onto both induced and non-induced LA or TSA plates and let dry before incubation at 37 °C overnight. Varying inducing and non-inducing conditions of the plates are listed in Table S4.

To confirm toxicity of the HPUFs and visualise the time-specific impact of toxHPUFs, the growth curves of the strains carrying the pRAB11N-HPUF plasmids were determined with and without induction. Three colonies of each strain were inoculated in a 1 mL TSB supplemented with Amp100 for *E. coli*, and TSB supplemented with Cm30 for *S. aureus* and incubated at 37 °C overnight with a 200 RPM shaking. Cells were resuspended and washed with an equal volume of TSB, and OD_{600} was measured. The washed cells were used as a starting inoculum after resuspending to an OD_{600} of 0.01 into fresh TSB, with and without the inducer (ATc 0.4 μM). The bacteria were grown in Bioscreen Honeycomb plates (Oy Growth Curves Ab Ltd., Helsinki, Finland) in triplicate. The OD_{600} was measured using the Bioscreen C MBR (Oy Growth Curves Ab Ltd., Helsinki, Finland) every 30 min for 16 h with settings of continuous shaking, high amplitude, and normal speed. The shaking was stopped 10 s before each OD_{600} measurement. The mean values and standard deviations were calculated using triplicate data points.

4.7. Genomic DNA Sequencing

Bacterial gDNA isolated from *E. coli* DH10B/pRAB11N-HPUF clones was sequenced at Novogene Company Ltd. Contigs were assembled using BV-BRC (https://www.bv-brc.org/app/Assembly2, accessed on 26 June 2023), and a nucleotide BLAST (Basic Local Alignment Search Tool, version 2.14.0, https://blast.ncbi.nlm.nih.gov/Blast.cgi, accessed on 26 June 2023) search was used to align the sequence assemblies with the individual pRAB11N-HPUF and *E. coli* DH10B genome sequences. Protein BLAST was used to align sequences to known proteins.

4.8. Structural and Functional Analysis of Toxic Proteins

Phyre2, HHpred, and AlphaFold2 were used to predict the functions and structures of the toxic hypothetical proteins. Comparisons were made between the sequence identities of the proteins and known protein structures, with cut-offs of 30% identity and confidence levels over 90% for Phyre2 and similar parameters for HHpred. Functional and structural protein database files were superimposed using the molecular visualisation system PyMOL utilising the 'super' function (The PyMOL Molecular Graphics System, version 2.5, Schrödinger, LCC). RMSD scores were calculated using PyMOL to measure structural alignment and overlap of the predicted protein structures.

Supplementary Materials: The following supporting information can be downloaded at: https://www.mdpi.com/article/10.3390/antibiotics12071213/s1, Figure S1: Relative joint sequence reads ratios for non-toxic genes from Stab21 phage; Figure S2: Toxicity drop test of *E. coli* DH10B/pRAB11N-HPUFs; Figure S3: Toxicity drop test of *S. aureus* RN4220/pRAB11N-HPUFs on various concentrations of antibiotic; Figure S4: Toxicity drop test of *S. aureus* RN4220/pRAB11N-HPUFs on different concentrations of inducer; Figure S5: Gel electrophoresis of *E. coli* DH10B/pRAB11N-toxHPUFs ATc tolerant mutant colony PCR products; Figure S6: ATc sensitive and tolerant *E. coli* DH10B/pRAB11N-toxHPUF toxicity screening; Figure S7: TetR sequence alignment of ATc sensitive pRAB11N-*g172*, *g187* and ATc tolerant pRAB11N-*g172*-T, *g187*-T; Figure S8: Predicted structures of the top 5 toxHPUFs; Figure S9: Superimposition of Gp081c with Phyre2 and HHPred functional models of *Enterobacter* phage 22 tail needle protein Gp26; Table S1: Details of the NGS assay; Table S2: Recombinant strains used in this project; Table S3: Primers and oligonucleotides used in this study; Table S4: Gene inducing and non-inducing pair conditions tested for *E. coli* and *S. aureus* toxicity drop test using recombinant strains.

Author Contributions: Conceptualisation, M.P., M.S. and X.W.; methodology, E.N., P.W., O.L. and Ö.Y.; software, E.N., P.W. and X.W.; validation, P.W. and O.L.; investigation, E.N., P.W., O.L. and Ö.Y.; writing—original draft preparation, E.N., P.W., O.L., Ö.Y., M.P., M.S. and X.W.; writing—review and editing, E.N., P.W., M.S. and X.W.; visualisation, E.N., P.W., O.L. and X.W.; supervision, M.P., M.S. and X.W.; resources, M.S.; project administration, M.S.; funding acquisition, M.S. and X.W. All authors have read and agreed to the published version of the manuscript.

Funding: This research was funded by the Academy of Finland (grant number 288701), and by Jane and Aatos Erkko Foundation to M.S. (decision 2016). Additionally, X.W. received a personal grant from the Jane and Aatos Erkko Foundation (grant number 200050).

Institutional Review Board Statement: Not applicable.

Informed Consent Statement: Not applicable.

Data Availability Statement: Not applicable.

Acknowledgments: We thank Pentti Kuusela from HUSLAB for kindly providing the plasmid pCU1.

Conflicts of Interest: The authors declare no conflict of interest.

References

1. Coates, A.R.M.; Halls, G.; Hu, Y. Novel Classes of Antibiotics or More of the Same? *Br. J. Pharmacol.* **2011**, *163*, 184–194. [CrossRef] [PubMed]
2. Mulani, M.S.; Kamble, E.E.; Kumkar, S.N.; Tawre, M.S.; Pardesi, K.R. Emerging Strategies to Combat ESKAPE Pathogens in the Era of Antimicrobial Resistance: A Review. *Front. Microbiol.* **2019**, *10*, 539. [CrossRef]
3. World Health Organization. WHO Publishes List of Bacteria for Which New Antibiotics Are Urgently Needed. Available online: https://www.who.int/news/item/27-02-2017-who-publishes-list-of-bacteria-for-which-new-antibiotics-are-urgently-needed (accessed on 26 June 2023).
4. Loomba, P.S.; Taneja, J.; Mishra, B. Methicillin and Vancomycin Resistant *S. sureus* in Hospitalized Patients. *J. Glob. Infect. Dis.* **2010**, *2*, 275–283. [CrossRef] [PubMed]
5. Wang, J.-T.; Hsu, L.-Y.; Lauderdale, T.-L.; Fan, W.-C.; Wang, F.-D. Comparison of Outcomes among Adult Patients with Nosocomial Bacteremia Caused by Methicillin Susceptible and Methicillin Resistant *Staphylococcus aureus*: A Retrospective Cohort Study. *PLoS ONE* **2015**, *10*, e0144710. [CrossRef] [PubMed]
6. Wan, X.; Hendrix, H.; Skurnik, M.; Lavigne, R. Phage-Based Target Discovery and Its Exploitation towards Novel Antibacterial Molecules. *Curr. Opin. Biotechnol.* **2021**, *68*, 1–7. [CrossRef]
7. Liu, J.; Dehbi, M.; Moeck, G.; Arhin, F.; Bauda, P.; Bergeron, D.; Callejo, M.; Ferretti, V.; Ha, N.; Kwan, T.; et al. Antimicrobial Drug Discovery through Bacteriophage Genomics. *Nat. Biotechnol.* **2004**, *22*, 185–191. [CrossRef]

8. Singh, S.; Godavarthi, S.; Kumar, A.; Sen, R. A Mycobacteriophage Genomics Approach to Identify Novel Mycobacteriophage Proteins with Mycobactericidal Properties. *Microbiology* **2019**, *165*, 722–736. [CrossRef]
9. Oduor, J.M.O.; Kiljunen, S.; Kadija, E.; Mureithi, M.W.; Nyachieo, A.; Skurnik, M. Genomic Characterization of Four Novel *Staphylococcus* Myoviruses. *Arch. Virol.* **2019**, *164*, 2171–2173. [CrossRef]
10. Sharma, M. Lytic Bacteriophages: Potential Interventions against Enteric Bacterial Pathogens on Produce. *Bacteriophage* **2013**, *3*, e25518. [CrossRef]
11. Kasurinen, J.; Spruit, C.M.; Wicklund, A.; Pajunen, M.I.; Skurnik, M. Screening of Bacteriophage Encoded Toxic Proteins with a Next Generation Sequencing-Based Assay. *Viruses* **2021**, *13*, 750. [CrossRef]
12. Nyhamar, E. Identification of Staphylococcus Bacteriophage Stab21 Toxic Gene Products Using *Escherichia coli* as a Host. Master's Thesis, University of Helsinki, Helsinki, Finland, 2022.
13. Zimmermann, L.; Stephens, A.; Nam, S.-Z.; Rau, D.; Kübler, J.; Lozajic, M.; Gabler, F.; Söding, J.; Lupas, A.N.; Alva, V. A Completely Reimplemented MPI Bioinformatics Toolkit with a New HHpred Server at Its Core. *J. Mol. Biol.* **2018**, *430*, 2237–2243. [CrossRef] [PubMed]
14. Oduor, J.M.O.; Kadija, E.; Nyachieo, A.; Mureithi, M.W.; Skurnik, M. Bioprospecting *Staphylococcus* Phages with Therapeutic and Bio-Control Potential. *Viruses* **2020**, *12*, 133. [CrossRef] [PubMed]
15. Guzman, L.M.; Belin, D.; Carson, M.J.; Beckwith, J. Tight Regulation, Modulation, and High-Level Expression by Vectors Containing the Arabinose PBAD Promoter. *J. Bacteriol.* **1995**, *177*, 4121–4130. [CrossRef] [PubMed]
16. Kelley, L.A.; Mezulis, S.; Yates, C.M.; Wass, M.N.; Sternberg, M.J.E. The Phyre2 Web Portal for Protein Modeling, Prediction and Analysis. *Nat. Protoc.* **2015**, *10*, 845–858. [CrossRef]
17. Söding, J.; Biegert, A.; Lupas, A.N. The HHpred Interactive Server for Protein Homology Detection and Structure Prediction. *Nucleic Acids Res.* **2005**, *33*, W244–W248. [CrossRef]
18. Jumper, J.; Evans, R.; Pritzel, A.; Green, T.; Figurnov, M.; Ronneberger, O.; Tunyasuvunakool, K.; Bates, R.; Žídek, A.; Potapenko, A.; et al. Highly Accurate Protein Structure Prediction with AlphaFold. *Nature* **2021**, *596*, 583–589. [CrossRef]
19. Chothia, C.; Lesk, A.M. The Relation between the Divergence of Sequence and Structure in Proteins. *EMBO J.* **1986**, *5*, 823–826. [CrossRef]
20. Prestinaci, F.; Pezzotti, P.; Pantosti, A. Antimicrobial Resistance: A Global Multifaceted Phenomenon. *Pathog. Glob. Health* **2015**, *109*, 309–318. [CrossRef]
21. Schmelcher, M.; Donovan, D.M.; Loessner, M.J. Bacteriophage Endolysins as Novel Antimicrobials. *Future Microbiol.* **2012**, *7*, 1147–1171. [CrossRef]
22. Saier, M.H.J.; Reddy, B.L. Holins in Bacteria, Eukaryotes, and Archaea: Multifunctional Xenologues with Potential Biotechnological and Biomedical Applications. *J. Bacteriol.* **2015**, *197*, 7–17. [CrossRef]
23. Roach, D.R.; Donovan, D.M. Antimicrobial Bacteriophage-Derived Proteins and Therapeutic Applications. *Bacteriophage* **2015**, *5*, e1062590. [CrossRef]
24. Chaitanya, K.V. Structure and Organization of Virus Genomes. In *Genome and Genomics: From Archaea to Eukaryotes*; Springer: Singapore, 2019; pp. 1–30. ISBN 978-981-15-0702-1.
25. Ruiz, N.; Silhavy, T.J. How *Escherichia coli* Became the Flagship Bacterium of Molecular Biology. *J. Bacteriol.* **2022**, *204*, e0023022. [CrossRef]
26. Augustin, J.; Rosenstein, R.; Wieland, B.; Schneider, U.; Schnell, N.; Engelke, G.; Entian, K.D.; Götz, F. Genetic Analysis of Epidermin Biosynthetic Genes and Epidermin-Negative Mutants of *Staphylococcus epidermidis*. *Eur. J. Biochem.* **1992**, *204*, 1149–1154. [CrossRef]
27. Helle, L.; Kull, M.; Mayer, S.; Marincola, G.; Zelder, M.-E.; Goerke, C.; Wolz, C.; Bertram, R. Vectors for Improved Tet Repressor-Dependent Gradual Gene Induction or Silencing in *Staphylococcus aureus*. *Microbiology* **2011**, *157*, 3314–3323. [CrossRef] [PubMed]
28. Gossen, M.; Bujard, H. Anhydrotetracycline, a Novel Effector for Tetracycline Controlled Gene Expression Systems in Eukaryotic Cells. *Nucleic Acids Res.* **1993**, *21*, 4411–4412. [CrossRef]
29. Sierra, R.; Prados, J.; Panasenko, O.O.; Andrey, D.O.; Fleuchot, B.; Redder, P.; Kelley, W.L.; Viollier, P.H.; Renzoni, A. Insights into the Global Effect on *Staphylococcus aureus* Growth Arrest by Induction of the Endoribonuclease MazF Toxin. *Nucleic Acids Res.* **2020**, *48*, 8545–8561. [CrossRef] [PubMed]
30. Choi, K.-H.; Gaynor, J.B.; White, K.G.; Lopez, C.; Bosio, C.M.; Karkhoff-Schweizer, R.R.; Schweizer, H.P. A Tn7-Based Broad-Range Bacterial Cloning and Expression System. *Nat. Methods* **2005**, *2*, 443–448. [CrossRef] [PubMed]
31. Jie, J.; Chu, X.; Li, D.; Luo, Z. A Set of Shuttle Plasmids for Gene Expression in *Acinetobacter baumannii*. *PLoS ONE* **2021**, *16*, e0246918. [CrossRef]
32. Brok-Volchanskaya, V.S.; Kadyrov, F.A.; Sivogrivov, D.E.; Kolosov, P.M.; Sokolov, A.S.; Shlyapnikov, M.G.; Kryukov, V.M.; Granovsky, I.E. Phage T4 SegB Protein Is a Homing Endonuclease Required for the Preferred Inheritance of T4 TRNA Gene Region Occurring in Co-Infection with a Related Phage. *Nucleic Acids Res.* **2008**, *36*, 2094–2105. [CrossRef]

33. Braun, V.; Pilsl, H.; Gross, P. Colicins: Structures, Modes of Action, Transfer through Membranes, and Evolution. *Arch. Microbiol.* **1994**, *161*, 199–206. [CrossRef]
34. Corrigan, R.M.; Foster, T.J. An Improved Tetracycline-Inducible Expression Vector for *Staphylococcus aureus*. *Plasmid* **2009**, *61*, 126–129. [CrossRef] [PubMed]

antibiotics

MDPI

Article

Biosynthesized Silver Nanoparticles Derived from Probiotic *Lactobacillus rhamnosus* (AgNPs-LR) Targeting Biofilm Formation and Quorum Sensing-Mediated Virulence Factors

Amir Mahgoub Awadelkareem [1], Arif Jamal Siddiqui [2], Emira Noumi [2], Syed Amir Ashraf [1], Sibte Hadi [3], Mejdi Snoussi [2], Riadh Badraoui [2], Fevzi Bardakci [2], Mohammad Saquib Ashraf [4], Corina Danciu [5], Mitesh Patel [6,*] and Mohd Adnan [2,*]

[1] Department of Clinical Nutrition, College of Applied Medial Sciences, University of Ha'il, Ha'il P.O. Box 2440, Saudi Arabia
[2] Department of Biology, College of Science, University of Ha'il, Ha'il P.O. Box 2440, Saudi Arabia
[3] Department of Forensic Sciences, Naif Arab University for Security Sciences, Riyadh, Saudi Arabia
[4] Department of Medical Laboratory Science, College of Applied Medical Sciences, Riyadh ELM University, Riyadh, Saudi Arabia
[5] Department of Pharmacognosy, Faculty of Pharmacy, "Victor Babes" University of Medicine and Pharmacy, 2 Eftimie Murgu Square, 300041 Timisoara, Romania
[6] Department of Biotechnology, Parul Institute of Applied Sciences, Centre of Research for Development, Parul University, Vadodara 391760, India
* Correspondence: patelmeet15@gmail.com (M.P.); drmohdadnan@gmail.com (M.A.)

Abstract: In recent years, bacterial pathogens have developed resistance to antimicrobial agents that have created a global threat to human health and environment. As a novel approach to combating antimicrobial resistance (AMR), targeting bacteria's virulent traits that can be explained by quorum sensing (QS) is considered to be one of the most promising approaches. In the present study, biologically synthesized silver nanoparticles derived from *Lactobacillus rhamnosus* (AgNPs-LR) were tested against three Gram-negative bacteria to determine whether they inhibited the formation of biofilms and triggered the virulence factors controlled by QS. In *C. violaceum* and *S. marcescens*, a remarkable inhibition (>70%) of QS-mediated violacein and prodigiosin production was recorded, respectively. A dose-dependent decrease in virulence factors of *P. aeruginosa* (pyocyanin, pyoverdine, LasA protease, LasB elastase and rhamnolipid production) was also observed with AgNPs-LR. The biofilm development was reduced by 72.56%, 61.70%, and 64.66% at highest sub-MIC for *C. violaceum*, *S. marcescens* and *P. aeruginosa*, respectively. Observations on glass surfaces have shown remarkable reductions in biofilm formation, with less aggregation of bacteria and a reduced amount of extra polymeric materials being formed from the bacteria. Moreover, swimming motility and exopolysaccharides (EPS) was also found to reduce in the presence of AgNPs-LR. Therefore, these results clearly demonstrate that AgNPs-LR is highly effective in inhibiting the development of biofilms and the QS-mediated virulent traits of Gram-negative bacteria. In the future, AgNPs-LR may be used as an alternative to conventional antibiotics for the treatment of bacterial infections after careful evaluation in animal models, especially for the development of topical antimicrobial agents.

Keywords: quorum sensing; biofilms; *Lactobacillus rhamnosus*; *Chromobacterium violaceum*; *Serratia marcescens*; green antimicrobial agent

1. Introduction

As a global public health issue, antimicrobial resistance (AMR) is a growing problem that occurs when microorganisms such as bacteria, viruses, fungi, and parasites become resistant to antimicrobial drugs that have previously served as effective treatments for infections [1,2]. When bacteria become resistant to antibiotics, they can spread infections which are difficult to treat, which can result in prolonged illness, disability and even death as a result [3,4]. Multi-drug resistance (MDR) is a form of AMR in which microorganisms become resistant to multiple drugs, making it more difficult to treat infections [5]. This can happen when antibiotics are overused or misused, as well as when there is poor infection prevention and control in healthcare settings [6]. The current problem of AMR and MDR poses a serious problem to global health [7]. According to the World Health Organization (WHO), by 2050 if no action will be taken against drug-resistant infection, the number of deaths will rise to 10 million annually [8]. AMR and MDR also have significant economic impacts. A drug-resistant infection costs more to treat than a non-resistant infection due to the need for more expensive drugs and longer hospital stays [5]. AMR also affects agricultural productivity as it can lead to the loss of livestock and crops [9]. Efforts to address AMR and MDR require a multi-sectoral approach, including reducing unnecessary antibiotic use, improving prevention of infection and measures of prevention, developing new antimicrobial drugs and diagnostic tools, and promoting global cooperation and coordination [10–12].

As a strategy to combat the AMR epidemic, anti-infective drugs should be designed, which can target quorum sensing (QS)-regulated virulence factors and biofilm formation [13]. Quorum sensing is a process used by bacteria to communicate with one another through the release and detection of chemical signals called autoinducers. This process permits bacteria to coordinate their behaviour and synchronize their gene expression against the changed environmental conditions [14]. Biofilms are communities of microorganisms embedded in a protective extracellular matrix that adhere to surfaces. QS has a key role in the formation and maintenance of these communities. The eradication of biofilms is extremely difficult and they contribute to the development of antimicrobial resistance by providing a protective environment for bacteria to grow and exchange genetic material, including antibiotic resistance genes [15]. Quorum sensing inhibitors (QSIs) are compounds that can disrupt the communication process between bacteria and prevent the formation of biofilms and reducing the spread of bacterial infections. QSIs have shown promise as a potential strategy to inhibit AMR by reducing resistance to antibiotics in biofilms. Additionally, by preventing the formation of biofilms, QSIs can make bacteria more susceptible to antibiotic treatment, lowering the likelihood of the development of resistance. Several natural and synthetic QSIs have been identified and research is ongoing to develop more effective QSIs and explore their potential clinical applications [16,17]. However, in this regard it is imperative to note that QSIs alone are unlikely to be a promising one for addressing AMR and that a comprehensive approach that includes reducing unnecessary antibiotic use and improving infection prevention and control measures is necessary to combat this global public health challenge [18,19].

Recently, a lot of attention has been paid in finding ways to produce and use the nanomaterials, and the interest is growing every day. In terms of manufacturing nanoparticles, one of the methods to be considered is the bio-approach (green) [20]. Using microorganisms for synthesis of nanoparticles, for example, is referred to as nanoparticles synthesis by biological means. Nanoparticles are produced both by living and dead microorganisms, contribute greatly to nanoparticle production [21]. Material can be controlled at the molecular level using nanotechnology. Silver nanoparticles resulted in significant attention because of their antimicrobial properties, and these metal nanoparticles are being used in different fields such as industrial packaging, agriculture, medicine, cosmetics, and in the military [22]. An array of microorganisms such as *E. coli*, *S. aureus*, *P. aeruginosa*, *B. subtilis*, *V. cholera* and *S. typhus* may be susceptible to AgNPs as antimicrobial agents [22–24]. Hence, as an emerging method for discovering antibacterial involves using green synthesized nanoparticles to target bacterial biofilm and QS. Utilization of silver nanoparticles as an alternative antimicrobial agent has been suggested in previous studies and it may prove useful as an alternative [17]. Furthermore, it has become apparent in recent years that nanotechnology has grasped a lot of attention from scientists because of the possibility of its application to medicine, diagnostics, agriculture, bioremediation and many other fields [18]. Nano-scaled materials appear to exhibit better biological effects than their bulk counterparts because their chemical and physical properties are different at this scale, which is mainly why the nano-scaled materials shown improved biological activity [23]. In the future, nanotechnology is expected to have potential applications in different fields of health care, such as for the purposes of new drugs, for drug delivery and diagnostics, and for the creation of improved biomaterials [24].

Lactobacillus rhamnosus (*L. rhamnosus*) is a probiotic bacterium that has gained considerable attention in the field of medicine due to its potential health benefits. As a naturally occurring bacterium in the human gastrointestinal tract, *L. rhamnosus* has been extensively studied for its various applications in promoting and supporting human health. With its ability to positively influence the gut microbiota and modulate the immune system, *L. rhamnosus* has shown promising potential in the prevention and management of several medical conditions [25]. This strain is therefore given more importance nowadays for its health benefits, ability to defeat intestinal pathogens, maintain intestinal flora balance, and maintain intestinal barriers [26,27]. The strain also produced antimicrobial metabolites that had an antagonistic effect on harmful bacteria, including *E. coli* [28], *S. enterica* [29] and *S. aureus* [28]. In addition to this, several studies have also shown that *L. rhamnosus* has the ability to reduce the bioavailability of mycotoxins in the gastrointestinal tract as well [30]. Therefore, in the present study, *L. rhamnosus* was used in order to synthesize silver nanoparticles (AgNPs-LR). The synthesized AgNPs-LR were investigated for their broad-spectrum effect on inhibiting the virulence factors controlled by QS in bacterial pathogens namely, *C. violaceum*, *P. aeruginosa* and *S. marcescens* in conjunction with the suppression of biofilm development.

2. Materials and Methods

2.1. Strains of Bacteria and Growth Conditions

The strain of lactic acid bacteria (LAB), *Lactobacillus rhamnosus* MTCC-1423 (*L. rhamnosus*) and pathogenic Gram-negative bacterial strain *C. violaceum* MTCC-2656 (*C. violaceum*) *P. aeruginosa* MTCC-741 (*P. aeruginosa*) and *Serratia marcescens* MTCC-97 (*S. marcescens*) were collected from the Microbial Type Culture Collection (IMTECH, Chandigarh, India). The De Man, Rogosa and Sharpe (MRS) agar plate (HiMedia®, Mumbai, India) was used for the growth and maintenance of *L. rhamnosus*, whereas, Luria-Bertani agar (LB) (HiMedia®, Mumbai, India) was used for the bacterial pathogens. All the bacterial strains were stored at 4 °C for further use.

2.2. Biosynthesis of Silver Nanoparticles (AgNPs) Using L. rhamnosus (AgNPs-LR)

The active culture of *L. rhamnosus* was added into a fresh MRS media and incubated at 37 °C for overnight. Following incubation, the grown culture was centrifuged for 10 min. at 10,000 rpm and 4 °C to collect the culture supernatant. Then, culture supernatant (10 mL) was mixed with 0.1 mM silver nitrate solution (90 mL) and incubated at 30 °C for 24 h in dark condition. Observations were made of the colour change of AgNPs after 24 h of synthesis. As part of the characterization of the AgNPs-LR, UV-Vis, FTIR and TEM analysis were performed [31].

2.3. Characterization of AgNPs-LR

2.3.1. Ultraviolet-Vis Analysis

In order to characterize AgNPs-LR, a spectrophotometric analysis was performed as a first step. With a resolution of 1 nm, AgNPs-LR were scanned in the range of 300 to 700 nm [31]. The UV-Vis analysis was further used to determine the size of AgNPs-LR using Haiss equation, $d = \ln((\lambda SPR - \lambda 0)/L1)/L2$. Where λSPR is the wavelength at which maximum absorption occurs, λ0 is the wavelength at which minimum absorption occurs at the start of SPR, L1 and L2 are the values taken from the data fit of TEM vs. UV-Vis, whose values are L1 = 6.53 and L2 = 0.0216 [32].

2.3.2. FTIR Analysis

The potential interaction between the culture supernatant of *L. rhamnosus* and $AgNO_3$ was examined using Fourier Transform Infrared spectroscopy (FT-IR) (Bruker®, Billerica, MA, USA). The spectra were recorded from 500 to 4000 cm^{-1} [33].

2.3.3. Transmission Electron Microscopy (TEM)

Additionally, TEM measurements were performed on the AgNPs-LR for determining the size and shape. For TEM analysis, a JEM-1400 Plus, Jeol, India was used. By applying the AgNPs-LR sample on a grid made of carbon-coated copper and water content was then evaporated within a vacuum dryer for 1 h, TEM analysis was performed [34].

2.4. Antibacterial Activity of AgNPs-LA

The antibacterial activity of AgNPs-LR was tested using the agar well diffusion method against *C. violaceum*, *S. marcescens*, and *P. aeruginosa* [35]. A sterilized swab was used to streak the inoculum of the bacterial culture onto a MHB agar plate. With the help of a sterile Cork Borer, wells were punched and each well was filled with AgNPs-LR. Afterwards, zone of inhibition was determined after 24 h of incubation at 37 °C.

2.5. Determination of Minimum Inhibitory Concentration (MIC)

In order to evaluate the antibacterial efficacy of AgNPs-LR, the standard broth dilution assay was performed [36]. A series of two-fold dilutions of AgNPs-LR from 1698.7 µg/mL to 0.10 µg/mL concentrations were used to determine MICs in LB broth with active bacterial culture (10^8 CFU/mL, 0.5 McFarland standard). Only inoculated broth was used for the control, which was incubated at 37 °C for 24 h. MIC is defined as the lowest concentration of AgNPs-LR at which no visible growth can be seen in the tubes at the end of the experiment. In order to confirm the MIC value, a visual examination of the tubes was performed before and after incubation to determine the turbidity.

2.6. Assessment of the Quantity of Violacein Pigment in C. violaceum

Violacein production was quantitatively assessed according to standard procedure [37]. In brief, *C. violaceum* was grown for 18 h without and with varying sub-MIC concentrations of AgNPs-LR at 30 °C. For the separation of the insoluble pigment (violacein) from the bacterial cells, centrifugation of 1 mL of culture was carried out at 10,000 rpm for 5 min. To dissolve the pigment, the cell pellet was resuspended in 1 mL of DMSO and vortexed vigorously for 5 min. To spin down the bacteria debris, the suspension was again centrifuged. The UV-spectrophotometer (UV-2600, Shimadzu, Japan) at 585 nm was used for measuring the absorbance of the supernatant.

2.7. Assessment of the Quantity of Prodigiosin Pigment in S. marcescens

The production of prodigiosin pigment was assessed using LB medium according to the standard method [38]. The active culture of *S. marcescens* was added into sterile LB medium with and without AgNPs-LR and grown at 30 °C for overnight. After incubation, centrifugation of 2 mL of grown culture was performed for 10 min. at 10,000 rpm to collect the cell pellet. Acidified ethanol was used to dissolve the obtained cell pellet (96 mL ethanol + 4 mL 1 M HCl) by vigorous shaking at room temperature. After centrifuging the sample once again to remove debris, the absorbance of the supernatant was measured at 534 nm using a spectrophotometer (UV-2600, Shimadzu, Japan).

2.8. Assessment of QS-Mediated Virulence Factors of P. aeruginosa

2.8.1. Estimation of Pyocyanin

The synthesis of pyocyanin by *P. aeruginosa* was evaluated in LB broth with (sub-MICs) and without AgNPs-LR [39]. The active culture of *P. aeruginosa* was inoculated into a sterile LB medium with and without AgNPs-LR and incubated for overnight at 30 °C. To collect the culture supernatant, 5 mL of grown culture was centrifuged for 10 min. at

10,000 rpm after incubation. Chloroform (3 mL) was then used to extract the pyocyanin from the culture supernatant. The organic phase was collected and further extracted with 1.2 mL of 0.2 N HCl. At last, the absorbance of aqueous phase was taken at 520 nm via spectrophotometer (UV-2600, Shimadzu, Japan).

2.8.2. Assessment of Pyoverdine

As per the standard procedure, the levels of pyoverdine were analysed via performing the standard method [40]. The *P. aeruginosa* was grown overnight at 37 °C without and with sub-MIC amounts of AgNPs-LR. A centrifugation process was performed to obtain a supernatant that was free of cells. Then, 900 µL of 50 mM Tris-HCl (pH 7.4) was mixed with 100 µL of culture supernatant. A multi-mode microplate reader was used to measure the fluorescence emission signal (460 nm) of the sample.

2.8.3. Assessment of LasA Staphylolytic Assay

The *P. aeruginosa* culture supernatant was applied to boiled *S. aureus* cells to determine LasA protease activity [41]. To collect the cell pellets from *S. aureus*, centrifugation of culture was carried out at 8000 rpm for 5 min. After collecting the cell pellet, 0.02 M Tris-HCl (pH-8.5) was added and boiled for 10 min. After that, to adjust the absorbance of 0.8 at 595 nm, it was diluted with 0.02 M Tris-HCl. In the following step, a diluted suspension of *S. aureus* was added to the culture supernatants of *P. aeruginosa* grown with and without AgNPs-LR (sub-MICs) (9:1). Afterwards, the absorbance was measured at 595 nm.

2.8.4. Assessment of LasB Elastinolytic Activity

The measurements of elastolytic activity were carried out using the procedure mentioned by Adonizio et al., (2008) [42]. The method was based on the treatment of a grown *P. aeruginosa* culture with or without AgNPs-LR (sub-MICs). The supernatant was collected and added to 900 µL of a buffer containing 20 mg of elastin congo red (100 mM Tris, 1 mM $CaCl_2$, pH-7.5), containing 20 mg of elastin (Sigma®, Bengaluru, India). To remove the insoluble components (elastin Congo red), centrifugation was performed after 3 h of incubation at 37 °C. The absorbance of supernatant was measured at 495 nm.

2.8.5. Assessment of Rhamnolipid

The active culture of *P. aeruginosa* was added into sterile LB broth in the presence or absence of AgNPs-LR and incubated at 37 °C for 24 h. Ethyl acetate evaporation was used to extract rhamnolipids from culture supernatant. Using the modified method of Pinzon and Ju (2009) [43], an estimate of *P. aeruginosa* rhamnolipid production was made by dissolving the extracted rhamnolipid in chloroform. A suspension of rhamnolipids was prepared by adding 200 µL of methylene blue solution (0.025%) to 2 mL of solution. A vortexing step was performed for 5 min. and the mixture was incubated at room temperature for 15 min. For phase separation, 0.2 N HCl was added to new tubes containing the chloroform layer after incubation. The mixture was mixed well and left at room temperature for 10 min. By using 0.2 N HCl as blank, 200 µL of the acidic phase holding methylene blue was spectrophotometrically measured at 638 nm.

2.9. Determination of the Swimming Motility of P. aeruginosa and S. marcescens

The LB plate containing sub-MIC (1/2 MIC) of AgNPs-LR were spotted with 5 µL of the active culture of *P. aeruginosa* and *S. marcescens*. The control plate was not amended. Incubation was carried out overnight at 30 °C. At the end of incubation, swimming zone was observed in the control and treatment plates [44].

2.10. Assessment of Antibiofilm Activity

The glass test tubes were used to determine the antibiofilm effect of AgNPs-LR as the hydrophilic surface [45]. Briefly, sterilized LB medium (3 mL) was transferred to tubes containing 1 mL of active bacterial culture and 500 µL of AgNPs-LR (sub-MICs). In the following step, the contents of the tube were mixed thoroughly and then tubes were incubated at room temperature in a shaker for 72 h. After incubation, the planktonic cells were removed from the tubes and washed with PBS. Then, the formed biofilm inside the tubes was stained with crystal violet. After removing the excess dye via washing with PBS, the stained biofilm was dissolved in acetic acid and absorbance was determined using a spectrophotometer at 595 nm. As a control for the growth of biofilms, LB medium containing individual bacterial strains was used. Estimates of the percentage inhibition of biofilm was made as follows:

$$\text{O.D.}_{\text{control}} - \text{O.D.}_{\text{test}}/\text{O.D.}_{\text{control}} \times 100$$

2.11. Light Microscopic Assessment of Biofilm Inhibition

In brief, 60 μL of active culture of bacteria was added in 6-well plates consisting 3 mL of sterile culture medium and allow to grown overnight. Sterile glass coverslips (1 × 1 cm) were placed in the wells along with the respective sub-MIC values of AgNPs-LR. No treatment was administered to the control group. Following incubation of 24 h, the planktonic cells were removed via washing with PBS and then air dried at room temperature for 20 min. The biofilm was stained with crystal violet for 15 min. Afterwards, the slides were washed and air dried for 30 min. to remove any excess dye. In order to visualize the biofilms, a light microscope was used (Axioscope A1, Zeiss, Jena, Germany). Magnification was set at 40× for the images [46].

2.12. Assessment of Exopolysaccharide (EPS) Production

A staining assay using ruthenium red was conducted to determine AgNPs-LR activity in reducing EPS content in biofilms [47]. Each of the bacterial test strains (100 μL) and AgNPs-LR were incubated for 24 h at 37 °C. After incubation, planktonic cells were removed and the cell pellet was washed with sterile PBS (200 μL). In order to stain the biofilms formed by the adherent cells, 200 μL of ruthenium red (0.01%) (Sigma-Aldrich®, Bangalore, India). A well that was free of biofilm and a well containing ruthenium red served as a blank. For the next step, the plate was incubated for 1 h at 37 °C. The residual stain was then re-dispersed into a new microtiter plate and the absorbance measured at 450 nm. Amount of dye fixed to biofilm matrix measured as follows:

$$\text{Abs}_{\text{BF}} = \text{Abs}_{\text{B}} - \text{Abs}_{\text{S}}$$

where, Abs_{B} = absorbance of the blanks, and Abs_{S} = absorbance of the residual stain collected from the sample wells.

3. Results

3.1. Synthesis and Characterization of AgNPs-LR

As a result of adding 1 mL of culture supernatant into 10 mL of 0.1 mM silver nitrate solution (1:10), the biosynthesis of AgNPs-LR has been achieved. It was observed during the period of incubation that the colour changed from yellow to dark brown, while the intensity increased over the course of the period of incubation, as a result of a successful biosynthesis of AgNPs-LR. As a first step, UV-Vis analysis of AgNPs-LR was conducted in order to confirm their biosynthesis. According to spectroscopic measurements made after 24 h of synthesis of AgNPs-LR, absorption spectrum with a clear symmetry was observed with a highest absorption at 464 nm (Figure 1A). Bu using information available from the UV-Vis analysis and Haiss equation, we calculated the size of AgNPs-LR as 6.26 nm. By using FTIR spectrum, different functional groups can be identified, as a result of which silver ions are reduced and stabilizing silver nanoparticles. A spectrum of AgNPs-LR is shown in Figure 1B. As shown in the figure, there are several vibrational bands that can be observed in the spectrum, which indicates the existence of several functional groups. The vibrational bands at 3285.38 cm^{-1}, 2934.78 cm^{-1}, 2125.44 cm^{-1}, 1639.12 cm^{-1}, 1401.45 cm^{-1}, 1243.24 cm^{-1} and 551.64 cm^{-1} are hydroxyl, C-H/methylene, thiocyanate, alkanyl, carboxylate, aromatic ethers, respectively. Study of infrared spectroscopy suggested the predicted factor groups bind to metals with the most strength, and by coating particles, they can be prevented from agglomerating and maintained for a prolonged period of time. Furthermore, the TEM studies of the AgNPs-LR revealed that most of the nanoparticles were spherical and polyhedral in shape, as well as poly dispersed nanoparticles (Figure 1C–E). It was found that the diameter of the AgNPs-LR ranged from 5 to 70 nm.

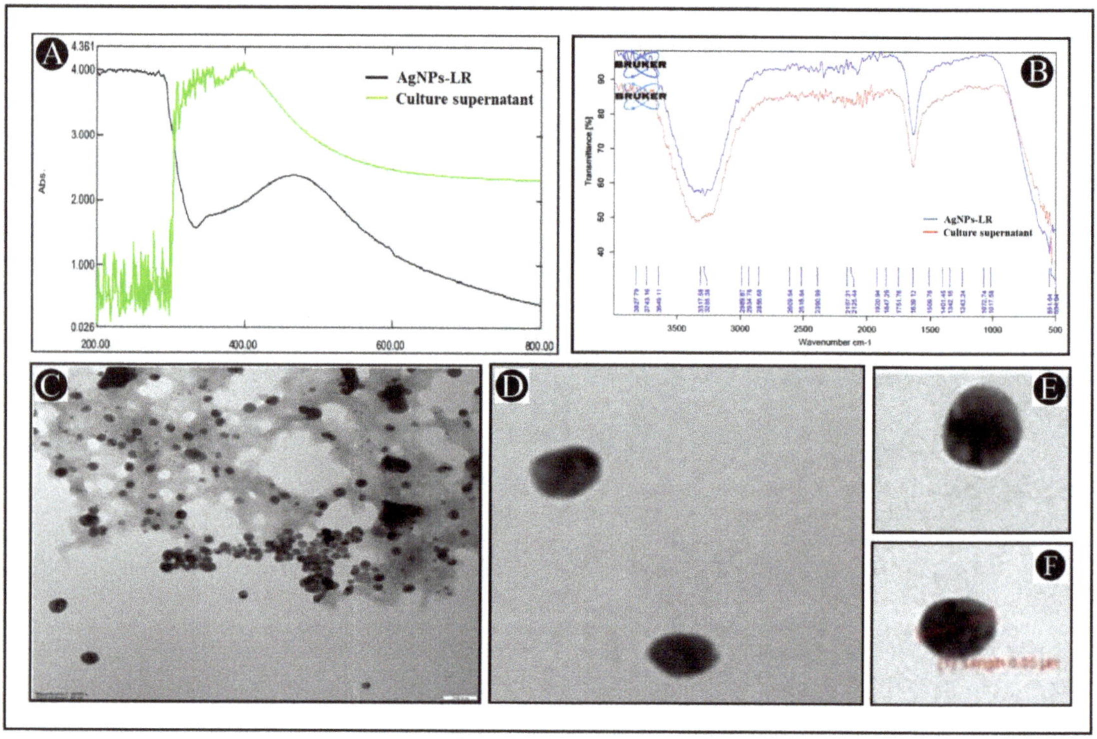

Figure 1. Characterization of AgNPs-LR. (**A**) UV-visible absorption spectra of AgNPs-LR. (**B**) FT-IR analysis of AgNPs-LR. (**C–F**) Morphological analysis of AgNPs-LR via TEM analysis.

3.2. *Antibacterial Potential of Biosynthesized AgNPs-LR*

Biosynthesized AgNPs-LR shown to possess antibacterial properties against all of the tested bacterial strains in well diffusion assays. Among the tested bacteria, *C. violaceum* showed the highest zone of inhibition, followed by *P. aeruginosa* and *S. marcescens* Figure 2. Additionally, a broth microdilution was employed in order to determine the MIC of AgNPs-LR. The AgNPs-LR had MIC values of 13.27 μg/mL against *C. violaceum*, 26.54 μg/mL against *P. aeruginosa* and 53.08 μg/mL against *S. marcescens*, respectively. In order to test the efficacy of biosynthesized AgNPs against formation of biofilm as well as QS-regulated virulence factors, the concentrations of AgNPs were below the inhibitory concentrations (sub-MICs).

3.3. *Inhibition of Inhibition of Virulence Factors of C. violaceum*

The AgNPs-LR has been checked for their preliminary anti-QS activity by determining their impact on *C. violaceum* pigment production. The pigment production in this strain is controlled by QS. Reduced pigment production can be considered as an indication of the presence of anti-QS activity. A treatment with 1/2, 1/4 and 1/8 MIC of AgNPs-LR in *C. violaceum* resulted in a 75.49%, 59.22% and 47.23% reduction in the synthesis of violacein, respectively (Figure 3A). This clearly indicates that green synthesized AgNPs-LR are capable of exhibiting anti-QS activity.

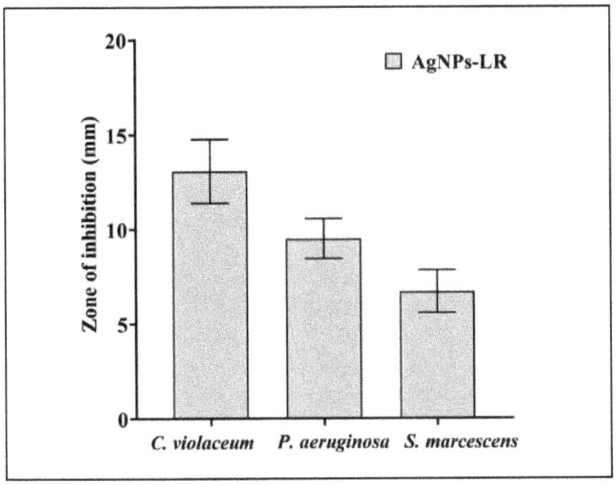

Figure 2. Antibacterial activity of AgNPs-LR against different Gram-negative bacterial pathogens. Values are represented as the mean ± SD of three independent experiments.

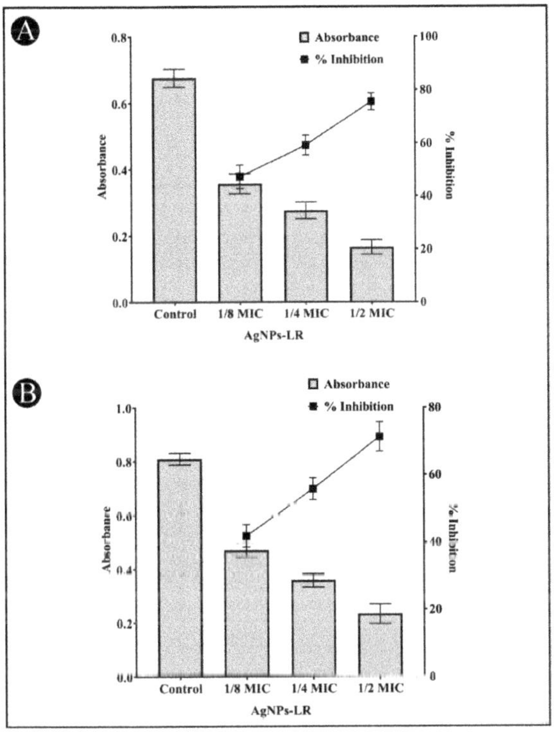

Figure 3. Anti-QS activity of AgNPs-LR against *C. violaceum* and *S. marcescens*. (**A**) An analysis of the quantitative inhibition of violacein in *C. violaceum* using AgNPs-LR. (**B**) An analysis of the quantitative inhibition of prodigiosin in *S. marcescens* using AgNPs-LR. Values are represented as the mean ± SD of three independent experiments. A secondary *y*-axis shows the percentage inhibition.

3.4. Inhibition of Virulence Factors of S. marcescens

AgNPs-LR were also tested for anti-QS activity against *S. marcescens* in an effort to determine whether they inhibit the broad spectrum of QS. *S. marcescens* produces a pink-red pigment called prodigiosin that is regulated via QS. As per Figure 3B, a range of sub-MICs of AgNPs-LR were found to reduced production of prodigiosin in *S. marcescens*. At the concentration of 1/2, 1/4 and 1/8 MIC, AgNPs-LR led to a 71.28%, 55.78% and 41.90% inhibition of prodigiosin, respectively.

3.5. Inhibition of Virulence Factors of P. aeruginosa

The virulence factor of *P. aeruginosa* mediated by QS was examined against AgNPs-LR. A blue-green pigment pyocyanin is produced by *P. aeruginosa* and is controlled by the communication between bacterial cells. The pigment production of the cells was gradually decreased following treatment with AgNPs-LR. A concentration of 1/2, 1/4 and 1/8 MIC reduced the pigment production of *P. aeruginosa* by 72.60%, 50.07% and 38.65% (Figure 4A). The pyocyanin contained in *P. aeruginosa* has been shown to be a significant contributor to its pathogenic potential through the interference with cellular functions of the host.

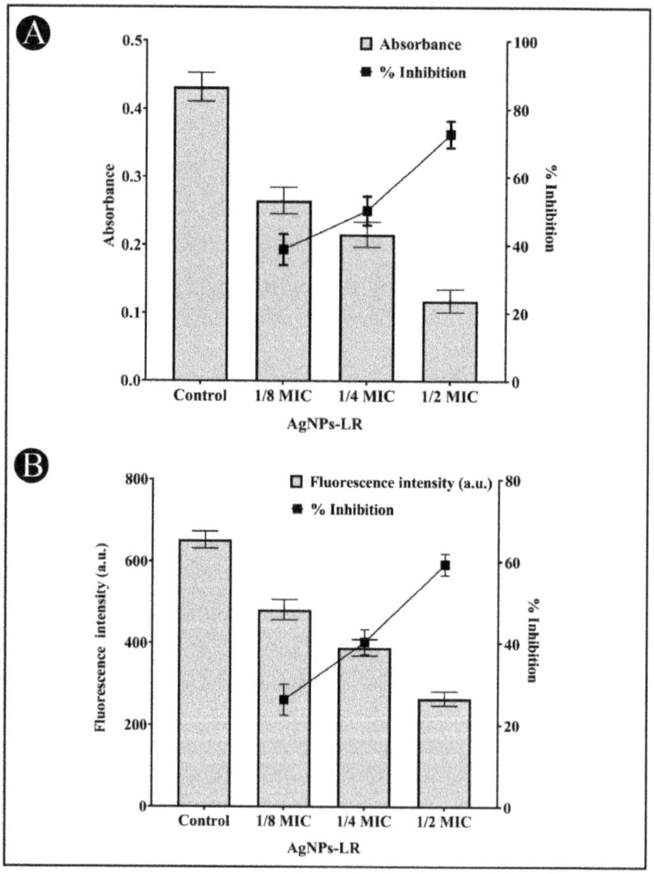

Figure 4. Anti-QS activity of AgNPs-LR against *P. aeruginosa*. (**A**) An analysis of the quantitative inhibition of pyocyanin production in *P. aeruginosa* using AgNPs-LR. (**B**) An analysis of the quantitative inhibition of pyoverdine production in *P. aeruginosa* using AgNPs-LR. Values are represented as the mean ± SD of three independent experiments. A secondary *y*-axis shows the percentage inhibition.

A pigment known as pyoverdine can also be produced by several strains of *P. aeruginosa* which are virulent. There was an inhibition of pyoverdine production in the supernatant by 59.30%, 40.28%, and 26.17%, respectively, when sub-MICs of AgNPs-LR is present (Figure 4B).

A virulent strain of bacteria produces proteolytic enzymes that cause damage to the tissues of the host upon successful infection. A staphylolytic assay was used to determine whether AgNPs-LR inhibit LasA protease activity. After treatment with sub-MICs of AgNPs-LR, LasA protease activity decreased by 62.41%, 41.55%, and 18.36%, respectively (Figure 5A).

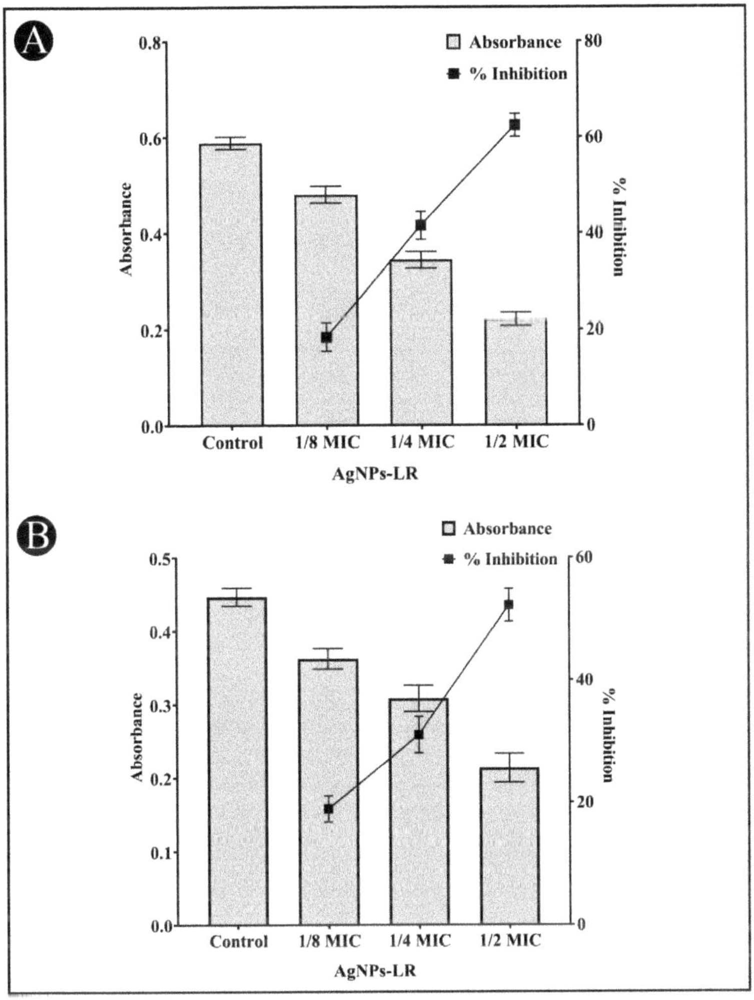

Figure 5. Anti-QS activity of AgNPs-LR against *P. aeruginosa*. (**A**) An analysis of the quantitative inhibition of LasA protease production in *P. aeruginosa* using AgNPs-LR. (**B**) An analysis of the quantitative inhibition of LasB elastase production in *P. aeruginosa* using AgNPs-LR. Values are represented as the mean ± SD of three independent experiments. A secondary *y*-axis shows the percentage inhibition.

An eleastase is a hydrolytic enzyme produced by bacteria during an infection that destroys and inhibit the host immune system. In the presence of AgNPs-LR, *P. aeruginosa* showed a concentration-dependent inhibition of its elastinolytic activity (Figure 5B).

In addition to maintaining the structure of biofilms, rhamnolipids play an important role in adhering bacterial cells to solid surfaces. Rhamnolipid production by *P. aeruginosa* is regulated by RhlR-RhlI QS. Following treatment with AgNPs-LR, rhamnolipid production was reduced (Figure 6). Rhamnolipid production was decreased by 55.86%, 42.76% and 31.82%, respectively, in the presence of sub-MICs of AgNPs-LR.

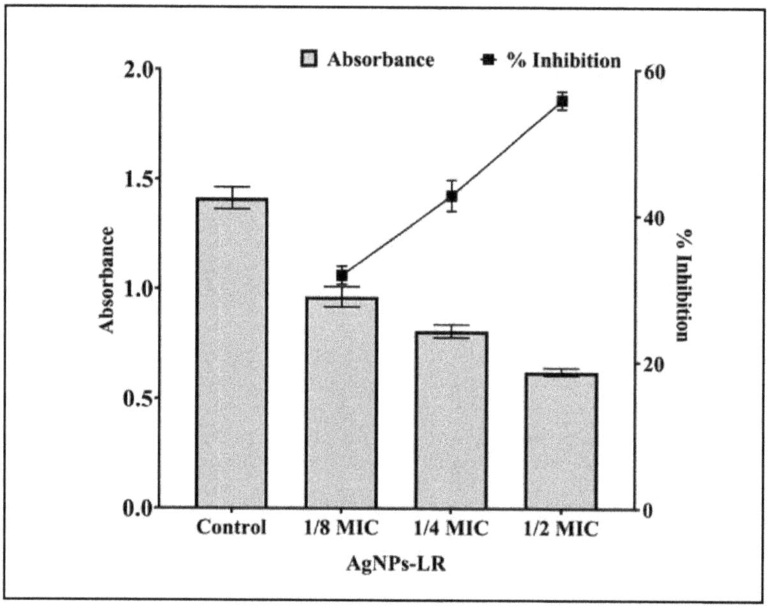

Figure 6. An analysis of the quantitative inhibition of rhamnolipid production in *P. aeruginosa* using AgNPs-LR. Values are represented as the mean ± SD of three independent experiments.

3.6. Quantitative Inhibition of the Formation of Biofilms

An AI-mediated QS phenomenon is often responsible for regulating the formation of a biofilm by regulating its mechanisms. The results obtained from the study on the effects of the AgNPs-LR on the formation of biofilms is shown in Figure 7A for all three bacteria tested. The development of bio-films of *C. violaceum* was inhibited by 72.56%, 55.37% and 42.70%, when 1/2, 1/4, and 1/8 MIC concentrations were used as treatment. The biofilm of *P. aeruginosa* was inhibited by 64.66%, 46.58% and 38.93% at sub-MICs. Similarly, when sub-MICs are present, the biofilms of *S. marcescens* decreased by 61.70%, 41.72%, and 36.50%, respectively.

3.7. Inhibition of EPS Production

The EPS matrix provides protection and support for the biofilm and is critical for its formation, stability, and function. EPS can help bacteria adhere to surfaces, create channels for nutrient flow, and provide protection against antibiotics and other stressors. The present study found that EPS production decreased upon the treatment of AgNPs-LR as 62.84%, 48.84% and 36.83% in *C. violaceum*, 56.91%, 43.12% and 31.77% in *P. aeruginosa* and 52.80%, 42.68% and 29.67% in *S. marcescens* at sub-MICs, respectively (Figure 7B).

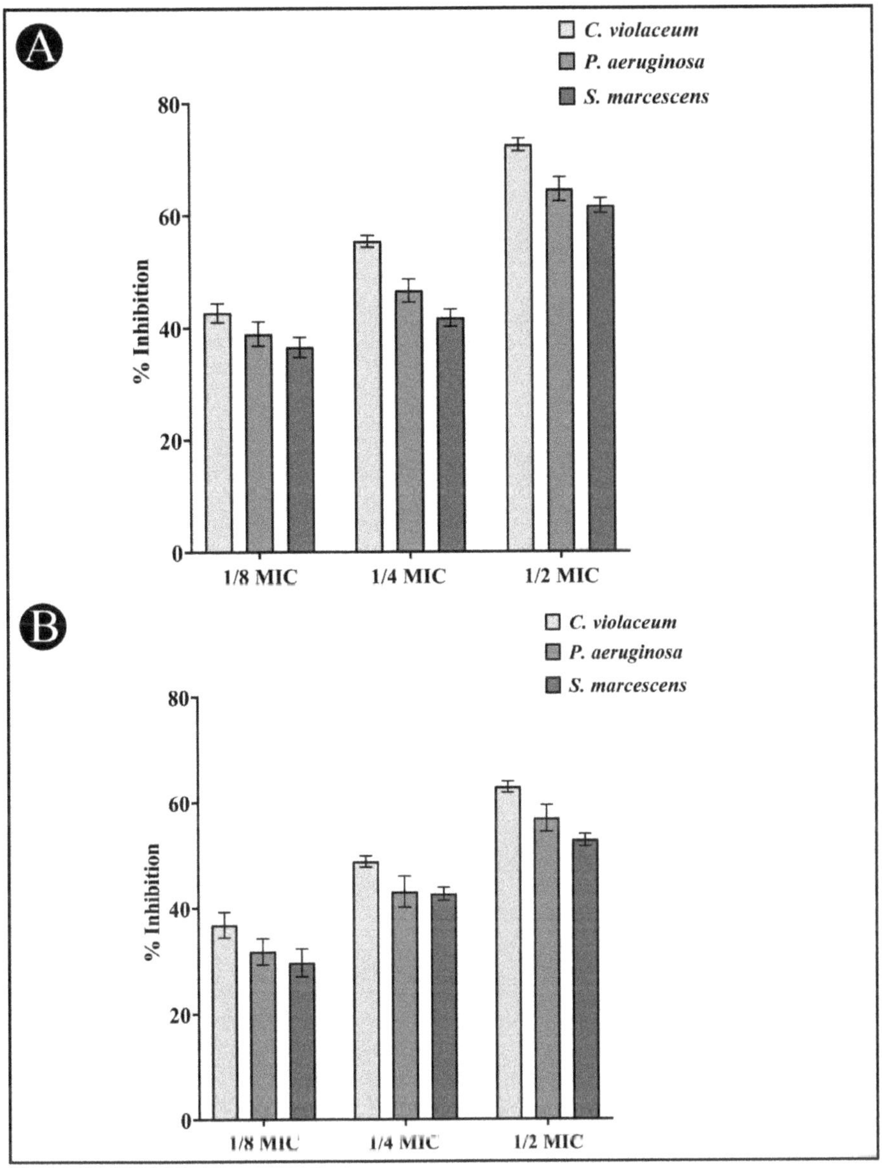

Figure 7. Anti-biofilm and EPS inhibition activity of AgNPs-LR against different Gram-negative bacterial pathogens. (**A**) An analysis of the quantitative inhibition of biofilm production using AgNPs-LR. (**B**) An analysis of the quantitative inhibition of EPS production using AgNPs-LR. Values are represented as the mean ± SD of three independent experiments.

3.8. Analysis of Biofilm Inhibition on Glass Surfaces Using Microscope

Using a microscopy technique, it was possible to perform a further evaluation of the inhibition of biofilms. For the purpose of examining a change in the biofilm architecture, the test bacteria were cultured without and with the maximum sub-MIC of AgNPs-LR in order to visualize biofilm architecture changes. All the tested bacteria displayed a dense cluster of cells on the glass coverslips, as can be seen from the light microscopy images

(Figure 8A–E). With AgNPs-LR treatment, cells were seen in a scattered form on the glass surface and were significantly reduced in clustering.

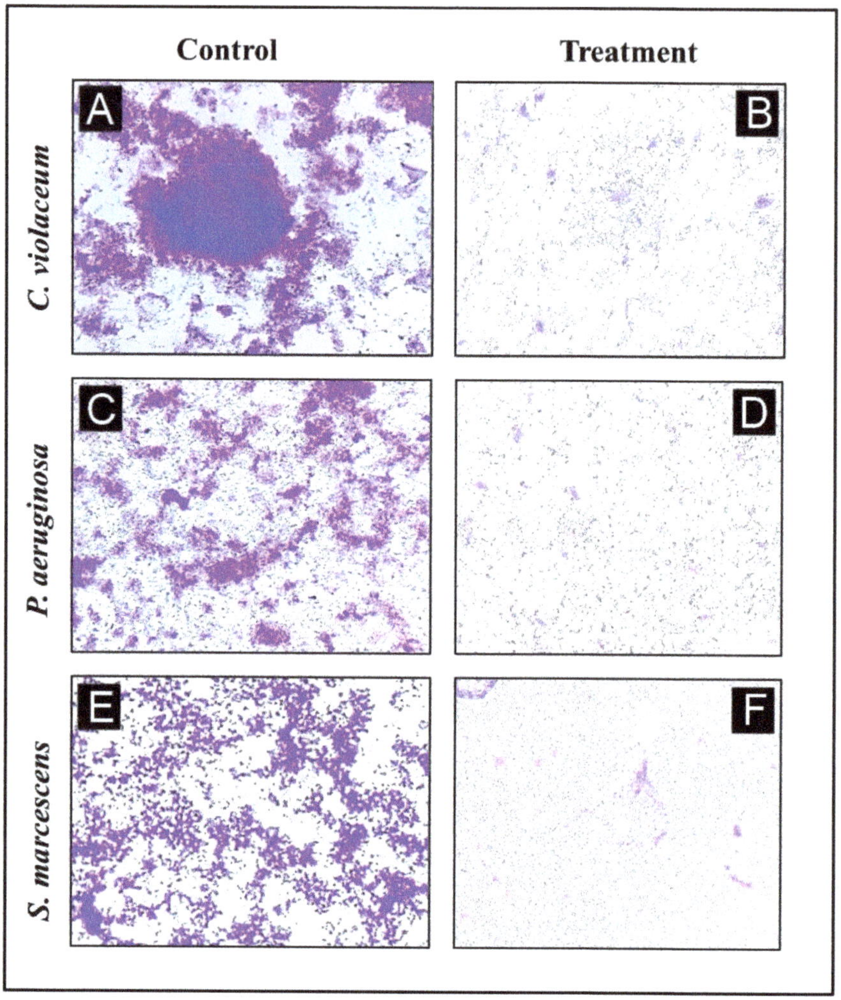

Figure 8. A representative light micrograph of a biofilm showing the effects of AgNPs-LR at their highest sub-MICs. (**A**) Control of *C. violaceum*, (**B**) Treatment of *C. violaceum* with 1/2 MIC, (**C**) Control of *P. aeruginosa*, (**D**) Treatment of *P. aeruginosa* with 1/2 MIC, (**E**) Control of *S. marcescens*, (**F**) Treatment of *S. marcescens* with 1/2 MIC.

3.9. Inhibition of Swimming Motility

QS has a very important role in controlling the movement of *P. aeruginosa* and *S. marcescens*, a crucial factor in determining the spread of infection in a host. It is also considered as a crucial factor in the pathogenicity of both bacteria, so it is an important factor in virulence. In Figure 9A–D, it is shown that the control *P. aeruginosa* and *S. marcescens* swims across the entire Petriplate after overnight incubation. Whereas, there was a decrease in the zone of swimming in the treatment plates.

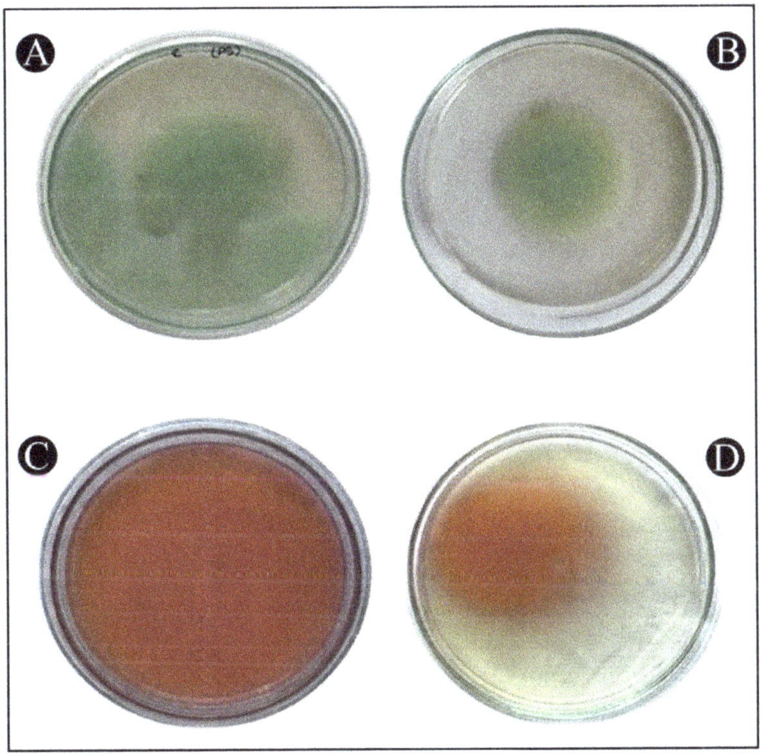

Figure 9. The inhibition of the swimming motility of *P. aeruginosa* and *S. marcescens* by AgNPs-MK. (**A**) Control of *P. aeruginosa*, (**B**) Treatment of *P. aeruginosa* with 1/2 MIC, (**C**) Control of *S. marcescens*, (**D**) Treatment of *S. marcescens* with 1/2 MIC.

4. Discussion

In order to synthesize metal nanoparticles, there are a variety of approaches such as chemical, physical and biological methods that can be utilized. There are significant drawbacks associated with chemical synthesis, primarily the fact that dangerous and non-biodegradable by-products are formed, making them harmful for the environment. The concept of green synthesis is gaining increasing popularity because of its environmental benefits, such as minimizing waste production, using non-hazardous materials and enhancing its environmental friendliness [19]. Besides not causing disease, probiotic bacteria also prevent pathogenic bacteria from multiplying in animals' digestive system and increase intestinal microflora that is beneficial for the animal. There has been a growing market for probiotics in the majority of countries [48].

Using *L. rhamnosus* as a basis for the production of AgNPs, the purpose of the present study was to establish a simple, green, and inexpensive approach that could be utilized to synthesize AgNPs. A prepared sample of *L. rhamnosus* was transferred to a final concentration of 1 mM of silver nitrate in order to observe the formation of AgNPs-LR. The colour change in the sample indicated AgNPs-LR formation, which were then characterized using UV-Vis, FT-IR and TEM analysis. Analyzing AgNPs with UV-Vis is a common technique used to characterize the optical properties of these nanoparticles. The technique is based on the principle of interaction of light with the localized surface plasmon resonance of AgNPs [49]. Therefore, the electron transition that occurs at 464 nm during AgNPs synthesis can be interpreted as a result of the interaction between incident light and the localized surface plasmon resonance of the AgNPs. At 464 nm, the absorption peak suggests that the electron transition involved is primarily a dipole transition. In a dipole transition, the conduction electrons of the AgNPs are excited from the ground state to a higher energy state by absorbing a photon with a specific energy corresponding to the wavelength of 464 nm [50–52]. FT-IR analysis of AgNPs is a technique utilized to determine the chemical composition and bonding properties of these nanoparticles. This technique is based on principle of the interaction of infrared radiation with the molecular vibrations of the nanoparticles [53]. Whereas, TEM analysis was performed to characterize the size, shape and distribution of synthesized AgNPs.

Previously, an iron oxide nanoparticle has been synthesized by Torabian et al. [54] using the green synthesis approach. Upon synthesis, iron oxide nanoparticles were found to be around 15 nm in size. Nanoparticles had round to spherical shape and they found its application in drug delivery or therapy as safe, effective and inexpensive [54]. By synthesizing AgNPs from the supernatant filtrate of *L. acidophilus*, Rajesh et al. [55] designed eco-friendly antibacterial components. Using electron microscopy, they determined that the particles had spherical shapes with sizes ranging from 4–50 nm. According to their report, AgNPs showed antibacterial properties when used against *Klebsiella pneumoniae* by causing cytolysis and destroying the membrane of the bacterial cell [55]. A further study conducted by Nithya et al. [56] examined the antimicrobial efficacy of AgNPs synthesized from *Brevibacterium linens* against multidrug-resistant clinical isolates and demonstrated that these nanoparticles were highly effective. As a result of the AgNPs incubated with *Escherichia coli* colonies for 3 h, it was observed that viable cells had decreased. In contrast, it can cause *Staphylococcus aureus* inhibition zones similar to those of Amikacin. Selenium nanoparticles (SeNP) with 50–80 nm size was prepared by Xu et al. [57] using *L. casei*. Furthermore, in mice infected with Enterotoxigenic *E. coli* K88, SeNP treatment resulted in lowering inflammatory cytokines and oxidative stress in the mice [57]. Using the probiotic *L. kimchicus* DCY51 isolated from traditional Korean kimchi, Markus et al. [58] synthesized gold nanoparticles (AuNPs). Synthesized AuNPs were found to be spherical structure with a size between 5–30 nm. The antioxidant properties of AuNP were demonstrated by its ability to remove free radicals [58]. The antimicrobial efficacy of AgNPs synthesized from one more probiotic *L. amylophilus* GV6 has been tested by Kumar et al. [59] using agar well plate assay against several bacterial pathogens such as, *B. subtilis* MTCC 121, *S. aureus MTCC 96*, *P. aeruginosa* MTCC 424, *K. pneumoniae* MTCC 109 and *E. coli* MTCC 43, which reported the 1.5 cm inhibition zone against *S. aureus* MTCC 96. Using two probiotic bacteria, *L. acidophilus* 58p and *L. plantarum* 92T, Garmasheva et al. [60] synthesized AgNPs and studied their antibacterial activity. The AgNPs obtained from *L. acidophilus* 58p were found more active against *E. coli*, *S. epidermidis*, *S. flexneri*, *K. pneumonia*, and *S. sonnei* than *L. plantarum* 92T AgNPs. In a similar study, Naseer et al. [61] synthesized AgNPs from *L. bulgaricus* and evaluated their antibacterial effectiveness against *S. aureus*, *S. epidermidis* and *S. typhi*. Gram-negative bacteria were found to be more susceptible than Gram-positive bacteria. A recent study by Sharma et al. [62] also synthesized safe, inexpensive and biocompatible AgNPs using four different probiotic isolates such as, *L. plantarum* F22, *L. paraplantarum* KM1, *L. pentosus* S6 and *L. crustorum* F11. Various bacterial and fungi pathogens viz., *B. cereus*, *L. monocytogenes*, antibiotic-resistant *S. aureus*, *P. aphanidermatum*, *P. parasitica* and *F. oxysporum* were also found to be susceptible to these AgNPs. Among them, AgNP synthesized by *L. crustorum* F11 showed maximum inhibition against all pathogens, with maximum activity against *S. aureus* (20 ± 0.61 mm) and *F. oxysporum* (23 ± 0.37).

The current study further explores the antibacterial, antibiofilm and anti-QS activities of biosynthesized AgNPs-LR. As a first step, biosynthesized AgNPs were tested against different bacteria pathogens using well diffusion assays. According to our results, the biosynthesized AgNPs-LR display the highest antibacterial activity against *C. violaceum*, *S. marcescens* and *P. aeruginosa*, respectively. As reported earlier, the high antibacterial activity of biosynthesized AgNPs resulting from reactive oxygen species production and the damage to membranes [63,64]. By virtue of the low MIC of biosynthesized AgNPs against bacterial pathogens, it is not necessary to use conventional antibiotics in conjunction with the biosynthesized AgNPs. Additionally, biosynthesized AgNPs showed higher susceptibility to *C. violaceum* and *P. aeruginosa* than *S. marcescens*. In general, each of these bacteria is capable of forming biofilms, which are difficult to eradicate even with conventional antibiotics available on the market, since their extracellular matrix also reveals resistance to both environmental factors and antibiotics [65,66]. The formation of biofilms contributes to pathogenesis, with almost 80% of infections attributed to biofilm formation [17]. Biofilms are responsible for reducing the efficiency of antibiotics by up to a thousand-fold, which places a burden on the health care system to treat infections. The AI often contributes to QS that controls the formation of a biofilm in a given environment. The synthesized AgNPs-LR were tested for their effect on the development of biofilms in all three bacterial pathogens and the results showed that they effectively inhibited the formation of biofilms at sub-MIC levels. It has been discovered that bacteria that form biofilms resist both chemical and physical therapy and their virulence genes are coordinated in their expression [67]. Previous studies found tobramycin resistance in biofilms of *P. aeruginosa* to be 1000 times higher than in planktonic bacteria [68]. A study carried out using AgNPs derived from the bark extract of *Holarrhena pubescens* reported that the AgNPs inhibited the development of biofilms of imipenem-resistant *P. aeruginosa* [69]. Additionally, AgNPs also inhibited the biofilm development of methicillin-resistant *S. aureus* and *P. aeruginosa* producing extended-spectrum beta-lactamases (EsbL) [70]. Histidine-capped AgNPs were also known to eradicate mature biofilm of *K. pneumoniae* by Chibber et al. [71].

The bacterial QS process is a unique way in which bacteria communicate between themselves, through cell density can be sensed by bacteria in their adjacent atmosphere and this in turn results in the activation or suppression of specific genes in the bacteria [72,73]. QS-dependent gene expression is responsible for many important bacterial characteristics such as physiology, virulence, and the formation of biofilms in bacteria. A huge attention has been given to research on QS because of its potential for human medicine over the past 15–20 years [74]. Thus, the current study also examined an inhibitory effect on QS of AgNPs-LR against *C. violaceum*, *P. aeruginosa* and *S. marcescens*.

Violacein production by *C. violaceum* is regulated by the QS system based on the density of bacteria in the population. Although, violacein itself is not usually considered a pathogenic factor, infections caused by *C. violaceum* can be serious and even life-threatening in individuals with compromised immune systems [75]. In these instances, violacein may help bacteria evade the immune system and establish infection by contributing to their virulence. In spite of the fact that cell-to-cell communication is critical to bacterial physiology and virulence, QS inhibitors have been shown to inhibit the production of violacein by *C. violaceum*, thus providing insights into the potential of QS inhibitors as therapeutic agents against bacterial infections [76].

Pyocyanin production in *P. aeruginosa* is also regulated by QS, just as violacein production. Pyocyanin is a blue-green pigment that is crucial for the pathogenesis of *P. aeruginosa* infections [77]. Pyocyanin plays a key role in *P. aeruginosa* infections by causing oxidative stress in the host. The pyocyanin pigment damages host cell membranes and contributes to the destruction of host tissues by generating reactive oxygen species (ROS). Aside from causing tissue damage and exacerbated infection, oxidative stress triggers inflammation [78]. The immune response to infection has also been interfered with by pyocyanin. Immune cells such as neutrophils and macrophages, which fight bacterial infections, are inhibited by it. As a result, *P. aeruginosa* infection that evades the immune system can become persistent [79,80]. Additionally, *P. aeruginosa* produces pyocyanin, a fluorescent green-yellow siderophore [81]. By facilitating iron acquisition, promoting bacterial growth, and stimulating the host immune response, it also plays an immense part in the pathogenesis of *P. aeruginosa* infections [82]. Furthermore, *P. aeruginosa* infections involve the production of a protease enzyme called Las A. Among the key factors in the pathogenesis of *P. aeruginosa* infection, it degrades host tissue proteins, interferes with host cell signaling, stimulates host immune responses, and promotes biofilm formation and detachment [83]. As for Las B, it is a zinc metalloprotease enzyme produced by *P. aeruginosa* that degrades host tissue proteins, including elastin, collagen, and fibronectin, during pathogenesis. This can result in tissue damage and destruction, which is then used by the bacterium to spread and colonize new sites within the host as a result of the damage [84]. Additionally, *P. aeruginosa* produces surface-active molecules known as rhamnolipids. Moreover, *P. aeruginosa* infections involve the activity of these molecules in a variety of ways. During infection by *P. aeruginosa*, it contributes to host cell lysis, promotes biofilm formation, stimulates the immune response, and aids bacterial adaptation to stress [85]. The QS is also responsible for the synthesis of prodigiosin, a bright red pigment produced by *S. marcescens*. The prodigiosin contributes to the pathogenesis of *S. marcescens* infections, as it is majorly responsible for the formation of biofilm, antimicrobial activity, immunomodulation, and cytotoxicity [86]. It is therefore possible to gain insights into the infections caused by pathogenic bacteria by regulating the activity of QS.

Furthermore, movement of bacteria by swimming is known as swimming motility that involves the rotation of flagella to propel the cell through liquid environments. Swimming motility plays a crucial role in the formation and spread of biofilms, as well as in the regulation of QS signaling pathways that are important for bacterial communication and virulence. Inhibition of swimming motility has therefore raised as a possible way for the development of antibiofilm and anti-QS agents. EPS inhibition is also an emerging strategy for development of antibiofilm and anti-QS agents [87]. The EPS matrix plays an important role for the development of biofilms, providing mechanical stability, protection against environmental stresses, and a barrier to antimicrobial agents. By targeting the EPS matrix or QS signaling pathways, it may be possible to prevent biofilm formation, make biofilms more susceptible to antimicrobial agents and disrupt a wide range of bacterial behaviors [88]. Accordingly, the results of this study clearly indicated that AgNPs-LR synthesized from *L. rhamnosus* played a broad-spectrum antibiofilm and anti-QS activity against Gram-negative pathogenic bacteria.

5. Conclusions

The biosynthesized AgNPs-LR demonstrated a remarkable reduction in multiple QS-regulated functions in Gram-negative bacteria, such as, *C. violaceum*, *P. aeruginosa*, and *S. marcescens*. In *C. violaceum*, there has been a significant decrease in the production of violacein pigments of more than 70%. Upon treatment with AgNPs-LR, *S. marcescens* virulent trait controlled by QS was also reduced by 70%. A dose-dependent inhibition of *P. aeruginosa* virulence factors was also observed with AgNPs-LR. All test bacteria were found to show a decrease in their ability to form biofilms at their respective sub-MICs by a dose-dependently manner. In addition, there was a notable reduction in the formation of biofilms on the surfaces of the coverslips, swimming motility as well as the production of EPS. As a result, it can be concluded that biosynthesized AgNPs-LR could be exploited for the treatment of skin infections resulting from topical application. In addition to this, medical implants/devices can also be coated with these materials in order to inhibit the bacterial adhesion and to prevent the formation of biofilms on the surfaces. However, there is a need to perform more *in-vivo* studies to determine the therapeutic efficacy of AgNPs-LR against infections caused by pathogens that are resistant to known antibiotics.

Author Contributions: Conceptualization, A.M.A., M.A. and M.P.; methodology, C.D., M.S., E.N., A.J.S., S.H. and S.A.A.; validation, C.D., M.S.A., M.S., F.B. and R.B.; formal analysis, C.D., M.P., M.A., M.S., F.B. and R.B.; investigation, C.D., S.A.A., A.J.S., M.S.A. and A.M.A.; data curation, M.P., F.B., A.M.A., S.A.A., S.H. and E.N.; writing—original draft preparation, A.M.A., M.P. and M.A.; writing—review and editing, F.B., M.S., M.S.A., S.H. and E.N.; software, M.A. and M.P.; visualization, M.P. and A.J.S.; supervision, M.A. and M.P.; project administration, M.A. All authors have read and agreed to the published version of the manuscript.

Funding: This research has been funded by Scientific Research Deanship at University of Ha'il-Saudi Arabia through project number RG-21093.

Institutional Review Board Statement: Not applicable.

Informed Consent Statement: Not applicable.

Data Availability Statement: All data generated or analyzed during this study are included in this article.

Acknowledgments: Authors are thankful to Scientific Research Deanship at University of Ha'il-Saudi Arabia for supporting this study through project number RG-21093.

Conflicts of Interest: The authors declare no conflict of interest. The funders had no role in the design of the study; in the collection, analyses, or interpretation of data; in the writing of the manuscript, or in the decision to publish the results.

References

1. Tanwar, J.; Das, S.; Fatima, Z.; Hameed, S. Multidrug Resistance: An Emerging Crisis. *Interdiscip. Perspect. Infect. Dis.* **2014**, *2014*, 541340. [CrossRef]
2. Aslam, B.; Wang, W.; Arshad, M.I.; Khurshid, M.; Muzammil, S.; Rasool, M.H.; Nisar, M.A.; Alvi, R.F.; Aslam, M.A.; Qamar, M.U. Antibiotic Resistance: A Rundown of a Global Crisis. *Infect. Drug Resist.* **2018**, *11*, 1645. [CrossRef] [PubMed]
3. Sabtu, N.; Enoch, D.A.; Brown, N.M. Antibiotic Resistance: What, Why, Where, When and How? *Br. Med. Bull.* **2015**, *116*, 105–113. [CrossRef]
4. Murray, C.J.L.; Ikuta, K.S.; Sharara, F.; Swetschinski, L.; Aguilar, G.R.; Gray, A.; Han, C.; Bisignano, C.; Rao, P.; Wool, E.; et al. Global Burden of Bacterial Antimicrobial Resistance in 2019: A Systematic Analysis. *Lancet* **2022**, *399*, 629–655. [CrossRef]
5. Dadgostar, P. Antimicrobial Resistance: Implications and Costs. *Infect. Drug Resist.* **2019**, *12*, 3903–3910. [CrossRef]
6. Giurazza, R.; Mazza, M.C.; Andini, R.; Sansone, P.; Pace, M.C.; Durante-Mangoni, E. Emerging Treatment Options for Multi-Drug-Resistant Bacterial Infections. *Life* **2021**, *11*, 519. [CrossRef] [PubMed]
7. Roca, I.; Akova, M.; Baquero, F.; Carlet, J.; Cavaleri, M.; Coenen, S.; Cohen, J.; Findlay, D.; Gyssens, I.; Heure, O.E. The Global Threat of Antimicrobial Resistance: Science for Intervention. *New Microbes New Infect.* **2015**, *6*, 22–29. [CrossRef]
8. World Health Organization. *Global Antimicrobial Resistance and Use Surveillance System (GLASS) Report: 2021*; World Health Organization: Geneva, Switzerland, 2021.
9. Mshana, S.E.; Sindato, C.; Matee, M.I.; Mboera, L.E.G. Antimicrobial Use and Resistance in Agriculture and Food Production Systems in Africa: A Systematic Review. *Antibiotics* **2021**, *10*, 976. [CrossRef] [PubMed]
10. Majumder, M.A.A.; Rahman, S.; Cohall, D.; Bharatha, A.; Singh, K.; Haque, M.; Gittens-St Hilaire, M. Antimicrobial Stewardship: Fighting Antimicrobial Resistance and Protecting Global Public Health. *Infect. Drug Resist.* **2020**, *13*, 4713–4738. [CrossRef]
11. Ranjalkar, J.; Chandy, S.J. India's National Action Plan for Antimicrobial Resistance–An Overview of the Context, Status, and Way Ahead. *J. Fam. Med. Prim. Care* **2019**, *8*, 1828. [CrossRef] [PubMed]
12. Sharma, P.; Towse, A. New Drugs to Tackle Antimicrobial Resistance: Analysis of EU Policy Options. *Available SSRN 2640028*. 2010. Available online: https://www.ohe.org/publications/new-drugs-tackle-antimicrobial-resistance-analysis-eu-policy-options/ (accessed on 4 April 2023).
13. Piewngam, P.; Chiou, J.; Chatterjee, P.; Otto, M. Alternative Approaches to Treat Bacterial Infections: Targeting Quorum-Sensing. *Expert Rev. Anti. Infect. Ther.* **2020**, *18*, 499–510. [CrossRef]
14. Davies, D.G.; Parsek, M.R.; Pearson, J.P.; Iglewski, B.H.; Costerton, J.W.; Greenberg, E.P. The Involvement of Cell-to-Cell Signals in the Development of a Bacterial Biofilm. *Science* **1998**, *280*, 295–298. [CrossRef] [PubMed]
15. López, D.; Vlamakis, H.; Kolter, R. Biofilms. *Cold Spring Harb. Perspect. Biol.* **2010**, *2*, a000398. [CrossRef] [PubMed]
16. Donlan, R.M. Biofilm Formation: A Clinically Relevant Microbiological Process. *Clin. Infect. Dis.* **2001**, *33*, 1387–1392. [CrossRef]
17. Schachter, B. Slimy Business—The Biotechnology of Biofilms. *Nat. Biotechnol.* **2003**, *21*, 361–365. [CrossRef]
18. Martins, N.; Rodrigues, C.F. Biomaterial-Related Infections. *J. Clin. Med.* **2020**, *9*, 722. [CrossRef] [PubMed]
19. Lasa, I.; Del Pozo, J.L.; Penadés, J.R.; Leiva, J. Biofilms Bacterianos e Infección. In *Anales del Sistema Sanitario de Navarra*; Gobierno de Navarra. Departamento de Salud: Pamplona, Spain, 2005, Volume 28, pp. 163–175.
20. Qais, F.A.; Khan, M.S.; Ahmad, I. Nanoparticles as Quorum Sensing Inhibitor: Prospects and Limitations. In *Biotechnological Applications of Quorum Sensing Inhibitors*; Springer: Berlin/Heidelberg, Germany, 2018; pp. 227–244.
21. Nagajyothi, P.C.; Cha, S.J.; Yang, I.J.; Sreekanth, T.V.M.; Kim, K.J.; Shin, H.M. Antioxidant and Anti-Inflammatory Activities of Zinc Oxide Nanoparticles Synthesized Using Polygala Tenuifolia Root Extract. *J. Photochem. Photobiol. B Biol.* **2015**, *146*, 10–17. [CrossRef]
22. Manikandan, R.; Manikandan, B.; Raman, T.; Arunagirinathan, K.; Prabhu, N.M.; Basu, M.J.; Perumal, M.; Palanisamy, S.; Munusamy, A. Biosynthesis of Silver Nanoparticles Using Ethanolic Petals Extract of Rosa Indica and Characterization of Its Antibacterial, Anticancer and Anti-Inflammatory Activities. *Spectrochim. Acta Part A Mol. Biomol. Spectrosc.* **2015**, *138*, 120–129. [CrossRef]
23. Mohanpuria, P.; Rana, N.K.; Yadav, S.K. Biosynthesis of Nanoparticles: Technological Concepts and Future Applications. *J. Nanoparticle Res.* **2008**, *10*, 507–517. [CrossRef]

24. Sre, P.R.R.; Reka, M.; Poovazhagi, R.; Kumar, M.A.; Murugesan, K. Antibacterial and Cytotoxic Effect of Biologically Synthesized Silver Nanoparticles Using Aqueous Root Extract of Erythrina Indica Lam. *Spectrochim. Acta Part A Mol. Biomol. Spectrosc.* **2015**, *135*, 1137–1144.
25. Nishiyama, K.; Sugiyama, M.; Mukai, T. Adhesion properties of lactic acid bacteria on intestinal mucin. *Microorganisms* **2016**, *4*, 34. [CrossRef]
26. Zhang, C.; Gui, Y.; Chen, X.; Chen, D.; Guan, C.; Yin, B.; Pan, Z.; Gu, R. Transcriptional homogenization of *Lactobacillus rhamnosus* hsryfm 1301 under heat stress and oxidative stress. *Appl. Microbiol. Biotechnol.* **2020**, *104*, 2611–2621. [CrossRef]
27. Matsubara, V.H.; Wang, Y.; Bandara, H.M.H.N.; Mayer, M.P.A.; Samaranayake, L.P. Probiotic lactobacilli inhibit early stages of *Candida albicans* biofilm development by reducing their growth, cell adhesion, and filamentation. *Appl. Microbiol. Biotechnol.* **2016**, *100*, 6415–6426. [CrossRef] [PubMed]
28. Li, N.; Pang, B.; Li, J.; Liu, G.; Xu, X.; Shao, D.; Jiang, C.; Yang, B.; Shi, J. Mechanisms for *Lactobacillus rhamnosus* treatment of intestinal infection by drug-resistant *Escherichia coli*. *Food Funct.* **2020**, *11*, 4428–4445. [CrossRef]
29. Zhang, W.; Zhu, Y.H.; Yang, G.Y.; Liu, X.; Xia, B.; Hu, X.; Su, J.H.; Wang, J.F. *Lactobacillus rhamnosus* GG affects microbiota and suppresses autophagy in the intestines of pigs challenged with *Salmonella Infantis*. *Front. Microbiol.* **2018**, *8*, 2705. [CrossRef]
30. Assaf, J.C.; Khoury, A.E.; Chokr, A.; Louka, N.; Atoui, A. A novel method for elimination of aflatoxin M1 in milk using *Lactobacillus rhamnosus* GG biofilm. *Int. J. Dairy Technol.* **2019**, *72*, 248–256. [CrossRef]
31. Syame, S.M.; Mansour, A.S.; Khalaf, D.D.; Ibrahim, E.S.; Gaber, E.S. Green Synthesis of Silver Nanoparticles Using Lactic Acid Bacteria: Assessment of Antimicrobial Activity. *World's Vet. J.* **2020**, *10*, 625–633. [CrossRef]
32. Haiss, W.; Thanh, N.T.; Aveyard, J.; Fernig, D.G. Determination of size and concentration of gold nanoparticles from UV−Vis spectra. *Anal. Chem.* **2007**, *79*, 4215–4221. [CrossRef] [PubMed]
33. Adebayo-Tayo, B.C.; Popoola, A.O. Biogenic Synthesis and Antimicrobial Activity of Silver Nanoparticle Using Exopolysaccharides from Lactic Acid Bacteria. *Int. J. Nano Dimens.* **2017**, *8*, 61.
34. Sintubin, L.; De Windt, W.; Dick, J.; Mast, J.; Van Der Ha, D.; Verstraete, W.; Boon, N. Lactic Acid Bacteria as Reducing and Capping Agent for the Fast and Efficient Production of Silver Nanoparticles. *Appl. Microbiol. Biotechnol.* **2009**, *84*, 741–749. [CrossRef]
35. Shameli, K.; Ahmad, M.B.; Yunus, W.M.Z.W.; Ibrahim, N.A.; Rahman, R.A.; Jokar, M.; Darroudi, M. Silver/Poly (Lactic Acid) Nanocomposites: Preparation, Characterization, and Antibacterial Activity. *Int. J. Nanomed.* **2010**, *7*, 573–579. [CrossRef] [PubMed]
36. Biedenbach, D.; Lob, S.; Badal, R.; Sahm, D. Variability of Susceptibility and Multidrug Resistance among *K. pneumoniae* from IAI in Asia/Pacific Countries–SMART 2012–2013. *Int. J. Antimicrob. Agents PO BOX* **2015**, *211*, 1000.
37. Matz, C.; Deines, P.; Boenigk, J.; Arndt, H.; Eberl, L.; Kjelleberg, S.; Jürgens, K. Impact of Violacein-Producing Bacteria on Survival and Feeding of Bacterivorous Nanoflagellates. *Appl. Environ. Microbiol.* **2004**, *70*, 1593–1599. [CrossRef] [PubMed]
38. Slater, H.; Crow, M.; Everson, L.; Salmond, G.P.C. Phosphate Availability Regulates Biosynthesis of Two Antibiotics, Prodigiosin and Carbapenem, in *Serratia* via Both Quorum-sensing-dependent And-independent Pathways. *Mol. Microbiol.* **2003**, *47*, 303–320. [CrossRef]
39. Essar, D.W.; Eberly, L.E.E.; Hadero, A.; Crawford, I.P. Identification and Characterization of Genes for a Second Anthranilate Synthase in *Pseudomonas aeruginosa*: Interchangeability of the Two Anthranilate Synthases and Evolutionary Implications. *J. Bacteriol.* **1990**, *172*, 884–900. [CrossRef] [PubMed]
40. Ankenbauer, R.; Sriyosachati, S.; Cox, C.D. Effects of Siderophores on the Growth of *Pseudomonas aeruginosa* in Human Serum and Transferrin. *Infect. Immun.* **1985**, *49*, 132–140. [CrossRef]
41. Kessler, E.; Safrin, M.; Olson, J.C.; Ohman, D.E. Secreted LasA of *Pseudomonas aeruginosa* is a Staphylolytic Protease. *J. Biol. Chem.* **1993**, *268*, 7503–7508. [CrossRef]
42. Adonizio, A.; Kong, K.-F.; Mathee, K. Inhibition of Quorum Sensing-Controlled Virulence Factor Production in *Pseudomonas aeruginosa* by South Florida Plant Extracts. *Antimicrob. Agents Chemother.* **2008**, *52*, 198–203. [CrossRef]
43. Pinzon, N.M.; Ju, L.-K. Analysis of Rhamnolipid Biosurfactants by Methylene Blue Complexation. *Appl. Microbiol. Biotechnol.* **2009**, *82*, 975–981. [CrossRef]
44. Kumar, L.; Chhibber, S.; Harjai, K. Zingerone Inhibit Biofilm Formation and Improve Antibiofilm Efficacy of Ciprofloxacin against *Pseudomonas aeruginosa* PAO1. *Fitoterapia* **2013**, *90*, 73–78. [CrossRef]
45. Ghaima, K.K.; Rasheed, S.F.; Ahmed, E.F. Antibiofilm, Antibacterial and Antioxidant Activities of Water Extract of *Calendula officinalis* Flowers. *Int. J. Biol. Pharm. Res.* **2013**, *4*, 465–470.
46. Musthafa, K.S.; Ravi, A.V.; Annapoorani, A.; Packiavathy, I.S.V.; Pandian, S.K. Evaluation of Anti-Quorum-Sensing Activity of Edible Plants and Fruits through Inhibition of the N-Acyl-Homoserine Lactone System in *Chromobacterium violaceum* and *Pseudomonas aeruginosa*. *Chemotherapy* **2010**, *56*, 333–339. [CrossRef] [PubMed]
47. Borucki, M.K.; Krug, M.J.; Muraoka, W.T.; Call, D.R. Discrimination among *Listeria monocytogenes* Isolates Using a Mixed Genome DNA Microarray. *Vet. Microbiol.* **2003**, *92*, 351–362. [CrossRef] [PubMed]
48. Guandalini, S. Probiotics for Prevention and Treatment of Diarrhea. *J. Clin. Gastroenterol.* **2011**, *45*, S149–S153. [CrossRef]
49. Ahmed, S.; Ikram, S. Silver Nanoparticles: One Pot Green Synthesis Using *Terminalia arjuna* Extract for Biological Application. *J. Nanomed. Nanotechnol.* **2015**, *6*, 309.

50. Tsuji, T.; Iryo, K.; Watanabe, N.; Tsuji, M. Preparation of silver nanoparticles by laser ablation in solution: Influence of laser wavelength on particle size. *Appl. Surface Sci.* **2002**, *202*, 80–85. [CrossRef]
51. Murphy, C.J.; Jana, N.R. Controlling the aspect ratio of inorganic nanorods and nanowires. *Adv. Mat.* **2002**, *14*, 80–82. [CrossRef]
52. Sastry, M.; Mayya, K.S.; Bandyopadhyay, K. pH Dependent changes in the optical properties of carboxylic acid derivatized silver colloidal particles. *Colloids Surf. A Physicochem. Eng. Asp.* **1997**, *127*, 221–228. [CrossRef]
53. Sondi, I.; Goia, D.V.; Matijević, E. Preparation of Highly Concentrated Stable Dispersions of Uniform Silver Nanoparticles. *J. Colloid Interface Sci.* **2003**, *260*, 75–81. [CrossRef]
54. Torabiana, P.; Ghandeharia, F.; Fatemib, M. Asian Journal of Green Chemistry. *Asian J. Green. Chem.* **2017**, *2*, 89–97.
55. Rajesh, S.; Dharanishanthi, V.; Kanna, A.V. Antibacterial Mechanism of Biogenic Silver Nanoparticles of *Lactobacillus acidophilus*. *J. Exp. Nanosci.* **2015**, *10*, 1143–1152. [CrossRef]
56. Nithya, R.; Ragunathan, R. Synthesis of Silver Nanoparticles Using a Probiotic Microbe and Its Antibacterial Effect against Multidrug Resistant Bacteria. *Afr. J. Biotechnol.* **2012**, *11*, 11013–11021.
57. Xu, C.; Guo, Y.; Qiao, L.; Ma, L.; Cheng, Y.; Roman, A. Biogenic Synthesis of Novel Functionalized Selenium Nanoparticles by Lactobacillus Casei ATCC 393 and Its Protective Effects on Intestinal Barrier Dysfunction Caused by Enterotoxigenic *Escherichia coli* K88. *Front. Microbiol.* **2018**, *9*, 1129. [CrossRef] [PubMed]
58. Markus, J.; Mathiyalagan, R.; Kim, Y.-J.; Abbai, R.; Singh, P.; Ahn, S.; Perez, Z.E.J.; Hurh, J.; Yang, D.C. Intracellular Synthesis of Gold Nanoparticles with Antioxidant Activity by Probiotic *Lactobacillus kimchicus* DCY51T Isolated from Korean Kimchi. *Enzym. Microb. Technol.* **2016**, *95*, 85–93. [CrossRef] [PubMed]
59. Kumar, K.K.; Mahalakshmi, S.; Harikrishna, N.; Reddy, G. Production, characterization and antimicrobial activity of silver nanoparticles produced by *Lactobacillus amylophilus* GV6. *European J. Pharm. Med. Res.* **2016**, *3*, 236242.
60. Garmasheva, I.; Kovalenko, N.; Voychuk, S.; Ostapchuk, A.; Livins'ka, O.; Oleschenko, L. Lactobacillus species mediated synthesis of silver nanoparticles and their antibacterial activity against opportunistic pathogens in vitro. *BioImpacts BI* **2016**, *6*, 219. [CrossRef]
61. Naseer, Q.A.; Xue, X.; Wang, X.; Dang, S.; Din, S.U.; Jamil, J. Synthesis of silver nanoparticles using *Lactobacillus bulgaricus* and assessment of their antibacterial potential. *Braz. J. Biol.* **2021**, *82*, e232434. [CrossRef]
62. Sharma, S.; Sharma, N.; Kaushal, N. Comparative Account of Biogenic Synthesis of Silver Nanoparticles Using Probiotics and Their Antimicrobial Activity Against Challenging Pathogens. *BioNanoScience* **2022**, *12*, 833–840. [CrossRef]
63. Kalaiyarasan, T.; Bharti, V.K.; Chaurasia, O.P. Retracted Article: One Pot Green Preparation of Seabuckthorn Silver Nanoparticles (SBT@ AgNPs) Featuring High Stability and Longevity, Antibacterial, Antioxidant Potential: A Nano Disinfectant Future Perspective. *RSC Adv.* **2017**, *7*, 51130–51141. [CrossRef]
64. Kora, A.J.; Arunachalam, J. Assessment of Antibacterial Activity of Silver Nanoparticles on *Pseudomonas aeruginosa* and Its Mechanism of Action. *World J. Microbiol. Biotechnol.* **2011**, *27*, 1209–1216. [CrossRef]
65. Otto, M. Staphylococcal Biofilms. In *Bacterial Biofilms*; Springer: Berlin/Heidelberg, Germany, 2008; pp. 207–228.
66. Gupta, P.; Chhibber, S.; Harjai, K. Subinhibitory Concentration of Ciprofloxacin Targets Quorum Sensing System of *Pseudomonas aeruginosa* Causing Inhibition of Biofilm Formation & Reduction of Virulence. *Indian J. Med. Res.* **2016**, *143*, 643.
67. Pompilio, A.; Crocetta, V.; De Nicola, S.; Verginelli, F.; Fiscarelli, E.; Di Bonaventura, G. Cooperative Pathogenicity in Cystic Fibrosis: Stenotrophomonas Maltophilia Modulates *Pseudomonas aeruginosa* Virulence in Mixed Biofilm. *Front. Microbiol.* **2015**, *6*, 951. [CrossRef] [PubMed]
68. Nickel, J.C.; Ruseska, I.; Wright, J.B.; Costerton, J.W. Tobramycin Resistance of *Pseudomonas aeruginosa* Cells Growing as a Biofilm on Urinary Catheter Material. *Antimicrob. Agents Chemother.* **1985**, *27*, 619–624. [CrossRef] [PubMed]
69. Ali, K.; Ahmed, B.; Dwivedi, S.; Saquib, Q.; Al-Khedhairy, A.A.; Musarrat, J. Microwave Accelerated Green Synthesis of Stable Silver Nanoparticles with *Eucalyptus globulus* Leaf Extract and Their Antibacterial and Antibiofilm Activity on Clinical Isolates. *PLoS ONE* **2015**, *10*, e0131178. [CrossRef]
70. Ali, S.G.; Ansari, M.A.; Khan, H.M.; Jalal, M.; Mahdi, A.A.; Cameotra, S.S. Antibacterial and Antibiofilm Potential of Green Synthesized Silver Nanoparticles against Imipenem Resistant Clinical Isolates of *P. aeruginosa*. *Bionanoscience* **2018**, *8*, 544–553. [CrossRef]
71. Chhibber, S.; Gondil, V.S.; Sharma, S.; Kumar, M.; Wangoo, N.; Sharma, R.K. A Novel Approach for Combating *Klebsiella pneumoniae* Biofilm Using Histidine Functionalized Silver Nanoparticles. *Front. Microbiol.* **2017**, *8*, 1104. [CrossRef]
72. Miller, M.B.; Bassler, B.L. Quorum Sensing in Bacteria. *Annu. Rev. Microbiol.* **2001**, *55*, 165–199. [CrossRef]
73. Jiang, Q.; Chen, J.; Yang, C.; Yin, Y.; Yao, K. Quorum Sensing: A Prospective Therapeutic Target for Bacterial Diseases. *BioMed Res. Int.* **2019**, *2019*, 2015978. [CrossRef]
74. Gajdács, M.; Spengler, G. The Role of Drug Repurposing in the Development of Novel Antimicrobial Drugs: Non-Antibiotic Pharmacological Agents as Quorum Sensing-Inhibitors. *Antibiotics* **2019**, *8*, 270. [CrossRef]
75. Abraham, W.-R. Controlling Pathogenic Gram-Negative Bacteria by Interfering with Their Biofilm Formation. *Drug Des. Rev.* **2005**, *2*, 13–33. [CrossRef]
76. Vijay, K.; Sakshi, S.; Divya, P. Recent Research Advances on *Chromobacterium violaceum*. *Asian Pac. J. Trop. Med.* **2017**, *10*, 810–818.
77. Lau, G.W.; Hassett, D.J.; Ran, H.; Kong, F. The Role of Pyocyanin in *Pseudomonas aeruginosa* Infection. *Trends Mol. Med.* **2004**, *10*, 599–606. [CrossRef] [PubMed]

78. De Vleesschauwer, D.; Cornelis, P.; Höfte, M. Redox-Active Pyocyanin Secreted by *Pseudomonas aeruginosa* 7NSK2 Triggers Systemic Resistance to Magnaporthe Grisea but Enhances *Rhizoctonia solani* Susceptibility in Rice. *Mol. Plant-Microbe Interact.* **2006**, *19*, 1406–1419. [CrossRef] [PubMed]
79. Usher, L.R.; Lawson, R.A.; Geary, I.; Taylor, C.J.; Bingle, C.D.; Taylor, G.W.; Whyte, M.K.B. Induction of Neutrophil Apoptosis by the *Pseudomonas aeruginosa* Exotoxin Pyocyanin: A Potential Mechanism of Persistent Infection. *J. Immunol.* **2002**, *168*, 1861–1868. [CrossRef] [PubMed]
80. Manago, A.; Becker, K.A.; Carpinteiro, A.; Wilker, B.; Soddemann, M.; Seitz, A.P.; Edwards, M.J.; Grassmé, H.; Szabo, I.; Gulbins, E. *Pseudomonas aeruginosa* Pyocyanin Induces Neutrophil Death via Mitochondrial Reactive Oxygen Species and Mitochondrial Acid Sphingomyelinase. *Antioxid. Redox Signal.* **2015**, *22*, 1097–1110. [CrossRef]
81. Ringel, M.T.; Brüser, T. The Biosynthesis of Pyoverdines. *Microb. Cell* **2018**, *5*, 424. [CrossRef]
82. Meyer, J.-M.; Neely, A.; Stintzi, A.; Georges, C.; Holder, I.A. Pyoverdin Is Essential for Virulence of *Pseudomonas aeruginosa*. *Infect. Immun.* **1996**, *64*, 518–523. [CrossRef] [PubMed]
83. Coin, D.; Louis, D.; Bernillon, J.; Guinand, M.; Wallach, J. LasA, Alkaline Protease and Elastase in Clinical Strains of Pseudomonas Aeruginosa: Quantification by Immunochemical Methods. *FEMS Immunol. Med. Microbiol.* **1997**, *18*, 175–184. [CrossRef]
84. Casilag, F.; Lorenz, A.; Krueger, J.; Klawonn, F.; Weiss, S.; Häussler, S. The LasB Elastase of Pseudomonas Aeruginosa Acts in Concert with Alkaline Protease AprA to Prevent Flagellin-Mediated Immune Recognition. *Infect. Immun.* **2016**, *84*, 162–171. [CrossRef]
85. Caiazza, N.C.; Shanks, R.M.Q.; O'toole, G.A. Rhamnolipids Modulate Swarming Motility Patterns of *Pseudomonas aeruginosa*. *J. Bacteriol.* **2005**, *187*, 7351–7361. [CrossRef]
86. Mun, I.R.A.; Hussin, M.S.; Kadum, M.M. Study of Prodigiosin and Virulence Factor Producing by Multi Drug Resistance *Serratia marcescens* Isolated from Some of Baghdad Hospitals Environment. *Al-Mustansiriyah J. Sci.* **2008**, *19*, 1–9.
87. De La Fuente-Núñez, C.; Korolik, V.; Bains, M.; Nguyen, U.; Breidenstein, E.B.M.; Horsman, S.; Lewenza, S.; Burrows, L.; Hancock, R.E.W. Inhibition of Bacterial Biofilm Formation and Swarming Motility by a Small Synthetic Cationic Peptide. *Antimicrob. Agents Chemother.* **2012**, *56*, 2696–2704. [CrossRef] [PubMed]
88. Lin, Y.; Chen, J.; Zhou, X.; Li, Y. Inhibition of *Streptococcus mutans* Biofilm Formation by Strategies Targeting the Metabolism of Exopolysaccharides. *Crit. Rev. Microbiol.* **2021**, *47*, 667–677. [CrossRef] [PubMed]

antibiotics

MDPI

Review

A Comprehensive Review on Significance and Advancements of Antimicrobial Agents in Biodegradable Food Packaging

Ipsheta Bose [1,†], Swarup Roy [2,*], Vinay Kumar Pandey [3,4,†] and Rahul Singh [3,*]

1 School of Bioengineering and Food Technology, Shoolini University, Solan 173229, India; ipsheta18@gmail.com
2 Department of Food Technology and Nutrition, School of Agriculture, Lovely Professional University, Phagwara 144411, India
3 Department of Bioengineering, Integral University, Lucknow 226026, India; vinaypandey794@gmail.com
4 Department of Biotechnology, Axis Institute of Higher Education, Kanpur 209402, India
* Correspondence: swaruproy2013@gmail.com (S.R.); rahulsingh.jnu@gmail.com (R.S.)
† First and third author share equal first authorship.

Abstract: Food waste is key global problem and more than 90% of the leftover waste produced by food packaging factories is dumped in landfills. Foods packaged using eco-friendly materials have a longer shelf life as a result of the increased need for high-quality and secure packaging materials. For packaging purposes, natural foundation materials are required, as well as active substances that can prolong the freshness of the food items. Antimicrobial packaging is one such advancement in the area of active packaging. Biodegradable packaging is a basic form of packaging that will naturally degrade and disintegrate in due course of time. A developing trend in the active and smart food packaging sector is the use of natural antioxidant chemicals and inorganic nanoparticles (NPs). The potential for active food packaging applications has been highlighted by the incorporation of these materials, such as polysaccharides and proteins, in biobased and degradable matrices, because of their stronger antibacterial and antioxidant properties, UV-light obstruction, water vapor permeability, oxygen scavenging, and low environmental impact. The present review highlights the use of antimicrobial agents and nanoparticles in food packaging, which helps to prevent undesirable changes in the food, such as off flavors, colour changes, or the occurrence of any foodborne outcomes. This review attempts to cover the most recent advancements in antimicrobial packaging, whether edible or not, employing both conventional and novel polymers as support, with a focus on natural and biodegradable ingredients.

Keywords: biodegradable; biopolymers; antimicrobial agent; active packaging; food industry

1. Introduction

Food packaging is described as enclosing meals to defend them from tampering or infection from physical, chemical, and biological sources, where active packaging is considered the most desirable packaging system used for retaining meals products [1]. The four essential purposes of traditional food packaging are containment and communication, protection and preservation, convenience and marketing [2]. Food packaging has to meet some criteria, including legislation, protection, and plenty of different situations, since it is required to be innovative, clean to apply, and have an appealing design. One of the principal duties of packaging within the food enterprise is to guard the product from chemical, mechanical, and microbiological impact, and additionally maintain the freshness of the product and its dietary value. Good packaging prevents waste and guarantees that the meals keep their flavor until some stage in their shelf life. Despite its significance and the important function that packaging plays, it is often seen as, at best, incredibly superfluous, and, at worst, a critical waste of resources and an environmental menace. The world loses an astounding quantity of food every year. Globally, around USD 750 billion worth of food is frittered away each year throughout the entire supply chain, among which up to 25% of residential meal waste is because of packaging size or design, for example, meals spoiling because of loss of packaging, condiments sticking to the perimeter and bottom of packing containers, or the inability to pack bulk clean ingredients for well-timed consumption [3,4]. Packaging waste, that from non-biodegradable polymers in particular, has ended up generating a large part of municipal solid waste, which results in a number of growing environmental concerns.

A significant waste management difficulty is presented by the very evident source of litter composed of leftover packaging. The petroleum-based polymer polyethylene (PE), which is one of these materials, is most frequently utilized in packaging applications [5]. After being dumped on land or along the coast, petroleum-based polymers such as PE are incredibly resistant to biodegradation, resulting in various degrees of contamination. To cope with this problem, a whole lot of interest has been paid to developing biodegradable polymers from renewable resources in recent years [6]. Numerous studies have shown great possibilities of new food packaging technologies using biodegradable and bio-based packaging material [7]. To lessen the environmental impact and petro-dependence, non-biodegradable plastics can be replaced with biopolymer. Biopolymers are the most promising alternative to synthetic plastic material for packaging that fully decomposes or can be composted [8]. Similar to this, there is current interest in the development of novel and more complex methods to prevent food from becoming contaminated by pathogenic microorganisms as a result of antimicrobial packaging, which refers to packaging systems that can prevent or eliminate pathogenic microorganisms from existing in the food [7]. However, the demand for environmentally friendly, affordable, sustainable materials has given a variety of naturally occurring antimicrobial compounds a fresh, intriguing outlook.

The growing trend also brings us to a point where we need to focus on antimicrobial packaging because spoilage due to microbial growth is one of the major problems faced by the food industry. These types of microbial growth elevate the risk of food-borne diseases and also alter the nutritional properties of the food product. In this sense, applying natural antimicrobial compounds to the packaging material will create a better packaging technology. As we all know that food packaging innovations have gradually accelerated towards the development of intelligent packaging throughout the beginning of the current millennium, the general motive of this paper is to provide an overview of ongoing research and the latest technologies which show the perspective of the next generation of intelligent, active food packaging systems that will sense various changes in the packaging or its environment [7]. An important development trend for the evolution of packaging is the incorporation of extremely effective antibacterial nanoparticles, antifungals, and antioxidants to biodegradable and environmentally friendly green polymers [2]. Due to increased awareness and needs for sustainable active packaging that may maintain the quality and extend the shelf life of foods and products, the development of antimicrobial packaging has been advancing quickly. Antimicrobial agents, if infused into the packing film, will prevent or eradicate the pathogenic microorganisms that cause food spoilage and sickness [3]. The uses of this novel packaging method for food, however, are still few. Even if this idea gains popularity and appears promising on paper, it is difficult to manage how much of an active ingredient is released into food, and little research has attempted to address this issue [2]. One effective way for expanding the shelf life of packaged food goods is the inclusion of active ingredients into natural and synthetic polymers and the development of coatings/films [6]. Theoretically, antimicrobial drugs ought to be given out at a controlled rate. Additionally, to prevent negative effects on sensory and toxicological qualities, the concentration of the released antimicrobial agent should be neither too high nor too low [3]. The use of cutting-edge active packaging methods in conjunction with innovative antimicrobial drugs has gained popularity. Sorbic acid is known to prevent the germination of bacterial spores, and both fungal and bacterial cell development is inhibited by organic acids. The fundamental cause of the inhibitory effect of organic acids is the compound's entry into the plasma membrane in its protonated form. As a result, the acid will dissociate when it comes into contact with the higher pH inside the cell, releasing charged protons and anions that cannot flow through the plasma membrane. Additionally, the inhibiting effect of organic acids on yeasts may be brought on by the start of a stressful reaction that is so demanding that attempts to restore equilibrium and avoid other negative effects result in the depletion of resources [8].

By utilizing the various antimicrobial packaging solutions, sustainable active packaging that meets industry standards for higher safety and quality as well as a longer shelf life will be even better. By using renewable and biodegradable polymers rather than typical synthetic ones, antimicrobial packaging not only has a number of benefits but also protects the environment by lowering the amount of plastic pollution produced by humans. The World Wildlife Fund also noted in 2018 that almost 60% of the estimated 8 million tonnes of plastic that enter the oceans annually came from China, Indonesia, Malaysia, the Philippines, Thailand, and Vietnam [9]. The considerable amount of extremely hazardous emissions, composting management concerns, and changes in the carbon dioxide cycle are mostly to blame for this environmental threat. Therefore, this phenomenon has drawn the attention of numerous researchers who are working to produce sustainable, active packaging materials. As a result, packaging design should take user-friendliness and environmental sustainability into account in addition to shelf life, cost, and protection [10].

One effective method for extending the shelf life of packaged food goods is the inclusion of active chemicals into natural and synthetic polymers and the development of film or coatings. A variety of polymers, including agar, pullulan, carrageenan, alginate, cellulose acetate soy protein, and chitosan, have been implemented to create films that contain antibacterial ingredients [6]. The advantage of these biopolymers is their sustainability, renewability as well as biodegradability, which make them superior over the synthetic petrochemical-derived plastics [2]. Recent reports suggest the bio-based polymers or bioplastics are easily degradable in soil and sea water, although the rate of degradation is highly dependent on the type of polymers and the other fillers present in the composite [8]. Most of the bio-based polymers are highly biodegradable and their use in the packaging is not harmful to our environment nor for our health. In order to allow the integrated antimicrobial peptide to diffuse and protect against bacteria that may be present on the food surface, appropriate contact between the active packing material and the food product must be ensured [3].

Antimicrobial peptides are primarily incorporated into packaging materials using three different techniques: direct integration into polymer matrix, immobilization, and coating on the material's surface [11]. To ensure the proper protective function during the anticipated shelf life, a balance between the development of microbial kinetics and the controlled release rate should be created. Controlling the rate at which antimicrobial agents leak from packaging and then diffuse into food products is thus one of the most intriguing difficulties in the practical application of antimicrobial systems. The effectiveness of active packaging systems can be impacted by such polymer-specific characteristics as mass transport, permeability, sorption, and migration. Traditional polymers can be thermally combined with tiny antibacterial agents. In this instance, the polymeric material's amorphous zones could accommodate the antimicrobial chemicals without appreciably affecting the polymer's internal structure [12]. A rising number of people are interested in developing and using controlled-release strategies for such compounds by making slight adjustments to the chemical and physical characteristics of the hosting materials to make them meet the specifications for food packaging materials [13].

The summary of current developments and uses of antimicrobial biodegradable films in the packaging sector, as well as the development of nanotechnology to produce highly effective new, bio-based packaging solutions, are the main topics of this review. Because of this, the impact of appealing product packaging on consumer purchase behaviour is significant. The majority of consumers prefer the new, added value that modern packaging technology has over conventional packaging. To meet the rising demand for packaged, ready-to-eat foods, which is regarded as a major driver of future packaging trends, the integration of these responsive technologies into food packaging will have a significant impact on the food processing sectors.

In general, antimicrobial agents can inhibit microbial growth in a variety of ways, including by changing the structure of proteins through modification or denaturation; altering the proteins or lipids in cell membranes; preventing the synthesis of components of cell walls; hindering the replication, transcription, and translation of nucleic acids; and interfering with cellular metabolism. Particularly in the context of perishable foods, the antimicrobial agents included into packing materials greatly increase microbiological safety, shelf life, and quality [14]. Antimicrobial agents can change the structure and engineering characteristics of packaging materials, including their tensile strength, gas permeability, and optical, thermal, morphological, and physical properties [15]. Clarke et al. 2016, investigated the physical characteristics of produced gelatin-based films containing the antibacterial agents Articoat DLP 02 (AR), Artemix Consa 152/NL (AXE), Auranta FV (AFV), and sodium octanoate (SO) [16]. The prepared films reported values for thickness, color, and transparency that were significantly greater than those of the control films. The very first polymeric nanocomposite to hit the market was clay, a revolutionary material for food packaging, with MMT being the most popular type. According to reports, the nanoclay contained in food packaging films reduces the rate of gas transmission to maintain the freshness and extend the shelf life of foods that are susceptible to oxygen [17]. Strong antibacterial activity against foodborne pathogenic microorganisms was demonstrated using gelatin-based nanocomposite films mixed with specific organic fillers and nanometals such titanium dioxide (TiO_2), nanocopper (CuNPs), nanosilver (AgNPs), and zinc oxide nanoparticles (ZnO NPs). The active food packaging sector has a high potential for using the antibacterial gelatin-based nanocomposite films [18].

Innovative antimicrobial food packaging films are often made of bio-based polymers, which are biocompatible and safe for human consumption. The majority of them are edible and generally recognized as safe (GRAS)-classified. For instance, chitosan and cellulose are GRAS on the micron scale. Although nanocellulose shows little cytotoxicity, it may nevertheless affect the population of gut bacteria and change intestinal function by impairing nutritional absorption [19]. However, in addition to its benefits, nanotechnology also poses certain threats and has unfavorable effects on both the environment and people. The non-degradable and persistent character of nanomaterials is primarily responsible for their toxicological effects, whereas the advantageous elements of the unique properties of nanoparticles are provided by their tiny size and high surface area. However, it also has negative side effects, such as a high reactivity when interacting with biological elements [20]. Due to their high level of activity, nanoparticles can easily bypass blood arteries and membrane barriers, which could have a variety of hazardous effects. Additionally, given their small size and huge surface area, nanoparticles have unique biokinetic properties that may promote their migration from packing materials to food products as well as their likelihood of free movement and cell penetration in the body [21]. The toxicological concern of Ag, ZnO, and CuO nanoparticles is among the most studied and researched, as various studies indicate a strong relation between decreasing nanoparticle size and increasing phytotoxicity [22]. The toxicity of nanoparticles has been found to be inversely related to particle size, meaning that toxicity rises as particle size decreases. For instance, compared to silver nanoparticles with a diameter of 100 nm, 20 nm silver nanoparticles are more hazardous to lung tissue. Therefore, the transfer of nano-components from packaging to food may result in negative health effects. A few reports have also indicated that these components may be genotoxic and carcinogenic [23]. Studies on essential oils show that at the concentrations used in food packaging, they are not hazardous. There are some worries that when essential oils are used to prevent pathogenic bacteria, they may also have a harmful effect on beneficial microorganisms [24]. Last but not least, before nanomaterials are actually commercialized, more research on the health and environmental safety of these materials is still required.

Numerous review articles on the use of antimicrobial compounds in packaging materials have recently been published that mainly highlight how well the substance reduces food spoilage and discuss how to include or use these ingredients in packaging materials. However, new developments in nanotechnology and the creation of biodegradable packaging material using different compounds have gained the limelight. In this review article, we briefly discuss various organic and chemical-based antimicrobial compounds which can be utilized in forming biodegradable packaging material, while highlighting recent research studies on the application of nanotechnology to build novel bio-based packaging solutions; this study assesses the current situation and applications of antimicrobial biodegradable films in the food packaging business.

2. Classification of Antimicrobial Agents

The main cause of food rotting is microbial infection. Food-borne microbial illnesses are treated using antimicrobial medicines. They are also utilized in the food packaging sector to create antimicrobial packaging films that protect food's structure, texture, color, and nutritional content. Food demand is increasing in tandem with population growth. Food waste must be stopped, and rotting must be avoided. The majority of the food spoils while being harvested, transported, and distributed. It is important to solve this significant issue. The most convenient technique to lessen food degradation and contamination is to add antibacterial agents. Each antimicrobial agent has a distinct mechanism and responds to various kinds of microbes in a different way. In this instance, the sorts of antimicrobials might sometimes place limitations on how they can be used. A suitably continuous, sticky, and cohesive matrix must be formed by at least one component during the production of antimicrobial films. A formulation like this includes a plasticizer (sorbitol, glycerol, and water), a pH-adjusting agent (acid, sodium hydroxide, and others), a film-forming agent (polymer), a solvent (ethanol, water, and others), and an antibacterial agent [11]. Depending on what the packaging material is being used for, different antimicrobial agents may be chosen. One of the most demanding methods for food preservation, food packaging, has undergone several alterations to support the characteristics and qualities of antibacterial materials. Due to historical reasons, low cost, and effective barrier properties, petrochemical polymers are currently the basis for the majority of food packaging materials. These polymers are not biodegradable, and they have already caused significant environmental problems in terms of short- and long-term contamination [12]. Antimicrobial packaging containing antimicrobial agents interacts with packed food in order to take effect, such as to inhibit, reduce, or retard microbial growth along with increasing shelf life of the food product [13]. Food-borne microbial diseases are treated with antimicrobial agents. They also benefit the food packaging sector, as they are utilized for the manufacture of antimicrobial packaging films which protect the structure, texture, color, and nutrient value of food. The antimicrobial packaging techniques fall into two categories. The first type is represented by packaging materials that allow for direct contact between the preserved food and an antimicrobial surface, allowing for the migration of active ingredients into the food. These containers are used for food that has been vacuum-sealed or wrapped in foil. The modified atmospheric packaging (MAP) is a second tactic that places the antimicrobial agent inside the package but out of direct contact with the food [14,15]. Bioactive agents can be added directly to packing compounds to create antimicrobial packaging, they can be coated onto packaging surfaces to create antimicrobial packaging, or they can be incorporated into films made of antimicrobial polymers [16]. Organic acids, enzymes, bacteriocins, fungicides, natural extracts, ions, ethanol, polyphenols, protein hydrolysates, and other substances can all be used as active agents [17,18].

In a recent research work it has been highlighted that there are a few salts and organic acids which possess strong antimicrobial properties; some agents include sorbic, benzoic, acetic, propionic, and ascorbic acids, and they can change the transport and permeability of membranes as well as the pH levels inside cells [19]. Essential oils and aqueous or alcoholic extracts from herbs, spices, and plants such as basil, eucalyptus, thyme, mustard, and clove lemon, horseradish, onion, garlic, rosemary, and oregano have been researched as antimicrobial agents [21,22]. In another study, a concept was proposed which says that bacterial infections, particularly those brought on by Gram-positive bacteria, can be prevented by lysozyme [23,24]. Its activity is explained by its capacity to hydrolyze the primary component of the cell wall, which results in the loss of intracellular components and bacterial death, which proves that enzymes can be used as an antimicrobial agent and can be incorporated in packaging.

3. Types of Antimicrobial Agent

3.1. Natural Antimicrobial Agent

There are several natural compounds which possess certain antibacterial activities. Some of these natural or organic compounds are used in the industry on a very large scale. One of the most significant sources of antimicrobial packaging is natural antibacterial agents. They are safe for health because they are natural. A crucial characteristic of antibacterial organic compounds is that they exhibit long life and high stability under specific conditions, such as heat, but they also have some drawbacks, such as weak mold-resistant activity; as a result, a large dosage is required when used professionally on an industrial scale. Some research has given a brief description of natural antimicrobial agents, the sources of some antimicrobial agents from animal and plant origins, the packaging materials in which they are frequently incorporated, the foods for which these packaging materials are also made, and the microorganisms active in these natural antimicrobial agents [25]. It also lists some antimicrobial agents' sources from animal, plant, and microbial origins [26].

3.2. Plant-Based Antimicrobial Agent

The food sector is employing practical methods, such as the utilization of multiple plant-based compounds as a natural antibacterial agent in polymeric materials, to fully capitalize on the advantages and benefits of each material while also overcoming the downsides and shortcomings of each component. Individual volatile molecules are called essential oils (EOs). The effects of plant extracts employed as antibacterial agents in the form of thin edible films on food products are significant. These chemicals extended the shelf life of packaged foods and reduced waste [27]. They are obtained specifically from aromatic plants. Some of the most effective natural extracts are ginger, garlic, oregano, thyme, cinnamon, clove, coriander, and more [28]. The antimicrobial actions on particular microbes are brought on by the presence of active chemicals in these substances, such as flavanols, terpenes, anthocyanins, phenolic acids, tannins, and stilbenes. Additionally, they could offer other health advantages, similar to dietary supplements [29]. Ground beef's shelf life was increased by up to 12 days using a composite made of PLA and nanocellulose infused with plant essential oils (*Mentha piperita* or *Bunium percicum*). Authors in [30] have created three-component composite films based on PLA blended with chitosan and packed with tea polyphenols in a range of molar ratios. The composite film made of PLA, tea polyphenols, and chitosan exhibits up to three times more strength. Thyme and tarragon are common plants that contain caffeic acid, which has a potent antibacterial, antiviral, and antifungal action. The phenolic structures of flavones only contain one carbonyl group. It should be noted that they are effective antibacterial compounds acting against a wide variety of microorganisms and are thought to be produced by plants in response to microbial infection.

In contrast to minor components like ketones and aldehydes, spice and herb extracts contain phenolic, terpene, and aliphatic alcohols with antimicrobial properties [31]. Besides the antimicrobial activity, they offer antioxidant activity and other medicinal effects [32]. From this perspective, using antimicrobial compounds originating from plant sources could be a great option, especially for food packaging. *Listeria*-infected cheese can be preserved for 24 days using starch films that have been infused with clove leaf oil. Clove leaf oil performs a variety of functions, including enhancing tensile strength and elongation break as well as reducing *L. monocytogenes* proliferation, acting as a UV barrier, and scavenging free radicals [33]. The loss of plant-derived antimicrobial compounds during high-temperature processing and decreased antibacterial effectiveness are the current problems with plant-derived antimicrobial compounds [34]. Plants that contain phytochemicals are generally essential, especially those that have therapeutic advantages [35–39]. Due to rising consumer demand for safer food additives, numerous studies and evaluations have been carried out in photochemistry about natural antimicrobial agents. Table 1 describes the sources of some antimicrobial agents from plant origins.

Table 1. Active compound isolated/extracted from natural antimicrobial agents.

Natural Extract	Active Compounds	Antimicrobial Action	Reference
Oregano	Carvacrol and thymol	*Salmonella* enteric, mold and yeast, and mesophilic aerobic bacteria	[40]
Clove and thyme	Eugenol and thymol	*Escherichia coli*	[41]
Eucalyptus radiata	eucalyptol	Gram-negative bacteria	[42]
Grapefruit seed	phenolic compounds	*Pseudomonas fluorescence* and *Escherichia coli*	[43]
Apricot kernels	oleic acid	*Escherichia coli* and *Bacillus subtilis*	[44]
cinnamon	cinnamaldehyde	*R. nigricans* and *S. aureus*	[45]
Basil	Chavicol and eugenol	*L. curvatus* and *S. cerevisiae*	[46]
Tea polyphenols	Polyphenols	*Escherichia coli* and *Staphylococcus aureus*	[47]
Mentha rotundifolia L.	Ferulic acid	*Salmonella typhimurium*, *Escherichia coli*, *S. aureus*	[48]
Olive leaf extract	polyphenolic compounds	*Escherichia coli* and *L. innocua*	[49]
Chitosin	polycationic compounds	*S. aureus*, *Listeria monocytogenes*, and *Enterococcus faecalis*	[50]
Bacteriocins	Peptide	*Micrococcus luteus*, *S. aureus*, and *Bacillus cereus*	[51]
Cellulose		*Staphylococcus aureus*, *Escherichia coli*, and *Candida albicans*.	[52]
Starch		*Escherichia coli*	[53]
Lysozyme		Gram-positive bacteria	[54]

3.3. Animal and Microbe-Based Antimicrobial Agent

Mostly natural agents derived from plants were discussed in the previous section. In this section, antimicrobial agents derived from animal and microorganisms are briefly discussed. Today, a variety of strategies are employed to increase the effectiveness and production of natural antibacterial agents. These methods have enhanced the effectiveness of natural antibacterial agents and ensured the safety of food packaging. Pathogens are currently a big hazard to the food business. Dealing with the condition is highly challenging because the infections have rapid growth rates and develop a resistance to the antibacterial agents. In this situation, researchers put forth a lot of effort to overcome this problem. Hossain et al. 2017, in their study, explained that probiotics are the live microbes that are provided to humans and animals [50]. They act as the antibacterial agents in the intestinal tract and can fight harmful microbes in the ingested food. Bacteriocins from microorganisms (natamycin and nisin), as well as lactoferrin and lysozyme enzyme from animals, are natural preservatives used in food packaging [51]. In the twenty-first century, animal-derived antimicrobial agents are frequently employed in food packaging. The hypothetical study leads to the conclusion that sea cucumber is very significant from a medical and dietary standpoint. It is believed to have been used in the past to treat wounds, and current research suggests that it possesses antibacterial and antioxidant qualities. In most of Asia's regions today, it is employed in the food and pharmaceutical industries [52]. Next to cellulose, lignin is the second-most prevalent renewable and biodegradable natural resource. It includes a variety of functional groups in varying proportions, giving room for chemical modification and polarity adjustment to produce compatibility with suitable polymeric matrices [53]. The literature has determined that a variety of polymeric substances derived from animals, such as chitosan, protein hydrolysates, bioactive peptides, whey protein, etc., display innate antibacterial activity. Various bacteria, including *Escherichia coli, Bacillus cereus, Salmonella typhimurium, Staphylococcus aureus* and *Listeria monocytogenes*, as well as mold and yeast, including *Rhizoctonia solani, Botrytis cinerea, Fusarium oxysporum*, and *Candida lambica*, have shown antagonistic behavior toward chitosan [54]. Natural antimicrobials, such as bacteriocins, have a "green" nature and are well-known for their antimicrobial efficacies. In order to prevent synthetic antimicrobials from migrating into food, great effort has been paid to substituting naturally occurring antimicrobials with those found in synthetic ones. Bacteriocins are ribosomal-generated antimicrobial peptides made by bacteria that can prevent or eradicate other closely related bacteria from multiplying [55]. The various types of sustainable antimicrobial materials derived from animal and microorganism sources are updated, and future trends are examined, along with their compositions, traits, antimicrobial mechanisms, and food applications. Despite their impressive properties, more research is needed to confirm the materials' safety and effectiveness.

3.4. Chemical Antimicrobial Agent

As an antibacterial, organic acids and their salts are used in food packaging. Sorbic, propionic, lactic, acetic, and benzoic acids make up the majority of organic acids. By transferring nutrients and metabolizing them, they compromise the integrity of microorganisms' cell membranes and macromolecules [56]. Inorganic, organic, and biologically active compounds are among the antimicrobial agents employed in the creation of antimicrobial packaging materials [57]. The implementation of organic acids as antimicrobial agents in the food material depends on several characteristic properties of the acids, such as the chemical formula, physical form, pKa value, molecular weight, minimum inhibitory concentration, nature of the microorganism, buffering properties of the food, and acid–food exposure time [58]. These tests have shown that it is possible to make antimicrobial packaging from substances that are already used in the food business, typically in the form of a nanocomposite film. One of the biggest issues with the adoption of new technologies is the rise in production costs. With only minor changes to the production lines, the industry will adopt new technologies that can be reverse-engineered from the ones already in use. These adjustments may result from new rules, projections of higher earnings, shifts in public opinion and demand, or other factors [59]. The second most popular polysaccharide utilized to make edible films and biodegradable packaging is cellulose. It is available from a wide range of bacterial sources. Acidic hydrolysis can produce cellulose nanocrystals from bacterial cellulose (BC) from *Gluconacetobacter xylinus*. The factors limiting the applicability domains include the low mechanical performance and the lack of water resistance. The antimicrobial agent is applied to the cellulose to boost the added value of the packaging materials [60]. Organic acids, which are widely used in the industry for diverse purposes [61], can be generated by numerous microorganisms; the biological manufacture of organic acids via microbial fermentations has advantages over the chemical production techniques, such as cost-effectiveness, practicality, reliability, environmental friendliness, sustainability, and reduced carbon footprints (Table 2).

Table 2. Commonly used organic acids in the food industry.

Organic Acids	Antimicrobial Action	Reference
Malic acid	*L. monocytogenes*, *S. gaminara*	[62]
Phenyllactic acid	*E. cloacae*	[63]
Propionic acid	*E. coli* and *Salmonella*	[64]
Citric acid	*Sh. flexneri*	[65]
Sorbic acid	*Yeast* and *mold*	[66]
Oxalic acid	*Escherichia coli*	[67]
Acetic acid	*Shigella*	[68]
potassium sorbate	Bacteria and molds	[69]
Sodium citrate	*Listeria*, *bladder*, and *Escherichia coli*	[70]
Allyl isothiocyanate	*E. coli*	[71]

4. Potential Applications of Antimicrobial Packaging in Food

Antimicrobial agents are useful for many applications, including packaging and the pharmaceutical industry (Figure 1). Recently, there has been a huge growth in the need for biodegradable and renewable materials for packaging applications. There is a market demand for healthy and natural food products, and the strict guidelines to prevent infectious diseases that are spread by food; recalls have inspired researchers to develop new methods of delivering antimicrobials, which should lead to enhancing the food products' quality and safety over the course of storage. A promising type of active food packaging that is still in its infancy is antimicrobial packaging. Regulations for food packaging require a fresh strategy. Although promising, antimicrobial food packaging currently only has a few applications. This is as a result of the tested additives' status as authorized substances [71]. Furthermore, microbial activity is a major concern in the food packaging sector. Therefore, using antimicrobial agents or polymers to create barrier-enhanced or active packaging materials offers a desirable option for guarding against the growth and spread of microorganisms on food [72]. The use of an antimicrobial agent should be combined with biodegradable packaging materials for a more thorough approach. This is due to the fact that the use of biodegradable packaging films is currently a highly recognized global trend, particularly when the biodegradable components are generated from renewable resources. The application of antimicrobial agents in different food systems is briefly represented in Table 3.

Table 3. Antimicrobial agents' antimicrobial efficacy in various dietary products.

Antimicrobial Agent	Food Product	Targeted Microorganism	Reference
triclosan	Meat	*Triclosan*, *S. aureus*, *B. thermosphacta*	[73]
wasabi extract AM	Raw meat	*E. coli* and *S. aureus*, fungi *A. niger*, *P. italicum*.	[74]
Olive leaf extract	cheese	*S. aureus*	[75]
Grape seed extract	pork loin	*L. monocytogenes*, *E. coli*, *E. faecalis*, *E. faecium*, *S. typhimurium*, and *B. thermosphaceta B2*	[76]
Chitosan and cinnamaldehyde	vacuum-packed cured meat products (bologna, cooked ham, and pastrami)	*Enterobacteriaceae*, *Serratia liquefaciens*, and *Lactobacillus sakei*	[77]
Corn zein	Ready-to-eat chicken	*L. monocytogenes*	[78]
Pimento EOs	Beef muscle slices	*Pseudomonas* spp. and *E. coli* O157:H7	[79]

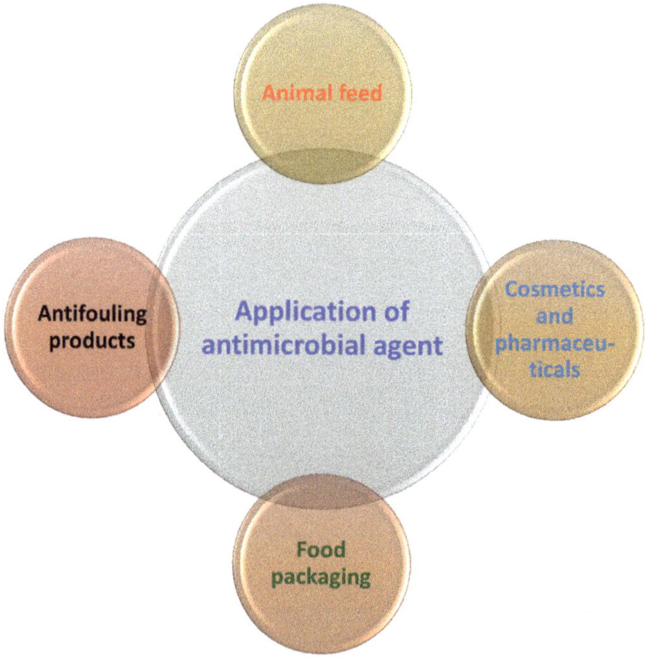

Figure 1. Various applications of antimicrobial agent.

Antimicrobial packaging is crucial for food packing as it may increase the shelf life and ensure food preservation. In terms of food product and food packaging films, antimicrobial packaging systems have offered various innovative technologies, among which one of the trending and most focused systems is the concept of active packaging. One of the most innovative active packaging technologies is antimicrobial packaging, which has several uses, including oxygen-scavenging packaging and moisture-controlling packaging [79]. In this sector, there is growing interest in edible packaging films due to environmental concerns of synthetic polymer-based packaging materials. The concept of biodegradable active packaging has been improved with edible packaging films with antibacterial coatings. On the surface of food goods, they have been employed to lessen and prevent the growth of germs through chemical and physical mechanisms. An antimicrobial packaging (AM) system seeks to safeguard packaged foods against various microbes [80].

Nanocrystalline cellulose (CNC) and cellulose nanofibers (CNFs) are biopolymers that are abundantly available in nature, biodegradable, non-toxic, and renewable. They can be extracted from lignocellulosic plants or produced by microbes. Nanocellulose (NC), which has a high surface-to-volume ratio and special physicochemical characteristics such as surface chemistry, high crystallinity, mechanical strength, and morphology in nanometer structures, enhances the packaging properties of nanocomposites such as coatings and nanofillers in films (81). On the other hand, the industry could also benefit from the creation of gelatin and other biodegradable films by using less water, solid waste, electricity, and emissions. Additionally, biopolymer-based films have a strong matrix and compatibility that makes it possible for antimicrobial and antioxidant agents to be incorporated into the film and perform their respective tasks for extending the shelf life, functionality, and safety of food products (82). Research was conducted earlier (83) to create smoke-flavored antimicrobial packaging using coconut fiber manufactured from *Litsea cubeba* oil at 0.03%, 0.06%, and 0.09% w/w mixed with wood smoking for 30, 45, and 60 min. The goal was to extend the shelf life of dried fish and check the antibacterial effect and smoky flavor. *Aspergillus niger* was completely prevented from sprouting on the outermost layer of dried fish by the prepared packaging material. Additionally, the treated packaging produced volatile compounds to keep dried fish fresh for at least 21 days at room temperature (30 °C) without the growth of bacteria or mold.

Future studies are likely to combine biopreservatives, biodegradable packaging materials, and naturally produced antimicrobial agents, which will highlight a wide variety of antimicrobial packaging in regards to food safety, longevity, and environmental friendliness. A helpful technology in antimicrobial packaging systems successfully charges the antimicrobial properties within the food packaging film medium and eventually produces it over the necessary period of time to kill the harmful microbes influencing food products [81]. The use of natural antibacterial chemicals is one of the new technologies that has gained popularity because it has no hazardous or unfavourable impacts on consumers. A study [82] has proven that the allyl isothiocyanate (AITC) from ground mustard seeds, when incorporated in designing active antimicrobial packaging, possesses the ability to inhibit the growth of microorganisms. PHB, PLGA, and starch derivatives all have properties that make them suitable for various antimicrobial packaging agents. In biomedical and food applications, they have been examined for both harmful and spoilage microorganisms under various testing settings [83]. The perfect AM polymer films should therefore satisfy a number of key requirements, with the ease and affordability of the AM film production process being the most crucial in the food business. Second, for long-term use and storage, the films must be chemically stable. As a water barrier and to preserve the AM effect during the packing period, the AM film must also be durable. It is crucial that the packaging materials for AM do not release dangerous particles into food and are safe to handle. However, due to factors including inadequate understanding regarding the effectiveness of AM in polymer films, economic impact, consumer acceptance, and a lack of particular rules surrounding active packaging, the development and deployment of natural AM active packaging is constrained.

The antimicrobial packaging system is a hurdle to preventing degradation of total quality of packaged food, providing protection against microorganisms. The application of preservative hurdles like low storage temperature, the addition of antimicrobials and/or antioxidants, water activity, pH, and high-pressure processing with alternative packaging, such as modified atmospheres, has generally shown the potential to further extend the shelf life of food products, as diagrammatically represented in the above Figure 2. The Figure 2 describes the hurdle technology in terms of moisture barrier, oxygen barrier and antimicrobial barrier to improve the life span of packed food. Contrary to popular belief, biodegradable packaging can be created from both bio-based and plant-based materials. The strength and molecular makeup of a material's polymer chain determine its capacity to degrade, not its origin [84]. In addition to serving as packaging, biodegradable packaging has a number of uses in the food industry, including extending the shelf life of packaged foods and slowing the growth of microorganisms that come into direct contact with food. In addition to being antibacterial, the packaging is also sanitizing and self-sterilizing. In order to increase shelf life and guarantee the microbial safety of fresh and minimally processed produce during storage, a number of antimicrobial packaging systems have been created. These systems deliver a continuous and controlled release of the active antimicrobial substances into the package [85]. A recent study created antibacterial and antiviral films, where silver ions were successfully integrated into polylactide acid (PLA) films [86]. These films have been utilized to package lettuce samples contaminated with Salmonella enterica. Six days of storage at 4 °C resulted in a 4 logCFU reduction in S. enterica in packaged lettuce. A polymer matrix capable of spreading antimicrobial chemicals uniformly is necessary for the production of antimicrobial packaging films. Although the scientific literature frequently reports on the antibacterial and antioxidant properties of nanomaterials and plant extracts in different polymer combinations [87], in order to do this, it has become more advantageous in recent years to produce antimicrobial films using biodegradable material as opposed to non-degradable material.

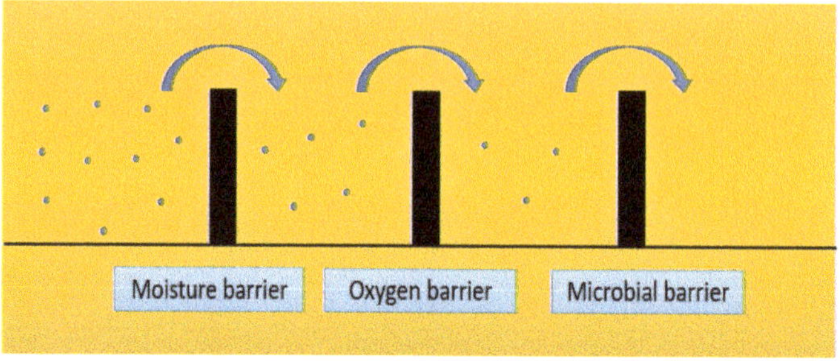

Figure 2. Hurdle technology in antimicrobial packaging system.

5. Nanotechnological Interventions of Green Antimicrobial Packaging

The purpose of packaging is to maintain the quality and texture, protect from contamination by germs, chemicals, and physical agents, and create a consumer-friendly presentation. Additionally, current approaches to environmentally friendly NP synthesis, based on the use of plant extracts and biomolecules as reducing and complexing agents in nanocomposite films, have demonstrated significant potential for palatable, biodegradable, and sustainable packaging [88]. A paradigm change from various chemical-based technologies to a greener and more sustainable approach has been brought about by growing environmental concerns. Recent discussions have focused on the development and potential of multifunctional nanocomposites based on antimicrobial agents in both the academic and industrial sectors. Nanotechnologies are rising very fast and gaining great popularity to support the benefits of the preservation of foods [89]. Nanoparticle-infused inorganic and metal oxides are also being explored. Due to their high stability and effective antibacterial properties, metal oxide-based nanoparticles such as ZnO, MgO, CuO, and TiO_2 have been investigated for use as antimicrobial agents in food packaging [90]. Recent green nanotechnological interventions combine biological sources, cleaner solvents, recyclable materials, and energy-saving procedures to create nanoparticles for use in food processing, packaging, and preservation (Figure 3). Many studies have already been conducted on various nanofillers derived from diverse sources, and more studies are being conducted to identify nanofiller-reinforced bionanocomposites that can be successfully applied for food packaging applications [91]. Additionally, a number of cutting-edge nanoencapsulation technologies have been created that use a number of biocompatible delivery systems as a carrier for a number of bioactive and nutritious components to enable regulated release and improved stability for food processing and preservation [92].

In the food packaging industry, new antimicrobial, antioxidant, and sustainable systems have been vigorously promoted as a viable eco-friendly alternative to conventional materials for improving the quality and safety of food products while minimizing or eliminating their negative environmental effects (Figure 4). The encouragement of more effective assembly and subsequent release of environmentally friendly active principles is made possible by the use of nanotechnologies, which also limits the usage of chemicals in terms of associated financial losses. Nanotechnology has the potential to completely alter the situation and satisfy the growing demand for global sustainability. Nevertheless, applying sustainable management measures that also take a nanotechnological approach to the full agri-food chain, from the plant to the food items, may be of interest.

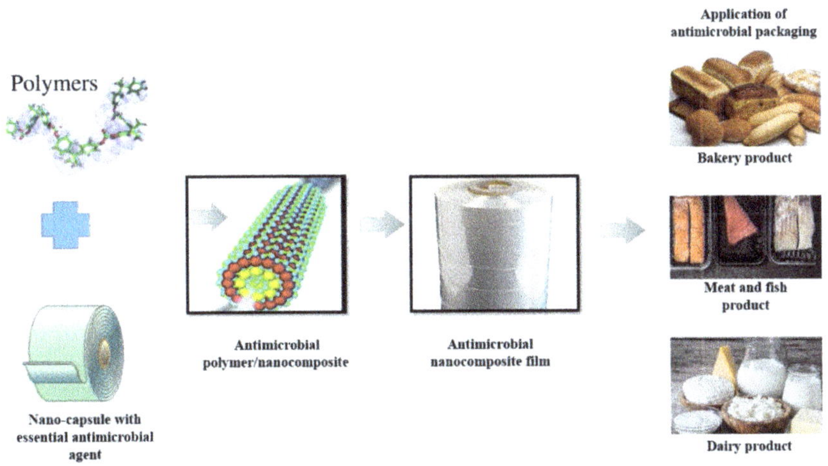

Figure 3. Preparation of nanostructured film incorporated with antimicrobial agent.

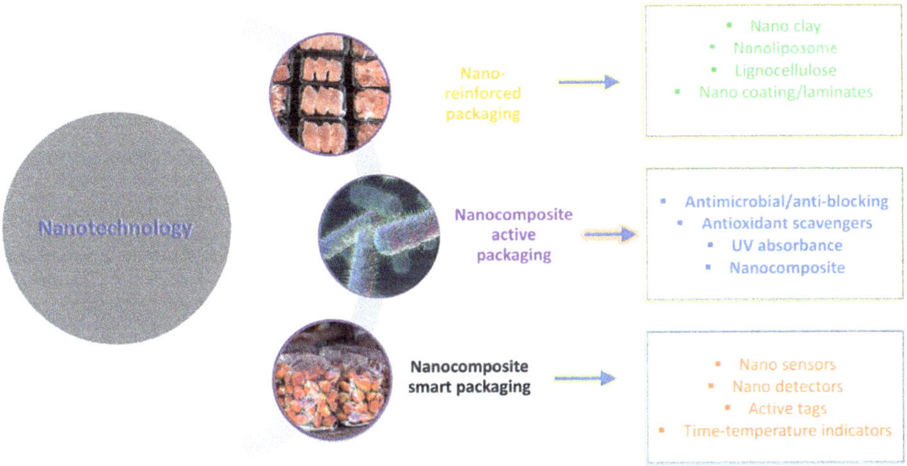

Figure 4. Application of nanotechnology in food packaging industry.

The usage of nanoparticles in food packaging, on the other hand, is anticipated to grow to USD 20 billion by 2020, according to the European Institute for Health and Consumer Protection [93]. The protection of the antimicrobial packaging against early inactivation in the food matrix and the regulated release of the drug, allowing a potential extension of shelf life, would be some benefits of nanotechnology [94]. As a result, nanotechnology has great promise for enhancing food safety and serving as an effective vehicle for the delivery and regulated release of natural antimicrobials [95,96]. Recently, the potential presented by a multifunctional system approach including sustainable supplies and greener methodologies was studied in connection to poly (lactic acid) (PLA)-based composites made using microcrystalline cellulose mixed with silver nanoparticles. Various stabilizing issues can be effectively solved by incorporating nanosized metals into biodegradable polymer matrices, which also allows for a controlled antibacterial effect [97]. The ability to make use of nanotechnology is considered compatible with the large-scale; roll-to-roll manufacturing of nanocomposite PLA films, as required by packaging technology, is provided by the simplicity of nanoparticle creation and the fact that they are obtained as a dispersion [98].

In the 1990s, research on the application of innovative packaging solutions, including those utilizing nanomaterials, nanocomposites, etc. [99], conducted a biological experiment against *Pseudomonas* spp. in which it was concluded that the suggested nanocomposites have strong antibacterial activity, making them a desirable nanomaterial.

6. Sustainable Contribution to the Society

The imminent threat that climate change poses to our society is constantly discussed in the media, but humanity's current use of resources is still not in line with the goal of sustainable development. In order to overcome the problems, changing how food is consumed is essential. A significant portion of the impact is attributable to agriculture and food production, and this is also true for food consumption. The enormous breakthrough that is globalization and the subsequent economic development are among the results of society's ongoing evolution and search for new solutions. Environmental considerations are now being given more weight in package development trends worldwide. Unfortunately, after being used, the packaging becomes waste, which can have a negative impact on the environment, which is why these concepts are also increasingly taken into account by companies from the packaging industry. In order to prevent the loss of goods, the packaging industry is intended to be transformed into one that is environmentally and socially conscious through the introduction of certain legislative requirements. According to SPA (an American organization, the Sustainable Packaging Coalition), packaging should be safe, effective, efficient, and cyclical [100]. Manufacturers are searching for novel solutions by developing creative biodegradable packaging materials or employing renewable raw materials in order to adapt the industry to the current requirements and changes. However, improving certain areas related to production, use, or disposal can sometimes be time- and labor-intensive, but not impossible.

Plastics are one of the most commonly utilized materials in the creation of packaging on a global scale, largely because of their adaptability and versatility. Contrary to popular belief, they are particularly well-suited for the creation of sustainable packaging since they offer protection, are long-lasting, and because of the package's light weight, they lower transportation costs and related greenhouse gas emissions. Additionally, they are easily moldable into any shape [101]. Unfortunately, they are often not managed properly after use and this is a global problem. Paper goods are utilized extensively in the creation of packaging all around the world in addition to plastics. They produce unit packaging, wrappings, labels, and, most importantly, transport packaging. Their biodegradability is their main selling point. Unfortunately, this process results in the production of methane, a greenhouse gas [102].

Sustainability is a multifaceted concept. In packaging, there are five fundamental categories as the cornerstones of sustainable packaging, i.e., society, environment, economy, development, and time, which are outlined in Figure 5 [103]. Due to the antimicrobials' absorption into the polymeric matrix, the previous non-compostable oil-derived polymers were replaced with antimicrobial biodegradable packaging materials, which presented additional issues. By improvising this, we can enhance the packaging system present on the market, but they should also be constantly improved and adapted to the changing requirements of the market, society, or the environment, as well as to the state and development of the packaging industry. More and more businesses are making efforts to transform the packaging sector into one that is socially and environmentally conscious. They take into account packaging from an economic, social, ethical, and environmental perspective. The answer for the various problems lies in rebuilding our industrial systems so that they are intrinsically sustainable rather than trying to mitigate their negative elements. More sustainable packaging will be a key component of such future systems.

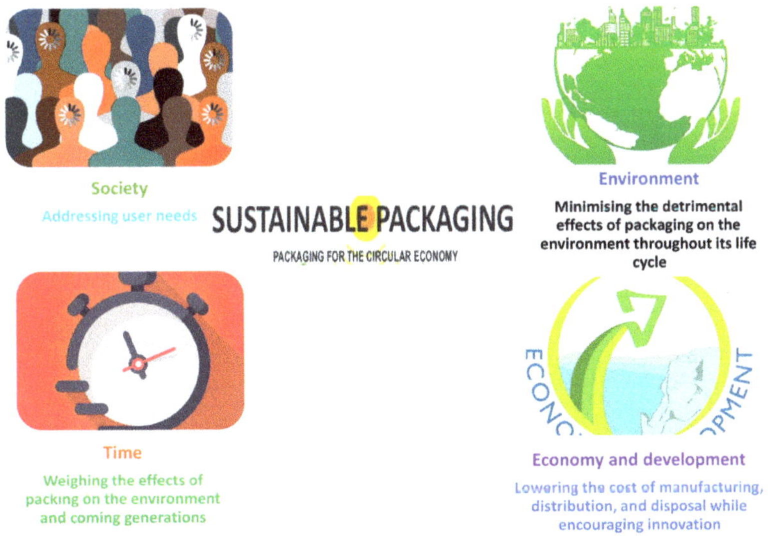
Society
Addressing user needs
SUSTAINABLE PACKAGING
PACKAGING FOR THE CIRCULAR ECONOMY
Environment
Minimising the detrimental effects of packaging on the environment throughout its life cycle
Time
Weighing the effects of packing on the environment and coming generations
Economy and development
Lowering the cost of manufacturing, distribution, and disposal while encouraging innovation

Figure 5. Sustainable packaging solution for the circular economy.

7. Conclusions and Future Prospects

Efficiency and innovation in packaging technologies have become a key component of the new regulations used to ensure food preservation and protection due to the constantly increasing demand for minimally processed food products and the resulting expansion of the market for those products. Due to the addition of the antimicrobial compounds into the polymeric matrix, compatibility between diverse components, and ease of degradation by heat and light, the antimicrobial biodegradable packaging materials that replaced conventional non-compostable oil-derived plastics presented new hurdles. The use of antimicrobial components in the packaging such as natural bioactive compounds, peptides, nanoparticles, etc., in food packaging helps to prevent undesirable changes in the food during storage, such as off flavors, color changes, or the occurrence of any foodborne outcomes. It also ensures controlled release over an extended period to improve the quality of food under observation and, overall, improves the quality in terms of value for money for the customers. While all of these antimicrobial packaging systems are somewhat successful at maintaining fresh and minimally processed produce's quality and ensuring its microbial safety, more research and development are required to increase the antimicrobial effectiveness of the current packaging technologies, find more potent natural antimicrobial compounds, increase the stability of natural antimicrobials in the packaging system, and guarantee the safety of their commercial application. When using nanoparticles in food products, thorough toxicity studies, safety precautions, and exploration of nano-based antimicrobial packaging techniques must be undertaken. The fundamental benefit of adding antimicrobial components to food packaging materials is that they gradually release into the food surface, allowing for continuous antibacterial activity and extending the shelf life of the food. However, more research on the in vitro and in vivo performances of this active packaging material is required in order to define regulation in this context. The development of techniques and technologies aimed at preserving food products and enhancing food safety and quality can still take advantage of this promising field. Future research is needed to increase the longevity and effectiveness of novel antimicrobial packaging materials because some antimicrobials (such as essential oils) have a high loss rate due to inherent volatilization. The limits of what is practical for sustainable packaging will continue to be pushed by advancements in design, production, and recycling technology. Researchers are working arduously to contribute to the most advanced solution for this issue.

Author Contributions: Conceptualization, I.B., R.S. and S.R.; software, I.B. and S.R.; validation, I.B., R.S., V.K.P. and S.R.; writing—original draft preparation, I.B., R.S., V.K.P. and S.R.; writing—review and editing, I.B. and S.R.; visualization, I.B. and S.R.; supervision, S.R. and R.S. All authors have read and agreed to the published version of the manuscript.

Funding: This research received no external funding.

Institutional Review Board Statement: Not applicable.

Informed Consent Statement: Not applicable.

Data Availability Statement: Not applicable.

Conflicts of Interest: The authors declare no conflict of interest.

References

1. Mahmud, N.; Islam, J.; Tahergorabi, R. Marine Biopolymers: Applications in Food Packaging. *Processes* **2021**, *9*, 2245. [CrossRef]
2. Zhang, W.; Roy, S.; Rhim, J.-W. Copper-based nanoparticles for biopolymer-based functional films in food packaging applications. *Compr. Rev. Food Sci. Food Saf.* **2023**, *22*, 1933–1952. [CrossRef] [PubMed]
3. Grzebieniarz, W.; Biswas, D.; Roy, S.; Jamróz, E. Advances in Biopolymer-Based Multi-Layer Film Preparations and Food Packaging Applications. *Food Packag. Shelf Life* **2023**, *35*, 101033. [CrossRef]
4. Singh, N.; Hui, D.; Singh, R.; Ahuja, I.P.S.; Feo, L.; Fraternali, F. Recycling of Plastic Solid Waste: A State of Art Review and Future Applications. *Compos. B Eng.* **2017**, *115*, 409–422. [CrossRef]
5. Zhong, Y.; Godwin, P.; Jin, Y.; Xiao, H. Biodegradable Polymers and Green-Based Antimicrobial Packaging Materials: A Mini-Review. *Adv. Ind. Eng. Polym. Res.* **2020**, *3*, 27–35. [CrossRef]
6. Ghosh, S.; Roy, S.; Naskar, J.; Kole, R.K. Plant-mediated synthesis of mono and bimetallic (Au-Ag) nanoparticles: Future prospects for food quality and safety. *J. Nanomater.* **2023**, *2023*, 2781667. [CrossRef]
7. Yadav, D.; Borpatra Gohain, M.; Karki, S.; Ingole, P.G. A Novel Approach for the Development of Low-Cost Polymeric Thin-Film Nanocomposite Membranes for the Biomacromolecule Separation. *ACS Omega* **2022**, *7*, 47967–47985. [CrossRef]
8. Mousavi Khaneghah, A.M.; Hashemi, S.M.B.; Limbo, S. Antimicrobial Agents and Packaging Systems in Antimicrobial Active Food Packaging: An Overview of Approaches and Interactions. *Food Bioprod. Process.* **2018**, *111*, 1–19. [CrossRef]
9. Ramakrishnan, R.; Kulandhaivelu, S.V.; Roy, S. Alginate/carboxymethyl cellulose/starch-based active coating with grapefruit seed extract to extend the shelf life of green chilli. *Ind. Crops Prod.* **2023**, *199*, 116752. [CrossRef]
10. Zhang, W.; Roy, S.; Ezati, P.; Yang, D.P.; Rhim, J.-W. Tannic acid: A green crosslinker for biopolymer-based food packaging films. *Trends Food Sci. Technol.* **2023**, *136*, 11–23. [CrossRef]
11. Santos, J.C.P.; Sousa, R.C.S.; Otoni, C.G.; Moraes, A.R.F.; Souza, V.G.L.; Medeiros, E.A.A.; Espitia, P.J.P.; Pires, A.C.S.; Coimbra, J.S.R.; Soares, N.F.F. Nisin and Other Antimicrobial Peptides: Production, Mechanisms of Action, and Application in Active Food Packaging. *Innov. Food Sci. Emerg. Technol.* **2018**, *48*, 179–194. [CrossRef]
12. Angane, M.; Swift, S.; Huang, K.; Butts, C.A.; Quek, S.Y. Essential Oils and Their Major Components: An Updated Review on Antimicrobial Activities, Mechanism of Action and Their Potential Application in the Food Industry. *Foods* **2022**, *11*, 464. [CrossRef] [PubMed]
13. Dıblan, S.; Kaya, S. Antimicrobials Used in Active Packaging Films. *Food Health* **2018**, *4*, 63–79. [CrossRef]
14. Paidari, S.; Ahari, H.; Pasqualone, A.; Anvar, A.; Beyk, S.A.Y.; Moradi, S. Bio-nanocomposites and their potential applications in physiochemical properties of cheese: An updated review. *J. Food Meas. Charact.* **2023**, *17*, 2595–2606. [CrossRef]
15. Malagurski, I.; Levic, S.; Nesic, A.; Mitric, M.; Pavlovic, V.; Dimitrijevic-Brankovic, S. Mineralized Agar-Based Nanocomposite Films: Potential Food Packaging Materials with Antimicrobial Properties. *Carbohydr. Polym.* **2017**, *175*, 55–62. [CrossRef] [PubMed]
16. Roy, S.; Priyadarshi, R.; Łopusiewicz, Ł.; Biswas, D.; Chandel, V.; Rhim, J.-W. Recent progress in pectin extraction, characterization, and pectin-based films for active food packaging applications: A review. *Int. J. Biol. Macromol.* **2023**, *239*, 124248. [CrossRef] [PubMed]
17. Ebrahimzadeh, S.; Biswas, D.; Roy, S.; McClements, D.J. Incorporation of essential oils in edible seaweed-based films: A comprehensive review. *Trends Food Sci. Technol.* **2023**, *135*, 43–56. [CrossRef]
18. Priyadarshi, P.; Roy, S.; Ghosh, T.; Biswas, D.; Rhim, J.-W. Antimicrobial nanofillers reinforced biopolymer composite films for active food packaging applications—A review. *Sustain. Mater. Technol.* **2022**, *32*, e00353. [CrossRef]
19. Khare, S.; De Loid, G.M.; Molina, R.M.; Gokulan, K.; Couvillion, S.P.; Bloodsworth, K.J.; Eder, E.K.; Wong, A.R.; Hoyt, D.W.; Bramer, L.M.; et al. Effects of Ingested Nanocellulose on Intestinal Microbiota and Homeostasis in Wistar Han Rats. *NanoImpact* **2020**, *18*, 100216. [CrossRef]
20. Chang, H.; Xu, J.; Macqueen, L.A.; Aytac, Z.; Peters, M.M.; Zimmerman, J.F.; Parker, K.K. High-throughput coating with biodegradable antimicrobial pullulan fibres extends shelf life and reduces weight loss in an avocado model. *Nat. Food* **2022**, *3*, 428–436. [CrossRef]

21. Nile, S.H.; Baskar, V.; Selvaraj, D.; Nile, A.; Xiao, J.; Kai, G. Nanotechnologies in Food Science: Applications, Recent Trends, and Future Perspectives. *Nano Micro. Lett.* **2020**, *12*, 45. [CrossRef] [PubMed]
22. Yang, Z.; Xiao, Y.; Jiao, T.; Zhang, Y.; Chen, J.; Gao, Y. Effects of Copper Oxide Nanoparticles on the Growth of Rice (*Oryza sativa* L.) Seedlings and the Relevant Physiological Responses. *Int. J. Environ. Res. Public Health* **2020**, *17*, 1260. [CrossRef] [PubMed]
23. Nehra, A.; Biswas, D.; Siracusa, V.; Roy, S. Natural Gum-Based Functional Bioactive Films and Coatings: A Review. *Int. J. Mol. Sci.* **2022**, *24*, 485. [CrossRef] [PubMed]
24. Abou Baker, D.H.; Al-Moghazy, M.; ElSayed, A.A.A. The In Vitro Cytotoxicity, Antioxidant and Antibacterial Potential of *Satureja hortensis* L. Essential Oil Cultivated in Egypt. *Bioorg. Chem.* **2020**, *95*, 103559. [CrossRef] [PubMed]
25. Gholami, P.; Dinpazhoh, L.; Khataee, A.; Orooji, Y. Sonocatalytic activity of biochar-supported ZnO nanorods in degradation of gemifloxacin: Synergy study, effect of parameters and phytotoxicity evaluation. *Ultrason. Sonochem.* **2019**, *55*, 44–56. [CrossRef]
26. Makaremi, M.; Yousefi, H.; Cavallaro, G.; Lazzara, G.; Goh, C.B.S.; Lee, S.M.; Solouk, A.; Pasbakhsh, P. Safely Dissolvable and Healable Active Packaging Films Based on Alginate and Pectin. *Polymers* **2019**, *11*, 1594. [CrossRef]
27. Ritchie, H.; Roser, M.; Plastic Pollution. Our World Data. 2018. Available online: https://ourworldindata.org/plastic-pollution?utm_source=newsletter (accessed on 1 May 2023).
28. Vinod, A.; Sanjay, M.R.; Suchart, S.; Jyotishkumar, P. Renewable and Sustainable Biobased Materials: An Assessment on Biofibers, Biofilms, Biopolymers and Biocomposites. *J. Clean. Prod.* **2020**, *258*, 120978. [CrossRef]
29. Syngai, G.G.; Ahmed, G. Lysozyme: A Natural Antimicrobial Enzyme of Interest in Food Applications. In *Enzymes in Food Biotechnology*; Elsevier: Amsterdam, The Netherlands, 2019; pp. 169–179.
30. Jha, K.; Kataria, R.; Verma, J.; Pradhan, S. Potential Biodegradable Matrices and Fiber Treatment for Green Composites: A Review. *AIMS Mater. Sci.* **2019**, *6*, 119–138. [CrossRef]
31. Thyavihalli Girijappa, Y.G.; Mavinkere Rangappa, S.; Parameswaranpillai, J.; Siengchin, S. Natural Fibers as Sustainable and Renewable Resource for Development of Eco-friendly Composites: A Comprehensive Review. *Front. Mater.* **2019**, *6*, 226. [CrossRef]
32. Mustapha, F.A.; Jai, J.; Hamidon, F.; Md Sharif, Z.I.M., Yusof, N.M. Antimicrobial Agents from Malaysian Plants and Their Potential Use in Food Packaging Material: Review. *Chem. Eng. Res. Bull.* **2017**, *19*, 57–66. [CrossRef]
33. Kamarudin, S.H.; Rayung, M.; Abu, F.; Ahmad, S.; Fadil, F.; Karim, A.A.; Norizan, M.N.; Sarifuddin, N.; Mat Desa, M.S.Z.; Mohd Basri, M.S.; et al. A Review on Antimicrobial Packaging from Biodegradable Polymer Composites. *Polymers* **2022**, *14*, 174. [CrossRef]
34. Ghasemi, M.; Khataee, A.; Gholami, P.; Soltani, R.D.C.; Hassani, A.; Orooji, Y. In-Situ electro-generation and activation of hydrogen peroxide using a CuFeNLDH-CNTs modified graphite cathode for degradation of cefazolin. *J. Environ. Manag.* **2020**, *267*, 110629. [CrossRef]
35. Talebi, F.; Misaghi, A.; Khanjari, A.; Kamkar, A.; Gandomi, H.; Rezaeigolestani, M. Incorporation of Spice Essential Oils into Poly-lactic Acid Film Matrix with the Aim of Extending Microbiological and Sensorial Shelf Life of Ground Beef. *L.W.T.* **2018**, *96*, 482–490. [CrossRef]
36. Tiwari, B.K.; Valdramidis, V.P.; O'Donnell, C.P.; Muthukumarappan, K.; Bourke, P.; Cullen, P.J. Application of Natural Antimicrobials for Food Preservation. *J. Agric. Food Chem.* **2009**, *57*, 5987–6000. [CrossRef]
37. Sofi, S.A.; Singh, J.; Rafiq, S.; Ashraf, U.; Dar, B.N.; Nayik, G.A. A Comprehensive Review on Antimicrobial Packaging and Its Use in Food Packaging. *Curr. Nutr. Food Sci.* **2018**, *14*, 305–312. [CrossRef]
38. Yang, S.; Cao, L.; Kim, H.; Beak, S.; Song, K.B. Utilization of Foxtail Millet Starch Film Incorporated with Clove Leaf Oil for the Packaging of Queso Blanco Cheese as a Model Food. *Starch-Stärke* **2018**, *70*, 1700171. [CrossRef]
39. Zaki, M.; HPS, A.K.; Sabaruddin, F.A.; Bairwan, R.D.; Oyekanmi, A.A.; Alfatah, T.; Danish, M.; Mistar, E.M.; Abdullah, C.K. Microbial treatment for nanocellulose extraction from marine algae and its applications as sustainable functional material. *Bioresour. Technol. Rep.* **2021**, *16*, 100811. [CrossRef]
40. Kwon, S.J.; Chang, Y.; Han, J. Oregano Essential Oil-Based Natural Antimicrobial Packaging Film to Inactivate Salmonella enterica and Yeasts/Molds in the Atmosphere Surrounding Cherry Tomatoes. *Food Microbiol.* **2017**, *65*, 114–121. [CrossRef] [PubMed]
41. Sharma, S.; Barkauskaite, S.; Duffy, B.; Jaiswal, A.K.; Jaiswal, S. Characterization and Antimicrobial Activity of Biodegradable Active Packaging Enriched with Clove and Thyme Essential Oil for Food Packaging Application. *Foods* **2020**, *9*, 1117. [CrossRef]
42. Luís, Â.; Duarte, A.; Gominho, J.; Domingues, F.; Duarte, A.P. Chemical Composition, Antioxidant, Antibacterial and Anti-quorum Sensing Activities of *Eucalyptus globulus* and *Eucalyptus radiata* Essential Oils. *Ind. Crops Prod.* **2016**, *79*, 274–282. [CrossRef]
43. Khah, M.D.; Ghanbarzadeh, B.; Roufegarinejad Nezhad, L.R.; Ostadrahimi, A. Effects of Virgin Olive Oil and Grape Seed Oil on Physicochemical and Antimicrobial Properties of Pectin-Gelatin Blend Emulsified Films. *Int. J. Biol. Macromol.* **2021**, *171*, 262–274. [CrossRef]
44. Priyadarshi, R.; Sauraj, B.; Kumar, B.; Deeba, F.; Kulshreshtha, A.; Negi, Y.S. Chitosan Films Incorporated with Apricot (*Prunus armeniaca*) Kernel Essential Oil as Active Food Packaging Material. *Food Hydrocoll.* **2018**, *85*, 158–166. [CrossRef]
45. Bahl, K.; Miyoshi, T.; Jana, S.C. Hybrid Fillers of Lignin and Carbon Black for Lowering of Viscoelastic Loss in Rubber Compounds. *Polymer* **2014**, *55*, 3825–3835. [CrossRef]
46. Chenni, M.; El Abed, D.; Rakotomanomana, N.; Fernandez, X.; Chemat, F. Comparative Study of Essential Oils Extracted from Egyptian Basil Leaves (*Ocimum basilicum* L.) Using Hydro-distillation and Solvent-Free Microwave Extraction. *Molecules* **2016**, *21*, 113. [CrossRef]

47. Ye, J.; Wang, S.; Lan, W.; Qin, W.; Liu, Y. Preparation and Properties of Polylactic Acid-Tea Polyphenol-Chitosan Composite Membranes. *Int. J. Biol. Macromol.* **2018**, *117*, 632–639. [CrossRef] [PubMed]
48. Moldovan, R.I.; Oprean, R.; Benedec, D.; Hanganu, D.; Duma, M.; Oniga, I.; Vlase, L. LC-MS Analysis, Antioxidant and Antimicrobial Activities for Five Species of Mentha Cultivated in Romania. *Dig. J. Nanomater. Biostruct.* **2014**, *9*, 559–566.
49. Duran, M.; Aday, M.S.; Zorba, N.N.D.; Temizkan, R.; Büyükcan, M.B.; Caner, C. Potential of Antimicrobial Active Packaging 'Containing Natamycin, Nisin, Pomegranate and Grape Seed Extract in Chitosan coating' to Extend Shelf Life of Fresh Strawberry. *Food Bioprod. Process.* **2016**, *98*, 354–363. [CrossRef]
50. Sundaram, J.; Pant, J.; Goudie, M.J.; Mani, S.; Handa, H. Antimicrobial and Physicochemical Characterization of Biodegradable, Nitric Oxide-Releasing Nanocellulose–Chitosan Packaging Membranes. *J. Agric. Food Chem.* **2016**, *64*, 5260–5266. [CrossRef]
51. Pisoschi, A.M.; Pop, A.; Georgescu, C.; Turcuş, V.; Olah, N.K.; Mathe, E. An Overview of Natural Antimicrobials Role in Food. *Eur. J. Med. Chem.* **2018**, *143*, 922–935. [CrossRef]
52. Nemeş, N.S.; Ardean, C.; Davidescu, C.M.; Negrea, A.; Ciopec, M.; Duţeanu, N.; Negrea, P.; Paul, C.; Duda-Seiman, D.; Muntean, D. Antimicrobial Activity of Cellulose Based Materials. *Polymers* **2022**, *14*, 735. [CrossRef]
53. Emolaga, C.S.; Paglicawan, M.A.; Bigol, U.P.; de Yro, P.A.N.; Sy, J.A.; Visaya, B.A.; Bauca, M.T.A. Preparation of Starch Nanocrystals with Antimicrobial Property. *MSF* **2022**, *1073*, 143–148. [CrossRef]
54. Irkin, R.; Esmer, O.K. Novel Food Packaging Systems with Natural Antimicrobial Agents. *J. Food Sci. Technol.* **2015**, *52*, 6095–6111. [CrossRef] [PubMed]
55. Hossain, M.I.; Sadekuzzaman, M.; Ha, S.D. Probiotics as Potential Alternative Biocontrol Agents in the Agriculture and Food Industries: A Review. *Food Res. Int.* **2017**, *100*, 63–73. [CrossRef] [PubMed]
56. Al-Hashimi, G.A.; Ammar, A.B.; Cacciola, F.; Lakhssassi, N. Development of a millet starch edible film containing clove essential oil. *Foods* **2020**, *9*, 184. [CrossRef]
57. Ali, G.; Sharma, M.; Salama, E.-S.; Ling, Z.; Li, X. Applications of chitin and chitosan as natural biopolymer: Potential sources, pretreatments, and degradation pathways. *Biomass-Convers. Biorefin.* **2022**, 1–15. [CrossRef]
58. Wen, P.; Zhu, D.H.; Wu, H.; Zong, M.H.; Jing, Y.R.; Han, S.Y. Encapsulation of Cinnamon Essential Oil in Electrospun Nanofibrous Film for Active Food Packaging. *Food Control* **2016**, *59*, 366–376. [CrossRef]
59. Sedayu, B.B.; Cran, M.J.; Bigger, S.W. A Review of Property Enhancement Techniques for Carrageenan-Based Films and Coatings. *Carbohydr. Polym.* **2019**, *216*, 287–302. [CrossRef]
60. Mandolini, M.; Campi, F.; Favi, C.; Germani, M. Manufacturing Processes Re-Engineering for Cost Reduction: The Investment Casting Case Study. In *International Design Engineering Technical Conferences and Computers and Information in Engineering Conference*; American Society of Mechanical Engineers: New York, NY, USA, 2019; p. V004T05A018. [CrossRef]
61. Motelica, L.; Ficai, D.; Ficai, A.; Oprea, O.C.; Kaya, D.A.; Andronescu, E. Biodegradable Antimicrobial Food Packaging: Trends and Perspectives. *Foods* **2020**, *9*, 1438. [CrossRef]
62. Coban, H.B. Organic Acids as Antimicrobial Food Agents: Applications and Microbial Productions. *Bioprocess Biosyst. Eng.* **2020**, *43*, 569–591. [CrossRef]
63. Liu, Y.; Liang, X.; Wang, S.; Qin, W.; Zhang, Q. Electrospun Antimicrobial Polylactic Acid/Tea Polyphenol Nanofibers for Food-Packaging Applications. *Polymers* **2018**, *10*, 561. [CrossRef]
64. Liu, L.; Zhu, Y.; Li, J.; Wang, M.; Lee, P.; Du, G.; Chen, J. Microbial Production of Propionic Acid from Propionibacteria: Current State, Challenges and Perspectives. *Crit. Rev. Biotechnol.* **2012**, *32*, 374–381. [CrossRef] [PubMed]
65. Song, X.; Wang, L.; Liu, L.; Li, J.; Wu, X. Impact of Tea Tree Essential Oil and Citric Acid/Choline Chloride on Physical, Structural and Antibacterial Properties of Chitosan-Based Films. *Food Control* **2022**, *141*, 109186. [CrossRef]
66. Eastoe, C.J. Stable Chlorine Isotopes in Arid Non-marine Basins: Instances and Possible Fractionation Mechanisms. *Appl. Geochem.* **2016**, *74*, 1–12. [CrossRef]
67. Kumar, R.; Chandar, B.; Parani, M. Use of Succinic & Oxalic Acid in Reducing the Dosage of Colistin Against New Delhi Metallo-β-lactamase-1 Bacteria. *Indian J. Med. Res.* **2018**, *147*, 97–101. [CrossRef] [PubMed]
68. Venugopal, V. *Marine Polysaccharides: Food Applications*; CRC Press: Boca Raton, FL, USA, 2016.
69. Jideani, V.A.; Vogt, K. Antimicrobial Packaging for Extending the Shelf Life of Bread—A Review. *Crit. Rev. Food Sci. Nutr.* **2016**, *56*, 1313–1324. [CrossRef]
70. Morey, A.; Bowers, J.W.J.; Bauermeister, L.J.; Singh, M.; Huang, T.S.; McKee, S.R. Effect of Salts of Organic Acids on *Listeria monocytogenes*, Shelf Life, Meat Quality, and Consumer Acceptability of Beef Frankfurters. *J. Food Sci.* **2014**, *79*, M54–M60. [CrossRef]
71. Huang, T.; Qian, Y.; Wei, J.; Zhou, C. Polymeric Antimicrobial Food Packaging and Its Applications. *Polymers* **2019**, *11*, 560. [CrossRef]
72. Sethi, S.; Gupta, S. Antimicrobial Spices: Use in Antimicrobial Packaging. In *Antimicrobial Food Packaging*; Elsevier: Amsterdam, The Netherlands, 2016; pp. 433–444.
73. Sung, S.Y.; Sin, L.T.; Tee, T.T.; Bee, S.T.; Rahmat, A.R.; Rahman, W.A.W.A.; Tan, A.; Vikhraman, M. Antimicrobial Agents for Food Packaging Applications. *Trends Food Sci. Technol.* **2013**, *33*, 110–123. [CrossRef]
74. Chana-Thaworn, J.; Chanthachum, S.; Wittaya, T. Properties and Antimicrobial Activity of Edible Films Incorporated with Kiam Wood (*Cotyleobium lanceotatum*) Extract. *L.W.T. Food Sci. Technol.* **2011**, *44*, 284–292. [CrossRef]

75. Kuorwel, K.K.; Cran, M.J.; Sonneveld, K.; Miltz, J.; Bigger, S.W. Antimicrobial Activity of Biodegradable Polysaccharide and Protein-Based Films Containing Active Agents. *J. Food Sci.* **2011**, *76*, R90–R102. [CrossRef]
76. Díaz-Montes, E. Polysaccharides: Sources, Characteristics, Properties, and Their Application in Biodegradable Films. *Polysaccharides* **2022**, *3*, 480–501. [CrossRef]
77. Gurav, R.; Bhatia, S.K.; Choi, T.R.; Hyun Cho, D.; Chan Kim, B.; Hyun Kim, S.; Ju Jung, H.; Joong Kim, H.; Jeon, J.M.; Yoon, J.J.; et al. Lignocellulosic Hydrolysate Based Biorefinery for Marine Exopolysaccharide Production and Application of the Produced Biopolymer in Environmental Clean-Up. *Bioresour. Technol.* **2022**, *359*, 127499. [CrossRef] [PubMed]
78. Mukurumbira, A.R.; Shellie, R.A.; Keast, R.; Palombo, E.A.; Jadhav, S.R. Encapsulation of Essential Oils and Their Application in Antimicrobial Active Packaging. *Food Control* **2022**, *136*, 108883. [CrossRef]
79. Trindade, M.A.; Nunes, C.; Coimbra, M.A.; Gonçalves, F.J.M.; Marques, J.C.; Gonçalves, A.M.M. Sustainable and Biodegradable Active Films Based on Seaweed Compounds to Improve Shelf Life of Food Products. In *Sustainable Global Resources of Seaweeds Volume 2: Food, Pharmaceutical and Health Applications*; Springer: Berlin/Heidelberg, Germany, 2022; pp. 235–252.
80. Matche, R.S.; Anup, G.J.; Mrudula, G. Development of Biodegradable Films from Marine Ingredients Incorporated with Natural Antimicrobial Agents for Food Packaging. *J. Packag. Technol. Res.* **2020**, *4*, 45–55. [CrossRef]
81. Firmanda, A.; Fahma, F.; Warsiki, E.; Syamsu, K.; Arnata, I.W.; Sartika, D.; Suryanegara, L.; Qanytah; Suyanto, A. Antimicrobial Mechanism of Nanocellulose Composite Packaging Incorporated with Essential Oils. *Food Control* **2023**, *147*, 109617. [CrossRef]
82. Suderman, N.; Isa, M.I.N.; Sarbon, N.M. The Effect of Plasticizers on the Functional Properties of Biodegradable Gelatin-Based Film: A Review. *Food Biosci.* **2018**, *24*, 111–119. [CrossRef]
83. Sinthupachee, A.; Matan, N.; Matan, N. Development of Smoke Flavour-Antimicrobial Packaging from Coconut Fibre Using Litsea Cubeba Essential Oil and Wood Smoke for Dried Fish Preservation and Reduction of PAH. *Food Control* **2023**, *148*, 109629. [CrossRef]
84. Aliabbasi, N.; Emam-Djomeh, Z.; Amighi, F. Active Food Packaging with Nano/Microencapsulated Ingredients. In *Application of Nano/Microencapsulated Ingredients in Food Products*; Elsevier: Amsterdam, The Netherlands, 2021; pp. 171–210.
85. Bahmid, N.A.; Pepping, L.; Dekker, M.; Fogliano, V.; Heising, J. Using Particle Size and Fat Content to Control the Release of Allyl Isothiocyanate from Ground Mustard Seeds for Its Application in Antimicrobial Packaging. *Food Chem.* **2020**, *308*, 125573. [CrossRef]
86. Mlalila, N.; Hilonga, A.; Swai, H.; Devlieghere, F.; Ragaert, P. Antimicrobial Packaging Based on Starch, Poly (3-Hydroxybutyrate) and Poly (Lactic-Co-Glycolide) Materials and Application Challenges. *Trends Food Sci. Technol.* **2018**, *74*, 1–11. [CrossRef]
87. Bouletis, A.D.; Arvanitoyannis, I.S.; Hadjichristodoulou, C. Application of Modified Atmosphere Packaging on Aquacultured Fish and Fish Products: A Review. *Crit. Rev. Food Sci. Nutr.* **2017**, *57*, 2263–2285. [CrossRef]
88. Ordoñez, R.; Atarés, L.; Chiralt, A. Biodegradable Active Materials Containing Phenolic Acids for Food Packaging Applications. *Compr. Rev. Food Sci. Food Saf.* **2022**, *21*, 3910–3930. [CrossRef] [PubMed]
89. Jung, J.; Zhao, Y. Antimicrobial Packaging for Fresh and Minimally Processed Fruits and Vegetables. In *Antimicrobial Food Packaging*; Elsevier: Amsterdam, The Netherlands, 2016; pp. 243–256.
90. Nakata, S.; Murata, K.; Hashimoto, W.; Kawai, S. Uncovering the Reactive Nature of 4-Deoxy-l-erythro-5-hexoseulose Uronate for the Utilization of Alginate, a Promising Marine Biopolymer. *Sci. Rep.* **2019**, *9*, 17147. [CrossRef] [PubMed]
91. Correa, M.G.; Martínez, F.B.; Vidal, C.P.; Streitt, C.; Escrig, J.; de Dicastillo, C.L. Antimicrobial Metal-Based Nanoparticles: A Review on Their Synthesis, Types and Antimicrobial Action. *Beilstein J. Nanotechnol.* **2020**, *11*, 1450–1469. [CrossRef] [PubMed]
92. Ceballos, R.L.; Von Bilderling, C.; Guz, L.; Bernal, C.; Famá, L. Effect of Greenly Synthetized Silver Nanoparticles on the Properties of Active Starch Films Obtained by Extrusion and Compression Molding. *Carbohydr. Polym.* **2021**, *261*, 117871. [CrossRef] [PubMed]
93. Hu, P.; Li, Z.; Chen, M.; Sun, Z.; Ling, Y.; Jiang, J.; Huang, C. Structural Elucidation and Protective Role of a Polysaccharide from *Sargassum fusiforme* on Ameliorating Learning and Memory Deficiencies in Mice. *Carbohydr. Polym.* **2016**, *139*, 150–158. [CrossRef] [PubMed]
94. Karki, S.; Gohain, M.B.; Yadav, D.; Ingole, P.G. Nanocomposite and bio-nanocomposite polymeric materials/membranes development in energy and medical sector: A review. *Int. J. Biol. Macromol.* **2021**, *193*, 2121–2139. [CrossRef]
95. Sarwar, M.S.; Niazi, M.B.K.; Jahan, Z.; Ahmad, T.; Hussain, A. Preparation and Characterization of PVA/nanocellulose/Ag Nanocomposite Films for Antimicrobial Food Packaging. *Carbohydr. Polym.* **2018**, *184*, 453–464. [CrossRef]
96. Pandhi, S.; Kumar, A.; Mishra, S.; Rai, D.C. Potential of Green Nanotechnology in Food Processing and Preservation. In *Handbook of Research on Food Processing and Preservation Technologies*; Apple Academic Press: Waretown, NJ, USA, 2021; pp. 135–161.
97. Broquá, J.; Zanin, B.G.; Flach, A.M.; Mallmann, C.; Taborda, F.G.D. Different Aspects of Chemical and Biochemical Methods for Chitin Production a Short Review. *J. Nanomed Nanosci. JNAN* **2018**, *10*, 1477–2577.
98. Brandelli, A.; Taylor, T.M. Nanostructured and Nanoencapsulated Natural Antimicrobials for Use in Food Products. In *Handbook of Natural Antimicrobials for Food Safety and Quality*; Woodhead Publishing Oxford: Cambridge, UK, 2015; pp. 229–257.
99. Duncan, T.V. Applications of Nanotechnology in Food Packaging and Food Safety: Barrier Materials, Antimicrobials and Sensors. *J. Colloid Interface Sci.* **2011**, *363*, 1–24. [CrossRef]
100. Roy, S.; Zhang, W.; Biswas, D.; Ramakrishnan, R.; Rhim, J.-W. Grapefruit Seed Extract-Added Functional Films and Coating for Active Packaging Applications: A Review. *Molecules* **2023**, *28*, 730. [CrossRef]

101. Bumbudsanpharoke, N.; Ko, S. Nano-food Packaging: An Overview of Market, Migration Research, and Safety Regulations. *J. Food Sci.* **2015**, *80*, R910–R923. [CrossRef] [PubMed]
102. Gheysari, H.; Mohandes, F.; Mazaheri, M.; Dolatyar, B.; Askari, M.; Simchi, A. Extraction of Hydroxyapatite Nanostructures from Marine Wastes for the Fabrication of Biopolymer-Based Porous Scaffolds. *Mar. Drugs* **2019**, *18*, 26. [CrossRef] [PubMed]
103. Sangroniz, A.; Sangroniz, L.; Gonzalez, A.; Santamaria, A.; del Rio, J.; Iriarte, M.; Etxeberria, A. Improving the Barrier Properties of a Biodegradable Polyester for Packaging Applications. *Eur. Polym. J.* **2019**, *115*, 76–85. [CrossRef]

antibiotics

MDPI

Review

Synthetic and Semisynthetic Compounds as Antibacterials Targeting Virulence Traits in Resistant Strains: A Narrative Updated Review

Dejan Stojković [1], Jovana Petrović [1], Tamara Carević [1], Marina Soković [1] and Konstantinos Liaras [2,*]

1 Department of Plant Physiology, Institute for Biological Research "Siniša Stanković"—National Institute of the Republic of Serbia, University of Belgrade, Bulevar Despota Stefana 142, 11000 Belgrade, Serbia; dejanbio@ibiss.bg.ac.rs (D.S.); jovana0303@ibiss.bg.ac.rs (J.P.); tamara.carevic@ibiss.bg.ac.rs (T.C.); mris@ibiss.bg.ac.rs (M.S.)

2 Department of Life and Health Sciences, School of Sciences and Engineering, University of Nicosia, 2417 Nicosia, Cyprus

* Correspondence: liarasn@gmail.com; Tel.: +30-6983396537

Abstract: This narrative review paper provides an up-to-date overview of the potential of novel synthetic and semisynthetic compounds as antibacterials that target virulence traits in resistant strains. The review focused on research conducted in the last five years and investigated a range of compounds including azoles, indoles, thiophenes, glycopeptides, pleuromutilin derivatives, lactone derivatives, and chalcones. The emergence and spread of antibiotic-resistant bacterial strains is a growing public health concern, and new approaches are urgently needed to combat this threat. One promising approach is to target virulence factors, which are essential for bacterial survival and pathogenesis, but not for bacterial growth. By targeting virulence factors, it may be possible to reduce the severity of bacterial infections without promoting the development of resistance. We discuss the mechanisms of action of the various compounds investigated and their potential as antibacterials. The review highlights the potential of targeting virulence factors as a promising strategy to combat antibiotic resistance and suggests that further research is needed to identify new compounds and optimize their efficacy. The findings of this review suggest that novel synthetic and semisynthetic compounds that target virulence factors have great potential as antibacterials in the fight against antibiotic resistance.

Keywords: antibiotic resistance; virulence factors; novel synthetic compounds; biofilms; antibacterial activity

1. Introduction

Antibiotic resistance is a major global health challenge, threatening the efficacy of currently available antibiotics [1]. The emergence and spread of multidrug-resistant bacteria underscore the urgent need for new antibacterial agents that can overcome resistance mechanisms [2]. Estimates indicate that, annually, over 2 million infections caused by resistants strains occur worldwide, with as many as approximately 30,000 fatal outcomes in the USA alone and USD 5 billion in health care assets allocated to this issue. At the beginning of the 21st century, a list of pathogenic microorganisms that showed different levels of resistance to antimicrobial agents was released, and it included *Enterococcus faecium*, *Staphylococcus aureus*, *Klebsiella pneumoniae*, *Acinetobacter baumannii*, *Pseudomonas aeruginosa*, and *Enterobacter* spp. The list is also known as the famous register of ESKAPE pathogens. Traditional antibiotics target bacterial growth, which can lead to the development of resistance through the acquisition of mutations or the transfer of resistance genes [3]. In contrast, compounds that target bacterial virulence traits, such as biofilm formation, quorum sensing, and motility, may be less prone to the development of resistance [4]. Bacterial infections remain a significant challenge in public health, and the emergence of antimicrobial resistance (AMR) has further complicated the treatment of bacterial infections [5]. Despite the availability of many antibiotics, the prevalence of bacterial infections caused by multidrug-resistant bacteria has increased alarmingly. One strategy to overcome AMR is to target the virulence traits of bacterial pathogens, which are distinct from traditional antibiotic targets [6]. Virulence factors are the attributes that enable pathogens to cause disease in a host, such as adhesion, invasion, colonization, and the secretion of toxins and enzymes [7]. Therefore, the inhibition of virulence factors is a promising approach to combating bacterial infections [8].

The virulence traits of resistant bacteria have received increasing attention in recent years. Biofilm formation is one of the important virulence factors that contribute to bacterial resistance [9]. Biofilms are complex communities of microorganisms that are encased in a self-produced extracellular matrix, which confers resistance to antibiotics and immune defense mechanisms [10]. Bacteria can cause disease by producing agents known as virulence traits, which are specific compounds produced by bacteria that allow them to evade the host's immune system response. Virulence traits such as quorum sensing, motility, and iron acquisition have also been reported to be involved in the pathogenicity and antibiotic resistance of bacterial pathogens. As well as adhesins, invasins, and antiphagocytic factors, toxins, hemolysins, and proteases are among the agents that cause harm to the host [11].

A variety of natural and synthetic compounds have been reported to possess antivirulence activity against resistant bacteria. Among them, azoles, indoles, thiophenes, glycopeptides, pleuromutilin derivatives, lactone derivatives, and chalcones have been found to exhibit promising antivirulence activity [12–15]. These compounds target various virulence factors and interfere with the pathogenicity of bacterial pathogens (Figure 1), thus enhancing the efficacy of antibiotics and reducing the emergence of resistance.

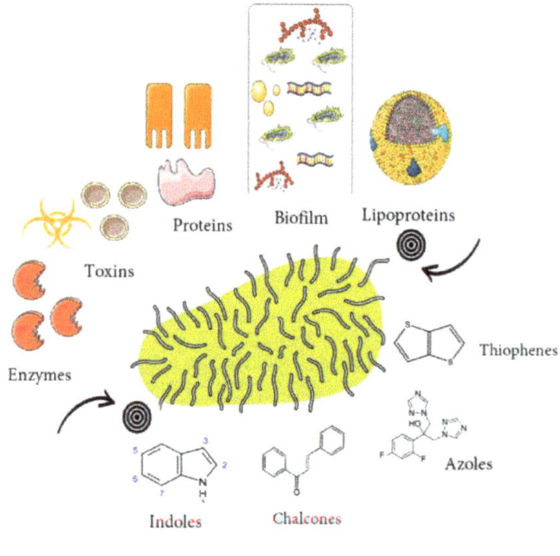

Figure 1. Group of compounds that target virulence traits in resistant bacteria.

Chalcones are a class of natural and synthetic compounds that have been shown to inhibit bacterial biofilm formation and quorum sensing [16]. Azoles, including pyrazoles, oxadiazoles, and triazoles, have been extensively studied as antifungal agents, but recent studies have shown that they also have antibacterial activity against resistant strains [17]. Coumarins have been found to inhibit bacterial quorum sensing and motility [18], while indoles and thiophenes have also shown potential as quorum sensing inhibitors [19]. Quinolines have been proposed as inhibitors of bacterial type II topoisomerases and have shown activity against multidrug-resistant bacteria [20]. Terpenoids, including triterpenoids and other scaffolds, have been mainly studied as semisynthetic analogues with promising antibacterial activity [21]. Glycopeptides, such as vancomycin and teicoplanin, have been widely used as antibiotics, but semisynthetic analogues have been developed to overcome resistance mechanisms [22]. Pleuromutilin derivatives, including retapamulin and lefamulin, have been approved for clinical use and have shown efficacy against resistant strains [23]. Finally, albocyclin and other lactone derivatives have shown activity against Gram-positive and Gram-negative bacteria, including resistant strains [24].

Targeting virulence traits is an attractive strategy to combat resistant bacteria. The use of compounds that target virulence factors can complement traditional antibiotic therapies, leading to enhanced efficacy and reduced resistance. Therefore, continuous research on the development of anti-virulence compounds and their mechanisms of action is crucial in the fight against AMR. In this review, we discuss recent studies on synthetic and semisynthetic compounds with antibacterial activity, focusing on their ability to target virulence traits in resistant strains. We also highlight the potential of these compounds to overcome antibiotic resistance mechanisms and suggest directions for future research. The presented review article mainly summarizes the progress in this field in the last 5 years, but its also covers some older important data. The fresh perspectives of compounds newly identified as potential therapeutics targeting virulence factors are presented, along with the established antimicrobial properties of certain novel compounds and the repurposing of existing antibacterial/antifungal therapeutics.

2. Indoles

Indoles, a widespread naturally occurring class of alkaloid compounds, are not only important bacterial intercellular signal molecules, but also a crucial component of the amino acid tryptophan. They are a particularly intriguing class of compounds covering a range of pharmacological activities, including antiinflammatory, antihistaminic, antitumor, antioxidative, and antidiabetic properties. Research covering this topic is quite important due to the versatile nature of indole compounds, which may lead to numerous chemical modifications, i.e., presenting possibilities for drug development. With respect to the subject of this review, their antibacterial potential, particularly their targeting of virulence factors, is thoroughly elaborated herein.

In the following section, we present the antibacterial potential of selected indole-derived compounds against clinically relevant strains, namely the causative agents of urinary and skin infections as well as gastroenteritis-causing bacteria. According to Balcerek et al. [25], commercial compounds, such as 5-halo-*1H*-indole-2-carboxylic acids, (Figure 2) were efficient against a panel of bacterial strains, particularly *Listeria monocytogenes*. The obtained results indicated that this activity may be used for the development of medicines in the treatment of listeriosis in cases when resistance/allergy is present. Along with these results, assays also showed that indol-2-one (Figure 2) with a morpholinosulfonyl component acted as a potent inhibitor of the DNA gyrase of both Gram-positive and Gram-negative bacteria, with activity against *S. aureus* even better than ciprofloxacin (IC_{50} values 18.75 μM and 26.43 μM, respectively) [26]. Furthermore, Alzahrani et al. [27] showed that novel derivatives of the compound thiazolo-indolin-2-one exerted rather promising antibacterial activity, with a noteworthy ability to affect virulence traits such as biofilm formation in *S. aureus* (ATCC 29213) and *P. aeruginosa* (biofilm inhibition concentration (BIC_{50}) of 1.95 μg/mL and 3.9 μg/mL, respectively). As for the ability to affect traits of *A. baumanii*, literature data indicate that d-pyrimido[4,5-*b*] indole derivatives show inhibitory potential against this pathogen in the range of 0.25–1 gmL^{-1} [28]. Furthermore, 3-amino indoles (Figure 2), 4-hydroxy-2-pyridone derivatives containing indolyl, 2-hydrazino2-imidazoline, and bis-indolyl methane Schiff bases have also been identified as potential antimicrobial agents that may also inhibit the growth of MDR *A. baumanii*. Recent research conducted by Raorane et al. [29] showed that halogenated indole 5-iodoindole (Figure 2) promptly affected the development and motility of *A. baumannii*, disrupted its biofilm formation, and eventually eradicated this pathogenic microorganism as effectively as ciprofloxacin and gentamicin. This was achieved via the development of ROS, which had a profound influence on the integrity of the plasma membrane, eventually leading to a loss of bacterial viability. Furthermore, the tested compound turned out to be verry effective against *Escherichia coli* and *S. aureus* but did not influence the viability of *P. aeruginosa*. According to Kim et al. [30], indole and its derivatives also proved efficient in the inhibiting single-species and multi-species biofilms of the acne-forming bacterial skin strains *Cutibacterium acnes* and *S. aureus*, with 3,3′-diindolylmethane as the most potent inhibitor. The obtained results indicated that indole-derived compounds may be useful in developing efficient skin treatments related to the tested bacteria.

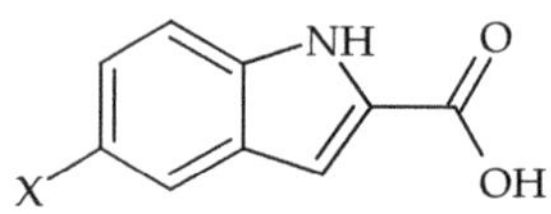

5-halo-1H-indole-2-carboxylic acid

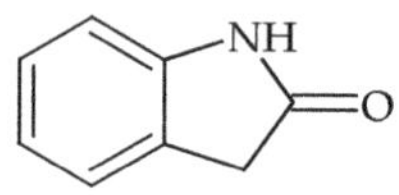

indol-2-one

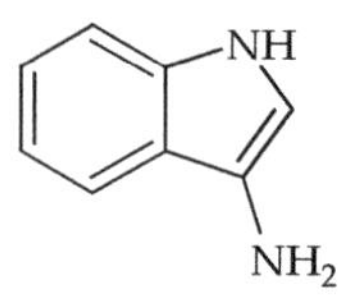

3-aminoindole

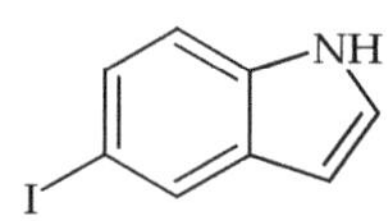

5-iodoindole

Figure 2. Chemical structures of 5-halo-*1H*-indole-2-carboxylic acid, indol-2-one, 3-amino indole, and 5-iodoindole.

The eradication of the nosocomial pathogen *Enterococcus faecalis* has been shown to be quite challenging in recent years, with biofilm development and resistance to antibiotics as the two main causes. Hence, new treatments are urgently needed, particularly those affecting these two traits. A study by Tatta et al. [31] showed that the indole terpenoid compound rhodethrin (Figure 3) in combination with chloramphenicol disrupted the overall formation of biofilm, which may lead to the easier and more effective treatment of vancomycin-resistant *E. faecalis*.

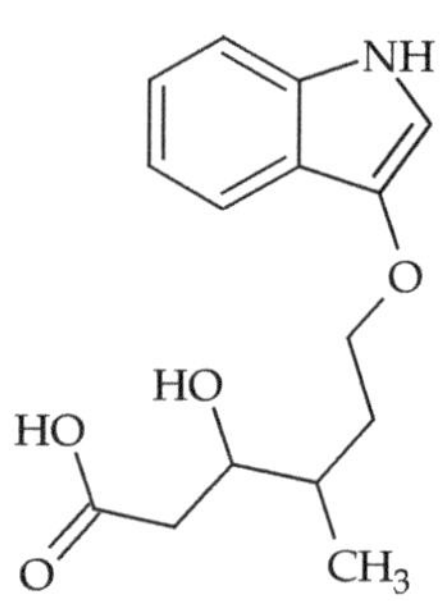

Rhodethrin

Figure 3. Chemical structure of rhodethrin.

Nosocomial urinary infections related to catheter application are most often caused by *Proteus mirabilis*. Due to biofilm development, they have been increasingly harder to treat, leading to a demand for novel and efficient treatments. Hence, Amer et al. [32] developed new Foley catheters impregnated with indole compounds (indole extract from the supernatant of the rhizobacterium *Enterobacter* sp. Zch127) in order to disrupt the biofilm formation of *Proteus mirabilis*. The results showed a reduction in the formation of biofilm of 60–70% in terms of biomass, which was confirmed by the expression of virulence genes responsible for biofilm formation, while genes that regulate the formation of capsular polysaccharides were not affected. The catheters were considered safe for use, since they had no cytotoxic effects on fibroblasts. Along with nosocomial *P. mirabilis*, uropathogenic *E. coli* is a common inhabitant of the human urinary tract, leading to recurrent infections. The recurrence rate depends on the pathogen's ability to infiltrate the urinary epithelium and evade host defense mechanisms. Boya et al. [33] demonstrated that 4-chloroindole, 5-chloroindole, and 5-chloro 2-methyl indole may profoundly impact biofilm formation at an average dose of 20 g/mL by as much as 67%, along with their ability to reduce bacterial motility, necessary for colony dispersal. A more in-depth study showed that the tested compounds affected the expression of genes related to adhesion and toxin production, which may be of importance in managing clinical manifestations of these health conditions.

Due to their ability to regulate internal environments by removing toxic substances, efflux pumps are an important target when considering the development of new drugs. According to Cernicchi et al. [34], indole derivatives could also have wide-ranging applications in this area, which could increase their use in clinical practice.

Along with the fact that indoles are highly active against pathogenic microorganisms of clinical relevance, they have also been shown to be very efficient in targeting virulence traits of *Agrobacterium tumefaciens*. This may be rather important with respect to the economy, since this microorganism is known as a plant pathogen causing significant lossess in various crops. As Ahmed et al. [35] demonstrated in their study, among 83 indole derivatives that were tested against *A. tumefaciens*, 4-chloroindole, 6-iodoindole, and 5-chloro-2-methyl indole inhibited its growth at doses as high as 50 μg mL^{-1}. Furthermore, they also affected virulence factors such as swimming motility, the production of exopolysaccharide and exoprotease, and cell surface hydrophobicity and biofilm formation.

Besides issues with various crops, the aquaculture sector also faces a serious problem resulting from bacterial infections. In terms of money, losses resulting from vibriosis—a disease caused by *Vibrio campbelli*—are quite substantial. This has inevitably led to the development of novel and sustainable strategies required for managing problems in the aquaculture industry. One of these is the evaluation of indole analogs' activity against *V. campbellii*, probably the main bacterial pathogens in aquaculture. Out of 44 tested compounds, 17 halogenated indoles (including 6-bromoindole, 7-bromoindole, 4-fluoroindole, 5-iodoindole, and 7-iodoindole) have been shown to affect the virulence traits of *V. campbellii*. Furthermore, they have been found to increase the survival of brine shrimp, used as a valid in vivo system model, by over 80% at 10 mM, as well as to affect virulence traits such as swimming motility and biofilm formation (at concentrations of 10 mM and 100 mM), whereas only mild inhibition was achieved with the tested concentrations regarding protease activity. The absence of hemolytic activity was observed using the tested concentrations [36]. Similar antibacterial virulence targeting activity was previously obtained for *Vibrio tasmaniensis* LGP32 and *Vibrio crassostreae* J2-9, used as two model infections of bivalves [36], which indicates that this strategy may be very useful in developing antivirulence therapy. The control of *Vibrio parahaemolyticus*, a potential cause of gastroenteritis brought on by the consummation of raw sea food, is also becoming increasingly important, since a certain amount of healthcare expenses have been directed towards treating this condition. In their study, Sathiyamoorthi et al. [37] demonstrated that halogenated indole derivatives (4-chloroindole, 7-chloroindole, 4-iodoindole, and 7-iodoindole) strongly influence some of the virulence factors of *V. parahaemolyticus*: for example, 4 chloroindole inhibited biofilm formation by 80% at a MIC of 50 g/mL, whereas 100 g/mL terminated its viability within the first 30 min of activity. As it turned out, the position of the halogenated substituent in indole core determines its extraordinary activity.

Though these results did not highlight the potential of indole compounds to target bacterial virulence factors, recent data published by Li et al. [38] showed that 5-methylindole instantly eradicated several bacterial strains, including *S. aureus*, *E.faecalis*, *E. coli*, *P. aeruginosa*, methicillin-resistant *S. aureus*, *K. pneumoniae*, and *Mycobacterium tuberculosis*.

3. Azoles

Azole derivatives are heterocyclic compounds comprised of a nitrogen atom and at least one other non-carbon atom (such as nitrogen, sulfur, or oxygen) as part of the ring. They encompass a wide number of derivatives, such as thiadiazole, oxadiazole, triazole, imidazole, isoxazole, and pyrazole. Mainly known as antifungal agents, azole derivatives demonstrate many other biological properties, including antidiabetic, immunosuppressant, antiinflammatory, and anticancer activities. Even though they were initially used for the treatment of fungal infections, various azole-containing compounds have been shown to inhibit the growth of bacteria as well, via a different mode of action. In fungi, azoles mainly inhibit the production of ergosterol—an essential component of the fungal plasma membrane—whereas in bacteria, their activity is based on the fact that the attachment of azole to bacterial flavohemoglobin (protein) eventually leads to the increasing production of ROS, which have fatal effects on bacterial viability [39].

Due to their versatility in chemical structure and biological activities, azoles have been widely investigated in pharmacochemistry, but they still present surprises. According to Srikanth et al. [28], azole compounds are highly efficient against *A. Baumanii*, which is of great importance considering that this multi-drug-resistant pathogenic microorganism belongs to the infamous ESKAPE group. In particular, naphthalimide-containing nitroimidazoles with decyl-piperazine exerted strong activity against *A. baumannii* (MIC 0.013 MmL^{-1}) and, combined with norfloxacin, eradicated even the resistant strains. Additionaly, ammonium containing imidazoles also showed antimicrobial potential. The same study demonstrated that the type of the modification as well as the substituent determines the level of antimicrobial properties. Thus, the presence of 4-Br-phenol modification increased activity against *A. baumanii*, whereas a hydrophobic *n*-butyl chain on the phenyl ring decreased activity against the same pathogen. The absence of a halogen molecule is generally reflected through a decrease in bioactivity.

Along with this growing trend of repurposing already available therapeutics, Olaifa et al. [40] also investigated the ability of itraconazole and fluconazole (Figure 4) to target specific virulence factors. The ability to disrupt biofilm formation in *A. baumanii* was demonstrated in the abovementioned study, which clearly indicated that azole compounds may very well be underinvestigated in terms of their antibacterial and virulence-targeting potential. This was also previously demonstrated by Qiu et al. [41]—using *Streptococcus mutans* clinical isolates as model organisms, clotrimazole and econazole (Figure 5) inhibited its growth at 12.5 and 25 mgL^{-1}, respectively. Furthermore, they were able to inhibit biofilm production, which undoubtedly demonstrated that these antifungal medicines may also target bacterial virulence factors.

Numerous data dealing with the antibacterial potential of antifungal drugs have been presented in the last two years. Even though these drugs do not target virulence factors, the results are noteworthy, favoring the repurposing of antifungal drugs as novel antibacterials. For example, Nasr et al. [42] demonstrated that a pyrazole derivative (der. 30) proved to be more effective against *Pneumocystis vulgaris* and *K. pneumoniae* than sulfisoxazole and gentamycin. Among 4-(4-formyl-3-phenyl-1*H*-pyrazol-1-yl)benzoic acid derivatives, some of the identified compounds showed antibacterial activity against *A. baumanii* with an MIC of 4 μg/mL [28]. Furthermore, according to Gomes et al. [43], of twenty-one freshly synthesized 1,4-naphthoquinones linked to 1,2,3-1*H*-triazoles, four (**9e**, **9h**, **9i** and **9j**) proved to possess antibacterial activity against *S. mutans* from oral cavities with IZs of 18.66–29.00 mm. The results also showed no toxic effects for these compounds, which possibly increases their potential for application in practice. 1,2,4-triazolidine-3-thiones (Figure 6) exerted antibacterial activity against the ESKAPE list of pathogenic bacteria. Furthermore, binaphthyl-1,2,3-triazole peptidomimetics were efficient against *A. baumannii* with an MIC of 4 g/mL. Along with this, cationic biaryl 1,2,3-triazolyl peptidomimetic derivatives moderately inhibited the growth of *A. baumannii* [28]. Antibacterial but not virulence-targeting activity was also demonstrated in a study by Sapijanskaite-Banevic et al. [44]. In order to create substituted 1-phenyl-5-oxopyrrolidine (Figure 6) derivatives with benzimidazole, oxadiazole, triazole, dihydrazone, and dithiosemicarbazide moieties in the structure, p-aminobenzoic acid (Figure 6) was employed. Using different assays, the antimicrobial activity of each drug was assessed in vitro against *S. aureus*, *Bacillus cereus*, *L. monocytogenes*, *Salmonella enteritidis*, *E. coli*, and *P. aeruginosa*. This work demonstrated the potent bactericidal effects of benzimidazoles and derivatives of amino acids, with some of the compounds exceeding the activity of ampicillin. In the field of medicinal chemistry, combining two or more pharmacological groups into a single molecule is a new approach to drug discovery [45]. As demostrated by Dawoud et al. [46], a novel group of heterocyclic compounds merged using a indazolylthiazole moiety was evaluated for their antimicrobial potential. The obtained results showed that four of the compounds exhibited antibacterial effects, with the strongest activity observed against *Streptococcus mutans* and *P. aeruginosa*. Furthermore, these novel compounds showed virulence-targeting activity, with high antibiofilm potential. Srikanth et al. [28] also suggested that aminothiazolyl berberine (Figure 6) affects the activity of the DNA gyrase of MDR *A. baumannii* strains, exerting remarkable activitiy at an MIC of 2 nmol/mL. Among oxazole/benzisoxazole-based compounds, N-(2-(1*H*-imidazol-4-yl)ethyl)-2-(2,3-dihydroxyphenyl)-*N*-hydroxy-5-methyloxazole-4-carboxamide showed antibacterial activity against *A. Baumannii*, with an MIC of 2 μg/mL (strains UNT190 and UNT197) [28].

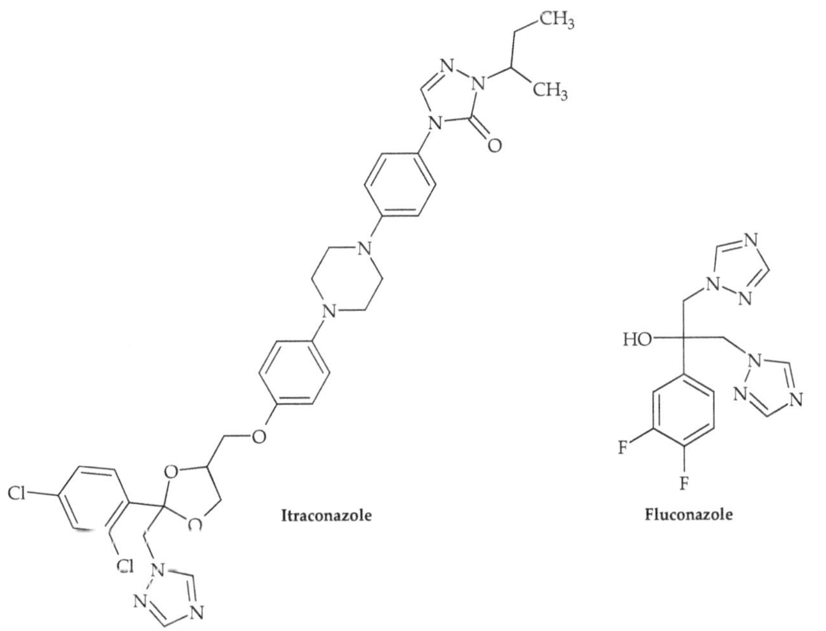

Figure 4. Chemical structures of itraconazole and fluconazole.

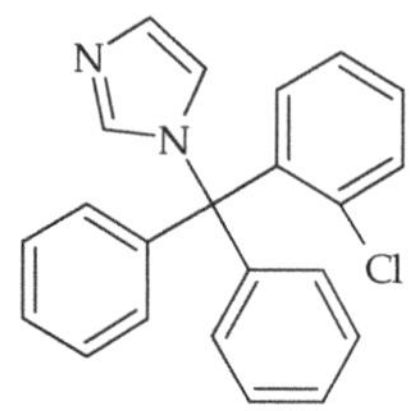

Clotrimazole

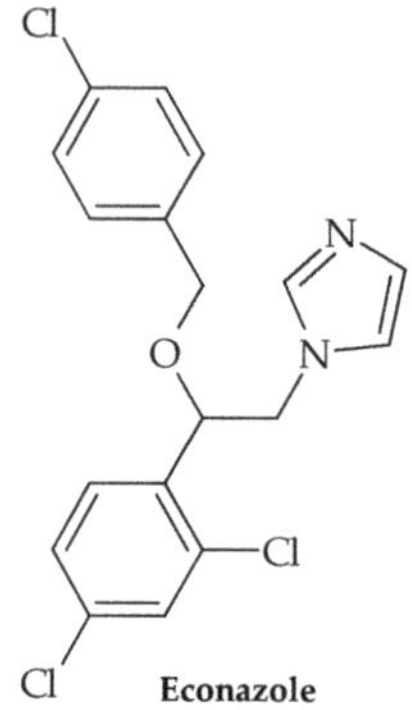

Econazole

Figure 5. Chemical structures of clotrimazole and econazole.

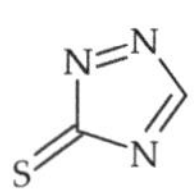

1,2,4-triazolidine-3-thione

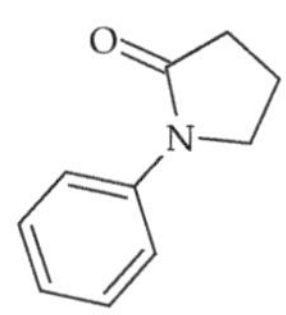

1-phenyl-5-oxopyrrolidine

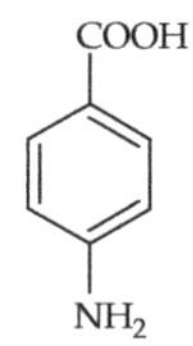

p-aminobenzoic acid

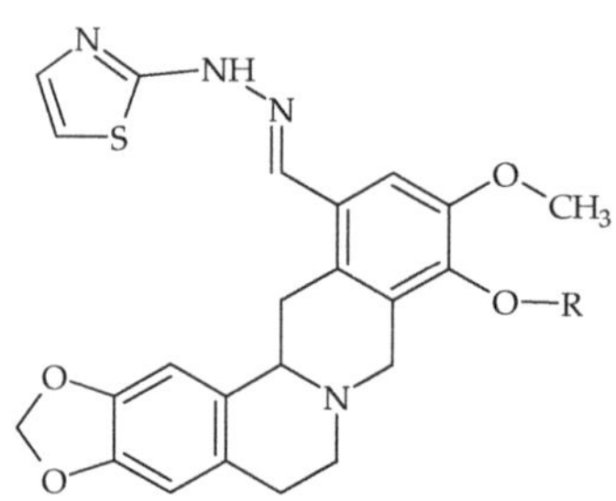

aminothiazolyl berberine derivatives

Figure 6. Chemical structures of 1,2,4-triazolidine-3-thione, 1-phenyl-5-oxopyrrolidine, p-aminobenzoic acid, and aminothiazolyl berberine.

4. Thiophenes

Thiophenes and related derivatives are rather versatile heterocyclic compounds with various applications in medicine and drug discovery. With a wide range of bioactive properties, they have been shown to possess remarkable anti-inflammatory, antianxiety, antimicrobial, antioxidant, and other activities. Furthermore, they have long been present on the market as commercial therapeutics, for example, tipeptidine, dorzolamide, and citizolam. However, only data relating to the scope of this review (i.e., antibacterial activity) are presented here. According to Rando et al. [47], 5,5′-dinitro-2-(2,3-diaza-4-(2′-tienyl)buta-1,3-dienyl)thiophene (Figure 7) possesses promising antituberculosis activity, as it inhibited the growth of pathogenic *Mycobacterium avium* and *M. kansasei*. This compound showed notable levels of mutagenicity as well, which limits its potential for application in clinical practice. Moreover, antimicrobial activity against *S. aureus* was observed by Scotti et al. [48], achieved by targeting RNA polymerase.

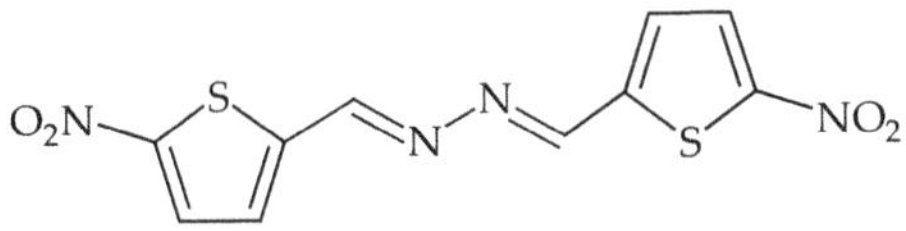

5,5′-dinitro-2-(2,3-diaza-4-(2′-tienyl)buta-1,3-dienyl)thiophene

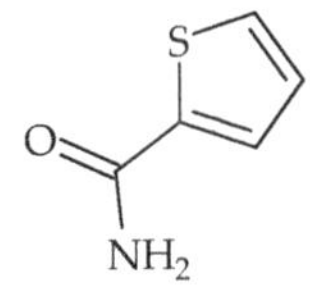

thiophene-2-carboxamide

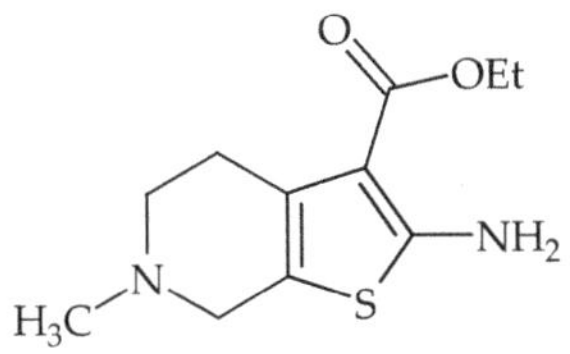

2-amino-3-carbethoxy-6-N-methylpiperidinothiophene

Figure 7. Chemical structures of 5,5′-dinitro-2-(2,3-diaza-4-(2′-tienyl)buta-1,3-dienyl)thiophene, 2-amino-3-carbethoxy-6-*N* methyl piperidino thiophene, and thiophene-2-carboxamide.

According to Ramalingam et al. [49], 2-amino-3-carbethoxy-6-*N* methyl piperidino thiophene (Figure 7) was used as a starting point for the synthesis of novel compounds to be tested for their antibacterial potential using the Kirby–Baurer method. Among the tested compounds, twelve were found to be potent against *B. subtilis* and *E. coli*.

The most recent research of Metwally et al. [50] indicated that thiophene-2-carboxamide (Figure 7) derivatives showed antibacterial properties, with *S. aureus*, *B. subtilis*, *E. coli*, and *P. aeruginosa* being the most susceptible to the activity of the tested compounds. While the results showed no indication of targeting virulence factors, the very fact that the novel synthesized compounds possessed microbicidal activity with no targeted virulence factors whatsoever suggests that there is still hope for old-fashioned drugs as antimicrobials.

The types of activity against pathogenic bacteria presented by indoles, azoles, and thiophenes are presented in Table 1.

Table 1. Selected compounds and their type of activity against pathogenic bacteria.

Group of Compounds	Compound	Bacteria	Type of Activity	Reference
Indole	5-halo-1*H*-indole-2-carboxylic acids	*Listeria monocytogenes*	Inhibits the growth of bacteria	[25]
Indole	indol-2-one with morpholinosulfonyl	*Staphylococcusaureus*	Inhibitor of DNA gyrase	[26]
Indole	thiazolo-indolin-2-one	*S. aureus* (ATCC 29213) *P. aeruginosa* (ATCC 9027)	Inhibits biofilm formation	[27]
Indole	d-pyrimido[4,5 b] indole	*Acinetobacter baumanii*	Inhibits the growth of bacteria	[28]
Indole	3-amino indoles	Multi-drug resistant *A. baumanii*	Inhibits the growth of bacteria	[28]
Indole	4-hydroxy-2-pyridone derivatives containing indolyl	Multi-drug resistant *A. baumanii*	Inhibits the growth of bacteria	[28]
Indole	2-hydrazino2-imidazoline	Multi-drug resistant *A. baumanii*	Inhibits the growth of bacteria	[28]
Indole	bis-indolyl methane	Multi-drug resistant *A. baumanii*	Inhibits the growth of bacteria	[28]

Table 1. *Cont.*

Group of Compounds	Compound	Bacteria	Type of Activity	Reference
Indole	5-iodoindole	*A. baumanii, Escherichia coli, S. aureus*	Inhibits the growth of bacteria, decreases motility, disrupts biofilm formation	[29]
Indole	3,3′-diindolylmethane	*Cutibacterium acnes S. aureus*	Inhibits the growth of bacteria	[30]
Indole	indole terpenoid compound rhodethrin	*Enterococcus faecalis*	Inhibits biofilm formation	[31]
Indole	indole extract from the supernatant of the rhizobacterium *Enterobacter* sp. Zch127	*Proteus mirabilis*	Inhibits biofilm formation	[32]
Indole	4-chloroindole, 5-chloroindole, 5-chloro 2-methyl indole	*E. coli*	Decreases bacterial motility, disrupts biofilm formation	[33]
Indole	4-chloroindole, 6-iodoindole, 5-chloro-2-methyl indole	*Agrobacterium tumefaciens*	Decreases swimming motility, the production of exopolysaccharide and exoprotease, and cell surface hydrophobicity and biofilm formation	[35]
Indole	indole	*V. tasmaniensis* LGP32 and *V. crassostreae* J2-9	Decreases swimming motility, inhibits biofilm formation	[36]
Indole	4-chloroindole, 7-chloroindole, 4-iodoindole, and 7-iodoindole	*V. parahaemolyticus*	Inhibits biofilm formation	[37]
Azole	naphthalimide-containing nitroimidazoles	*A. baumannii*	Inhibits the growth of bacteria	[28]
Azole	itraconazole and fluconazole	*A. baumannii*	Inhibits biofilm formation	[40]
Azole	clotrimazole, econazole	*Streptococcus mutans*	Inhibits biofilm formation	[41]
Azole	pyrazole 30	*Pneumocystis vulgaris Klebsiella pneumoniae*	Inhibits the growth of bacteria	[42]
Azole	1,4-naphthoquinones linked to 1,2,3-*1H*-triazoles—compounds (9e, 9h, 9i, and 9j)	*S. mutans*	Inhibits the growth of bacteria	[43]
Azole	binaphthyl-1,2,3-triazole peptidomimetics	*A. baumannii*	Inhibits the growth of bacteria	[28]
Azole	heterocycle compounds with indazolylthiazole moiety (compounds 2, 3, 7, and 8)	*S. mutans, P.aeruginosa*	Inhibits biofilm production	[46]
Azole	*N*-(2-(*1H*-imidazol-4-yl)ethyl)-2-(2,3-dihydroxyphenyl)-*N*-hydroxy-5-methyloxazole-4-carboxamide	*A. baumannii*	Inhibits the growth of bacteria	[28]

Table 1. *Cont.*

Group of Compounds	Compound	Bacteria	Type of Activity	Reference
Thiophene	5,5′-dinitro-2-(2,3-diaza-4-(2′-tienyl)buta-1,3-dienyl)thiophene	*Mycobacterium avium* *M. kansasei*	Inhibits the growth of bacteria	[47]
Thiophene	2 -amino-3-carbethoxy-6-*N* methyl piperidino thiophene	*B. subtilis* *E. coli*	Inhibits the growth of bacteria	[49]
Thiophene	thiophene-2-carboxamide	*S. aureus, B. subtilis, E. coli, P. aeruginosa*	Inhibits the growth of bacteria	[50]

5. Pleuromutilin Derivatives

Pleuromutilin (Figure 8), a diterpenoid secondary metabolite with a tricyclic structure, was initially discovered in *Pleurotus passeckerianus* and *P. mutilis* mushrooms in 1951 [51]. This compound and its derivatives demonstrated strong antibacterial efficacy against Gram-positive bacteria, mycoplasma, and chlamydia [52] by interacting with the peptidyl transferase core (PTC) of bacterial ribosomes and blocking protein synthesis [53,54].

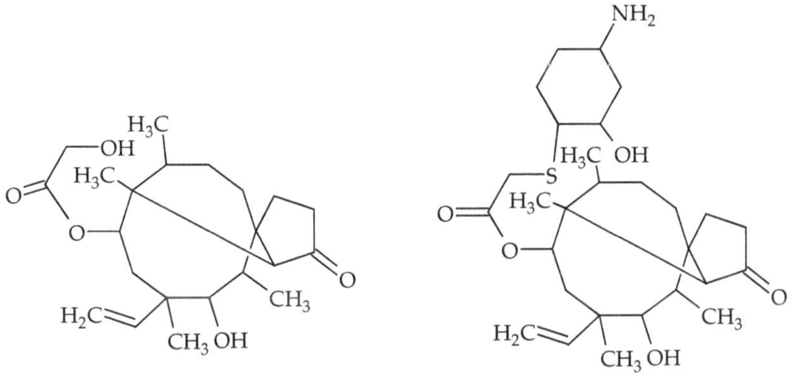

Pleuromutilin **Lefamulin**

Figure 8. Chemical structures of pleuromutilin and lefamulin.

Pleuromutilins bind to the PTC and compete for binding with the 16-atom macrolide and peptidyltransferase inhibitor carbomycin (but not with the 14-atom macrolide erythromycin) [55], inhibiting the formation of peptide bonds [56]. The X-ray crystallography of ribosome-drug complexes was used to identify the precise nature of pleuromutilin binding to the ribosome [57]

Four semi-synthetic derivatives of pleuromutilin have so far received approval for use in the treatment of infectious disorders, including lefamulin (Figure 8) for the treatment of adult community-acquired bacterial pneumonia (CABP) [58], tiamulin and valnemulin for use in veterinary medicine, and retapamulin for use as an antibiotic in the treatment of human skin infections [59,60]. Lefamulin is the only pleuromutilin derivative that has been demonstrated to inhibit the *S. aureus* cfr (chloramphenicol–florfenicol resistance gene) strain [61].

Chemists have worked very hard to create pleuromutilin derivatives due to its unique mechanism of action and promising antibacterial properties [62].

The gene cluster for pleuromutilin has been described and functionally characterized with regard to its production [63]. The creation of new pleuromutilin-based antibiotics will be aided by the identification of new pleuromutilin derivatives [64].

Lefamulin interferes with the peptidyl transferase center of the 50S ribosome by specifically binding at the A- and P-sites, blocking the formation of peptide bonds. This interferes with the production of bacterial proteins [54].

Lefamulin uses a special induced fit mechanism to close the binding pocket within the ribosome, ensuring the tight binding of the drug to the target site, even though this mechanism of action is similar to that of the oxazolidinones and can actually compete with the phenicols for the same binding site [54]. This is a unique strategy for preventing bacterial peptide chain elongation, especially with the creation of the first peptide bond; however, lefamulin is ineffective once elongation has begun [65]. With the exception of *M. pneumoniae*, lefamulin presents bacteriostatic characteristics against the majority of species [66]. Lefamulin has exhibited action against all aerobic Gram-positive organisms, except *E. faecalis* [54].

Likewise, methicillin-resistant *S. aureus* (MRSA), heterogeneous VISA (hVISA), vancomycin-resistant *S. aureus* (VRSA), penicillin-resistant *S. pneumoniae* (PRSP), MDR *S. pneumoniae*, and vancomycin-resistant *E. faecalis* (VRE) are among the resistant Gram-positive organisms against which lefamulin is effective [54,67,68].

Tiamulin and valnemulin (Figure 9) attach to the bacterial 50S ribosomal subunit to prevent protein synthesis. It has been shown that these medications interact with 23S RNA's domain V and are potent inhibitors of peptidyl transferase, leaving distinct chemical traces at the nucleotides A2058-9, U2506, and U2584-5. All of these nucleotides are at or near the PTC and have been linked to the binding of several antibiotics. The majority of them are well conserved both phylogenetically and functionally [69].

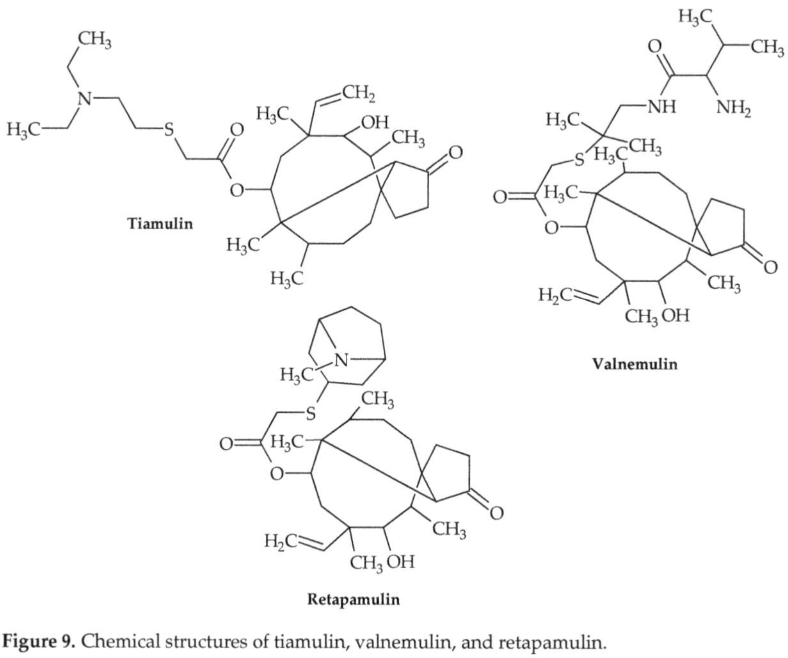

Figure 9. Chemical structures of tiamulin, valnemulin, and retapamulin.

These two compounds can bind alongside the macrolide erythromycin but compete with the macrolide carbomycin, which is a peptidyl transferase inhibitor, according to competitive footprinting. In order to impede the proper placement of the CCA ends of tRNAs for peptide transfer, these two chemicals interact with the rRNA in the peptidyl transferase slot on the ribosomes. Although ribosomal protein uL3 is located adjacent to the tiamulin binding site without coming into contact with the medication, tiamulin only interacts with rRNA residues [70]. Accordingly, tiamulin binds to the 50s subunit's A site, and the acetic acid tail extends to the P site, interfering with the formation of peptide bonds [70].

Retapamulin (Figure 9) is a pleuromutilin antibiotic that blocks the formation of the 50S ribosomal unit in bacteria, hence inhibiting the production of proteins [71]. It is effective against Gram-positive pathogens, and since 2007, a topical preparation has been licensed in the US for treating skin and soft tissue infections in adults and children older than 9 months [72].

Retapamulin has demonstrated remarkable in vitro and in vivo action against MRSA and MSSA strains of *S. aureus* in prior studies [73] and has also shown good outcomes against mupirocin-resistant MRSA [72].

6. Albocyclin and General Lactone Derivatives

A class of substances known as lactones is commonly present in nature [74]. Chemically, they can be categorized as variously sized intramolecular esters of hydroxycarboxylic acids. The most prevalent are the lactones with five- and six-membered rings due to the stability of the ring structure [75]. However, alternative ring sizes of lactones can also be extracted from natural sources or produced chemically [76].

Lactones are a very fascinating group that demonstrates various significant biological characteristics as a result of its diversity [77].

The main structure of the lactones group has recently been modified to create new analogs with stronger or different responses. These new analogs can exhibit a toxic effect on the cells of pathogenic bacteria and serve as an alternative to the widely used antibiotics [78].

It is known that bacteriostatic properties are exhibited by substances in which the lactone moiety is present in a small ring, e.g., xanthatin [79], a bicyclic lactone isolated from *Xanthium pensylvanicum* and *X. strumarium*, which is active against *S. aureus*, including MRSA-resistant methicillin strains [80].

Several strains of *Streptomyces* produce albocycline—a 14-membered macrolactone (Figure 10) [81]. This compound has shown in vitro antimicrobial activity against MRSA and VRSA equipotent to vancomycin [82,83]. Despite this, albocycline may represent a solution for the treatment of infections caused by *S. aureus* species.

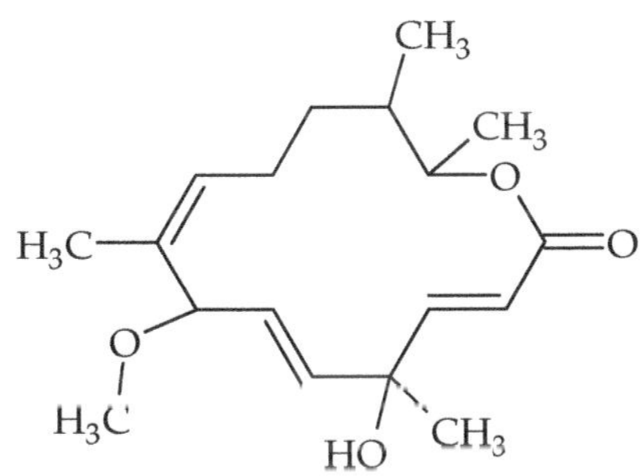

Albocycline

Figure 10. Chemical structure of albocycline.

A structural motif in the macrolide family of antibiotics, the 14-membered macrolactone of albocycline indicates that it targets the bacterial ribosome and thereby inhibits translation [84].

Albocycline, however, blocks the incorporation of radiolabeled *N*-acetylglucosamine ([3H]GlcNAc) into the peptidoglycan (PG), the protective polymer surrounding bacterial cells, according to research by Tomoda et al. The first component of bacterial PG production, N-acetylglucosamine (UDP-GlcNAc), accumulates as a result of albocycline's inhibition [82,85].

Due to albocycline's non-toxicity in mice and humans, in vivo investigations have suggested increased interest in the drug for potential therapeutic uses. Using human HepG2 hepatocellular liver cancer cells, the authors of [85] showed that albocycline was not harmful to human cells at a final concentration of less than 64 g/mL [83].

7. Glycopeptides

A class of non-ribosomal cyclic or polycyclic peptides known as glycopeptide antibiotics prevents the formation of Gram-positive bacterial cell walls. These substances function as substrate binders (of cell-wall precursors) as opposed to active-site enzyme inhibitors, unlike other antimicrobial classes [86–88].

By attacking lipid II (which represents a peptidoglycan-repeat unit that is related to the lipid transporter), glycopeptide antibiotics prevent Gram-positive bacteria from synthesizing PG. As a result, the lipid transporter shared by peptidoglycan and wall teichoic acid (WTA) biosynthesis, bactoprenol phosphate, cannot be recycled [89]. With each contributing almost 50% of the dry cell-wall weight, PG and WTA are two important parts of the cell wall. Through host attachment, colonization, infection, biofilm development, and the recruitment of penicillin-binding proteins (PBPs) to the septum during cell division, WTA plays a significant role in the pathogenicity of microbes [90]. Consequently, it serves as a desirable target for the creation of new antibiotics [89].

The oldest member of the class is vancomycin (Figure 11), while the more recent lipoglycopeptide derivatives oritavancin, teicoplanin, telavancin, and dalbavancin (Figures 12–15) were developed specifically to boost antibacterial activity, sometimes via secondary modes of action.

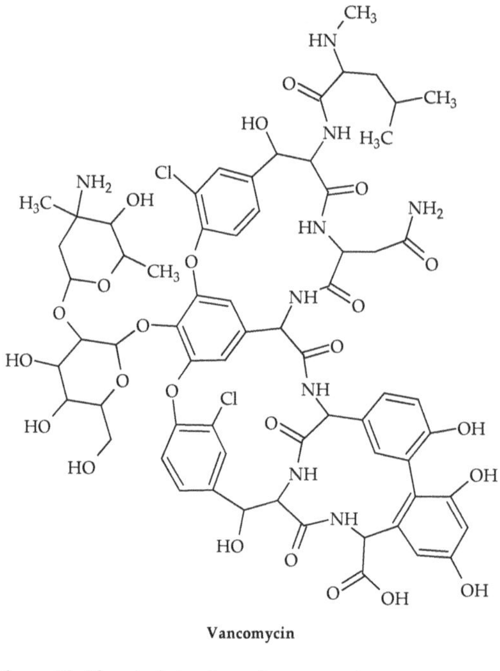

Vancomycin

Figure 11. Chemical structure of vancomycin.

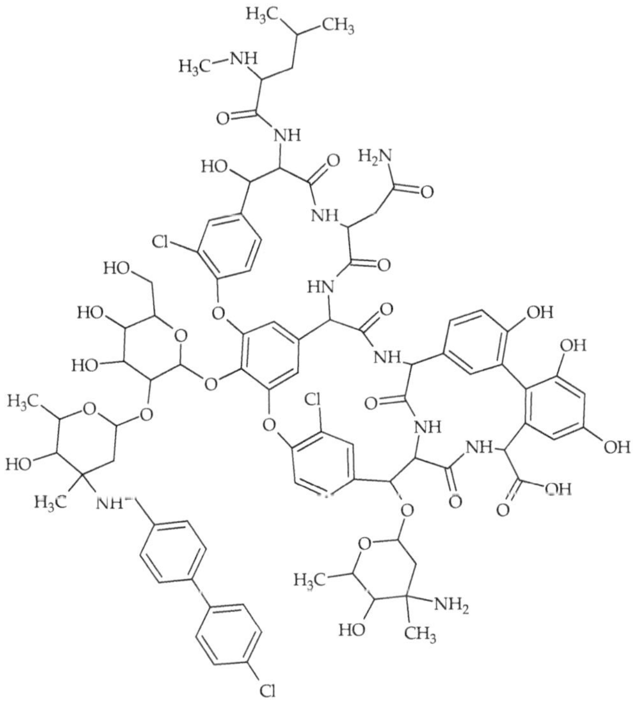

Oritavancin

Figure 12. Chemical structure of oritavancin.

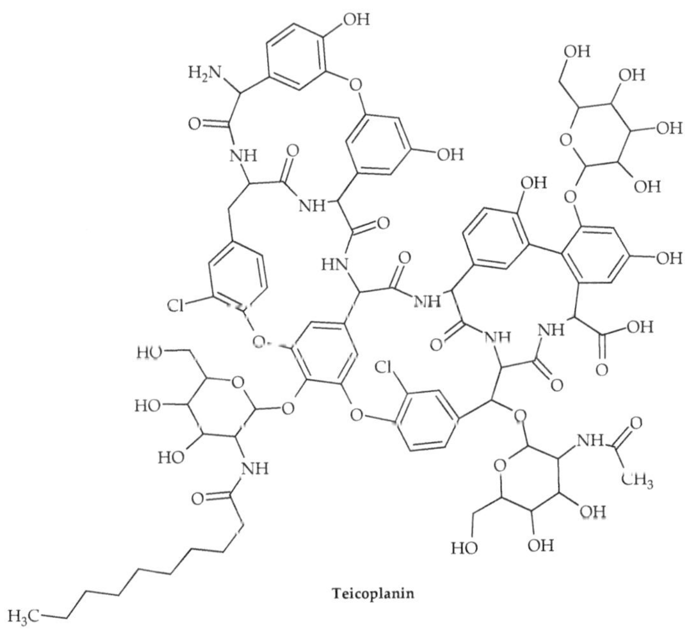

Teicoplanin

Figure 13. Chemical structure of teicoplanin.

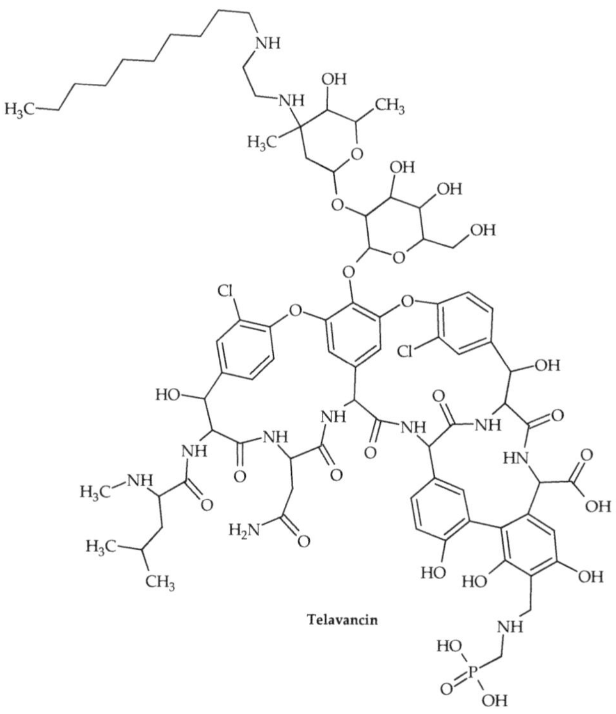

Figure 14. Chemical structure of telavancin.

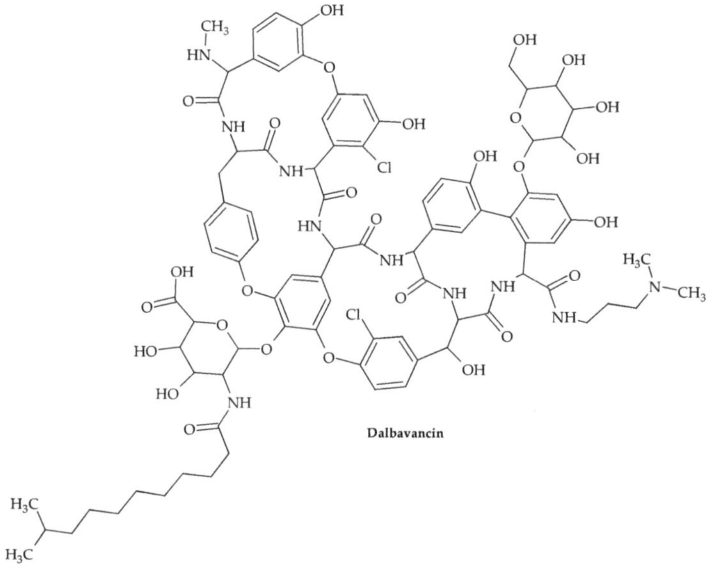

Figure 15. Chemical structure of dalbavancin.

The transglycosylation stage of PG production, which is necessary to replenish the lipid transporter, is prevented by glycopeptide antibiotic binding to lipid II. Therefore, for instance, when vancomycin is added to *S. aureus* during growth, Park's nucleotide, a cytoplasmic PG-precursor, accumulates [91]. Vancomycin binding to lipid II is an efficient way to suppress both PG and wall teichoic acid biosynthesis in *S. aureus* [89], since C55 is present in a surprisingly low number of copies per bacterium [92] and is a shared transporter needed in these processes [93].

Vancomycin is used to treat acute infections caused by Gram-positive organisms. By attaching to the D-Ala-D-Ala terminus of lipid II, a PG precursor tethered to the cell membrane by the lipid transporter bactoprenol-phosphate, vancomycin suppresses the formation of PG (C55-P). To stop C55-P regeneration, vancomycin-bound lipid II is sequestered from the PG biosynthesis transglycosylation step. Vancomycin's sequestration of lipid II causes the cytoplasmic buildup of Park's nucleotide [91], a cytoplasmic PG precursor, because C55 is present in bacteria in low concentrations [94]. When the dipeptide is swapped out for a depsipeptide D-Ala-D-Lac, vancomycin is unable to attach to the D-Ala-D-Ala terminus of lipid II in VRE [95].

As a result of investigating the structure–activity relationship of chloroeremomycin to combat vancomycin resistance, oritavancin was discovered [96], a semi-synthetic lipoglycopeptide that has potent antimicrobial effects against vancomycin-resistant organisms such as VRE and *S. aureus* resistant to vancomycin (VRSA) [97].

Oritavancin is currently a top therapeutic option for treating serious infections brought on by Gram-positive organisms that are multi-drug-resistant, such MRSA [89]. Oritavancin's chemical composition differs from vancomycin's due to the inclusion of a *N*-alkylated chlorobiphenyl side chain in the drug sugar's epivancosamine. In general, adding a hydrophobic side chain to the glycopeptide disaccharide greatly increases the medications' overall effectiveness and revives their activity against vancomycin-resistant bacteria. By using solid-state NMR to structurally characterize the binding site of these disaccharide-modified glycopeptides in *S. aureus* [98] and *E. faecium* [99] intact whole cells, it was discovered that the drug's hydrophobic side chain creates a secondary binding site. The lipoglycopeptides can target the cross-linked PG-bridge structure using this secondary binding site to aid in binding [100]. Oritavancin's binding to the developing PG prevents transpeptidase from effectively recognizing the PG template, which is necessary for effective PG cross-linking during cell-wall synthesis [101].

Teicoplanin is used to treat multidrug-resistant Gram-positive bacteria, such as MRSA and *Enterococci*, that are responsible for life-threatening infectious illnesses [102]. This glycopeptide antibiotic was initially isolated from *Actinoplanes teichomyceticus*, which was identified in 1978 from an Indian soil sample [103].

Teicoplanin shares structural similarities with vancomycin but differs in that it does not contain a lipid. Both antibiotics work by forming hydrogen bonds with the D-Ala-D-Ala C-terminus of the pentapeptide substrate to prevent the formation of the peptidoglycan chains that make up bacterial cell walls [104]. The hydrophobic lipid chain of this pentapeptide substrate is also known to interact with teicoplanin, placing the antibiotic next to the peptidoglycan [102,105].

Derivatives of teicoplanin have also been shown to form nanoscale aggregates in aqueous solution [106], thereby achieving increased binding power [107].

The oral and topical routes of administration for teicoplanin may result in poor permeability across the epithelial lining due to this concentration-dependent aggregation, and the aggregated form may reduce effective concentrations on certain sites, necessitating a higher dose and ultimately causing bacteria to develop resistance [108].

Another lipoglycopeptide derivative of vancomycin is telavancin (TD-6424). This was developed as a cutting-edge treatment for MRSA and other resistant Gram-positive bacterial infections [109]. The United States Food and Drug Administration (USFDA) granted telavancin approval in 2009 for the treatment of difficult skin and skin structure infections (cSSSIs) caused by Gram-positive bacteria, including MRSA, *S. aureus*, *Streptococcus agalactiae*, *S. pyogenes*, the *S. anginosus* group, and *E. faecalis* [110,111].

Two modes of action for telavancin have been suggested. Telavancin achieves bactericidal activity by interacting with the C-terminal *d*-alanyl-*d*-alanine residue on bacterial cell-wall peptidoglycan precursors, just like vancomycin. This interaction significantly alters the phases of cell-wall formation that include the polymerization of peptidoglycan (transglycosylation) and subsequent cross-linking (transpeptidation) [112]. Telavancin is 10-times more effective than vancomycin at inhibiting peptidoglycan production in intact MRSA cells because it strongly inhibits peptidoglycan generation at the transglycosylase stage.

Furthermore, a second mechanism of action has been mentioned. The depolarization of the bacterial cell membrane is involved, which affects how the cell membrane functions. Given that so few other glycopeptides are thought to function in this way, this dual method of action is of special importance [109]. The interaction of the lipophilic decylaminoethyl moiety of telavancin with the lipid bilayer of the bacterial cell membrane is thought to be the process by which telavancin disrupts cell membranes, albeit this is not fully understood [113]. Telavancin's affinity for lipid II, a molecule found in bacterial cell membranes, is facilitated by this lipophilic substance.

By disrupting the bacterial cell-wall transglycosylation pathway rather than the bacterial cell-wall transpeptidation mechanism, where vancomycin preferentially binds, telavancin is able to enter the bacterial cell with ease [114].

According to reports, lipid II binding is necessary for telavancin to cause membrane depolarization in *S. aureus*. This might not, however, accurately reflect the crucial phase of bacterial membrane disruption [115]. The loss of potassium ions and cytoplasmic adenosine triphosphate (ATP) may also be related to membrane depolarization. Telavancin's faster bactericidal impact compared to vancomycin may be caused by this alternative method of action, which only affects bacterial cell membranes and not mammalian cells [112].

Dalbavancin is a semisynthetic derivative of teicoplanin. It is active against most pathogenic Gram-positive organisms, including *Streptococcus* spp., *E. faecalis*, *E. faecium*, MSSA, MRSA, and vancomycin-intermediate *S. aureus*. However, it has poor activity against vancomycin-resistant *S. aureus* and VRE [116].

Similarly to vancomycin and other glycopeptides, dalbavancin inhibits cell-wall formation by interacting with the D-alanyl-D-alanine terminus in the bacterial cell-wall peptidoglycan and blocking cross-linking.

In the USA and Europe, acute bacterial skin and skin structure infections (ABSSSIs) are the only conditions for which dalbavancin is currently licensed [117].

8. Chalcones

Due to the hues of the majority of naturally occurring chalcones, the name "chalcone" was derived from the Greek word "chalcos", which means "bronze". 1,3-diaryl-2-propen-1-one (Figure 16), also referred to as chalconoid, is a chemical building block shared by all chalcone molecules. The trans isomer is thermodynamically more stable than the cis isomer. Through the use of plants and herbs for the treatment of many diseases, such as cancer, inflammation, and diabetes, chalcones have been applied therapeutically for thousands of years. Several chalcone-based substances have received clinical use authorization.

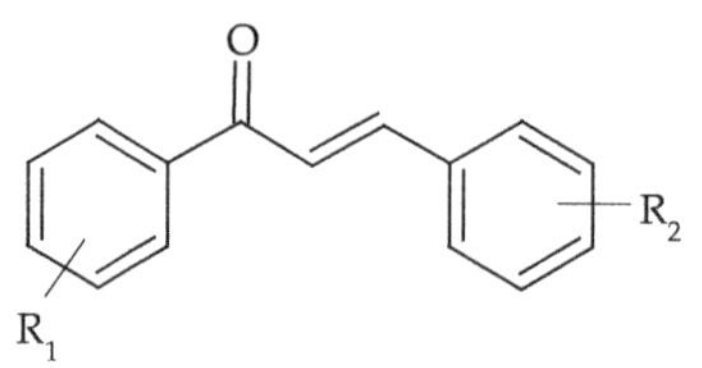

1,3-diaryl-2-propen-1-one

Figure 16. General structure of 1,3-diaryl-2-propen-1-ones.

Chalcones are a class of natural and synthetic compounds that have shown promising antivirulence properties against a variety of pathogenic bacteria. With the rise of antibiotic-resistant strains, there is an urgent need to develop alternative therapies that target virulence factors of bacteria, rather than traditional bactericidal approaches. In recent years, several studies have investigated the antivirulence potential of chalcones in resistant bacterial strains.

Several studies have investigated the activity of chalcones against multidrug-resistant *Pseudomonas aeruginosa* and found that they were able to inhibit the expression of virulence genes involved in quorum sensing, motility, and biofilm formation [118,119].

Furthermore, a study on *Acinetobacter baumannii*, a notorious multi-drug resistant pathogen, showed that chalcones exhibited significant antivirulence activity by modulating gene expression, biofilm formation, and virulence traits [120].

These studies suggested that chalcones have potential as antivirulence agents against resistant bacterial strains by targeting various virulence traits. However, further studies are needed to evaluate the efficacy of chalcones in vivo and their potential as a therapeutic option for antibiotic-resistant infections.

Overall, it can be concluded that, since virulence factors are essential for the infection of the host, techniques employed to prevent this process from initiating and search for novel bioactive compounds with these properties are rather appealing.

Along with the synthetic and hemi-synthetic compounds elaborated in this review article, numerous naturally derived compounds have also demonstrated great potential as efficient virulence-targeting compounds. Dehydroabietic acid showed considerable potential against several pathogenic microorganisms, especially *Pseudomonas syringae* pv. *actinidiae*, *Xanthomonas oryzae* pv. *oryzae*, and *Xanthomonas axonopodis* pv. citri [121]. Furthermore, for some natural compounds, a mode of action has even been proposed. For example, the exposure of *Serratia marcescens* to hordenine (25, 50, and 100 g/mL) reduced the synthesis of acyl-homoserine lactones and prevented the development of biofilms. It also increased the susceptibility of preformed biofilms to commercial antibiotic ciprofloxacin by lowering extracellular polysaccharide production and altering membrane permeability. Additionally, the presence of hordenine downregulated expression and affected genes associated with biofilm and QS [122], which may be explored in other matrices. Additionally, even though some compounds do not exert anti-QS activities per se, they can sometimes be easily modified into compounds that do exert various bioactivities, as was argued by Du et al. [123]. This comprehensive review article offered new research solutions; proposed novel strategies; and compared existing results, leading to new conclusions.

9. Future Perspectives

The use of novel synthetic and semisynthetic compounds that target virulence factors as antibacterials presents a promising avenue for combating antibiotic resistance. However, there are several challenges that need to be addressed in order to fully realize the potential of this approach. One of the challenges is the identification of new compounds with antibacterial potency that can target virulence factors. Despite recent progress in this area, many of the compounds that have been investigated are not yet ready for clinical use. The process of discovering, developing, and testing new compounds can be time-consuming and expensive, and there is a need for new screening methods and assays to identify potential candidates more efficiently. Another challenge is the optimization of the efficacy and safety of existing compounds. Many of the compounds that have been identified have shown promising results in vitro, but their efficacy in vivo and safety in humans need to be further evaluated. In addition, the development of resistance to these compounds is a potential concern, and efforts must be made to prevent or delay the emergence of resistance. Furthermore, there is a need for an improved understanding of the mechanisms of action of these compounds. Many of the compounds that target virulence factors have complex modes of action that are not yet fully understood. A deeper understanding of these mechanisms could lead to the development of more effective compounds, as well as the identification of new targets for antibacterial therapy.

There are ongoing clinical trials on novel antivirulence drugs that are trying to take the next steps forward within this area, evaluating the safety and efficacy of novel synthetic and semisynthetic compounds. These trials are being conducted by pharmaceutical companies, academic institutions, and government agencies around the world.

Despite the many challenges, the potential benefits of targeting virulence factors as a strategy to combat antibiotic resistance are significant. By reducing the severity of bacterial infections without promoting the development of resistance, this approach could help to extend the lifespan of existing antibiotics and reduce the need for new ones. In addition, the use of antibacterials that target virulence factors could help to reduce the burden of antibiotic-resistant infections, which are a major public health concern.

10. Conclusions

The development of novel antibacterials that target virulence factors is an area of active research aimed at addressing the global challenge of antibiotic resistance. The potential benefits of these compounds lie in their ability to attenuate bacterial pathogenesis without necessarily killing the bacteria, thus reducing selective pressure for resistance development. While the field is still in its early stages, the progress made so far is promising. The use of synthetic and semisynthetic compounds has emerged as an important strategy to combat antibiotic resistance. The compounds reviewed in this paper—chalcones, azoles, indoles, thiophenes, terpenoids, glycopeptides, pleuromutilin derivatives, and lactone derivatives—have shown potential as antibacterials mostly targeting virulence traits in resistant strains. Clinical trials evaluating the safety and efficacy of these compounds are ongoing, and their results will provide critical insights into the role of virulence-targeted antibacterials in the management of bacterial infections. However, given the complexity of bacterial pathogenesis and the evolution of resistance mechanisms, the development of novel antibacterials remains a challenging task. Further research is required to identify novel targets and to optimize the efficacy and safety of these compounds. Additionally, efforts are needed to overcome the regulatory and economic hurdles that often hinder the development and commercialization of novel antibacterial agents.

The development of novel antibacterials that target virulence factors offers a promising avenue for combating antibiotic resistance. While there is still much work to be carried out, the progress made so far suggests that these compounds have the potential to play an important role in the management of bacterial infections in the future.

Author Contributions: Conceptualization, D.S., K.L; investigation, D.S., J.P., T.C., M.S. and K.L.; resources, D.S and K.L.; writing—original draft preparation, D.S., J.P. and T.C.; writing—review and editing, M.S. and K.L. All authors have read and agreed to the published version of the manuscript.

Funding: This work was supported by the Ministry of Education, Science and Technological Development of the Republic of Serbia (451-03-68/2022-14/200007).

Institutional Review Board Statement: Not applicable.

Informed Consent Statement: Not applicable.

Data Availability Statement: Not applicable.

Conflicts of Interest: The authors declare no conflict of interest.

References

1. Piddock, L.J. Reflecting on the final report of the O'Neill review on antimicrobial resistance. *Lancet Infect. Dis.* **2016**, *16*, 767–768. [CrossRef]
2. Rasko, D.A.; Sperandio, V. Anti-virulence strategies to combat bacteria-mediated disease. *Nat. Rev. Drug Discov.* **2010**, *9*, 117–128. [CrossRef]
3. Zhang, F.; Cheng, W. The Mechanism of Bacterial Resistance and Potential Bacteriostatic Strategies. *Antibiotics* **2022**, *11*, 1215. [CrossRef]
4. Clatworthy, A.E.; Pierson, E.; Hung, D.T. Targeting virulence: A new paradigm for antimicrobial therapy. *Nat. Chem. Biol.* **2007**, *3*, 541–548. [CrossRef] [PubMed]
5. Fischbach, M.A.; Walsh, C.T. Antibiotics for emerging pathogens. *Science* **2009**, *325*, 1089–1093. [CrossRef] [PubMed]
6. Annunziato, G. Strategies to Overcome Antimicrobial Resistance (AMR) Making Use of Non-Essential Target Inhibitors: A Review. *Int. J. Mol. Sci.* **2019**, *20*, 5844. [CrossRef]

7. Dörr, T.; Lewis, K.; Vulic, M. SOS response induces persistence to fluoroquinolones in Escherichia coli. *PLoS Genet.* **2009**, *5*, e1000760. [CrossRef] [PubMed]
8. Flemming, H.C.; Wingender, J. The biofilm matrix. *Nat. Rev. Microbiol.* **2010**, *8*, 623–633. [CrossRef]
9. Kalia, V.C. Quorum sensing inhibitors: An overview. *Biotechnol. Adv.* **2013**, *31*, 224–245. [CrossRef]
10. Bhat, A.; Ahmad, I. Anti-virulence strategies: Stalling the micromachines of bacterial pathogens. *Front. Microbiol.* **2018**, *9*, 1456. [CrossRef]
11. Jeong, J.W.; Lee, K.Y.; Kim, J.S. Natural products as sources of new fungicides. *J. Microbiol. Biotechnol.* **2009**, *19*, 1263–1270.
12. Gutiérrez-Barranquero, J.A.; Reen, F.J.; McCarthy, R.R.; O'Gara, F. Deciphering the role of coumarin as a novel quorum sensing inhibitor suppressing virulence phenotypes in bacterial pathogens. *Appl. Microbiol. Biotechnol.* **2015**, *99*, 3303–3316. [CrossRef] [PubMed]
13. Frederich, M.; Tits, M.; Angenot, L. Potential antimalarial activity of indole alkaloids. *Trans R. Soc. Trop. Med. Hyg.* **2008**, *102*, 11–19. [CrossRef]
14. Singh, R.; Dubey, A.K. Lactone derivatives as potential antibacterial agents. *Med. Chem. Res.* **2018**, *27*, 1589–1611.
15. Okano, A.; Isley, N.A.; Boger, D.L. Peripheral modifications of [9]dodecanylglycylgramicidin A: Discovery of novel antimicrobial agents with high potency and selectivity against methicillin-resistant *Staphylococcus aureus* (MRSA). *J. Am. Chem. Soc.* **2017**, *139*, 944–955.
16. El-Messery, S.M.; Habib, E.E.; Al-Rashood, S.T.A.; Hassan, G.S. Synthesis, antimicrobial, anti-biofilm evaluation, and molecular modelling study of new chalcone linked amines derivatives. *J. Enzym. Inhib. Med. Chem.* **2018**, *33*, 818–832. [CrossRef]
17. Peng, X.M.; Cai, G.X.; Zhou, C.H. Recent developments in azole compounds as antibacterial and antifungal agents. *Curr. Top. Med. Chem.* **2013**, *13*, 1963–2010. [CrossRef]
18. Deryabin, D.; Inchagova, K.; Rusakova, E.; Duskaev, G. Coumarin's Anti-Quorum Sensing Activity Can Be Enhanced When Combined with Other Plant-Derived Small Molecules. *Molecules* **2021**, *26*, 208. [CrossRef]
19. Sethupathy, S.; Sathiyamoorthi, E.; Kim, Y.G.; Lee, J.H.; Lee, J. Antibiofilm and Antivirulence Properties of Indoles Against Serratia marcescens. *Front. Microbiol.* **2020**, *11*, 584812. [CrossRef]
20. Hooper, D.C.; Jacoby, G.A. Topoisomerase Inhibitors: Fluoroquinolone Mechanisms of Action and Resistance. *Cold Spring Harb. Perspect.Med.* **2016**, *6*(9), a025320. [CrossRef]
21. Cappiello, F.; Loffredo, M.R.; Del Plato, C.; Cammarone, S.; Casciaro, B.; Quaglio, D.; Mangoni, M.L.; Botta, B.; Ghirga, F. The Revaluation of Plant-Derived Terpenes to Fight Antibiotic-Resistant Infections. *Antibiotics* **2020**, *9*, 325. [CrossRef]
22. van Groesen, E.; Innocenti, P.; Martin, N.I. Recent Advances in the Development of Semisynthetic Glycopeptide Antibiotics: 2014–2022. *ACS Infect. Dis.* **2022**, *8*, 1381–1407. [CrossRef] [PubMed]
23. Shang, R.; Wang, S.; Xu, X.; Yi, Y.; Guo, W.; Liu, Y.; Liang, J. Chemical synthesis and biological activities of novel pleuromutilin derivatives with substituted amino moiety. *PLoS ONE* **2013**, *8*, e82595. [CrossRef] [PubMed]
24. Breijyeh, Z.; Karaman, R. Design and Synthesis of Novel Antimicrobial Agents. *Antibiotics* **2023**, *12*, 628. [CrossRef]
25. Balcerek, M.; Szmigiel-Bakalarz, K.; Lewańska, M.; Günther, D.; Oeckler, O.; Malik, M.; Morzyk-Ociepa, B. Experimental and computational study on dimers of 5-halo-1H-indole-2-carboxylic acids and their microbiological activity. *J. Mol. Struct.* **2023**, *1274*, 134492. [CrossRef]
26. Salem, M.A.; Ragab, A.; El-Khalafawy, A.; Makhlouf, A.H.; Askar, A.A.; Ammar, Y.A. Design, synthesis, in vitro antimicrobial evaluation and molecular docking studies of indol-2-one tagged with morpholinosulfonyl moiety as DNA gyrase inhibitors. *Bioorg. Chem.* **2020**, *96*, 103619. [CrossRef]
27. Alzahrani, Y.A.; Ammar, M.; Abu-Elghait, M.A.; Salem, M.; Assiri, T.E.; Ali, R. Development of novel indolin-2-one derivative incorporating thiazole moiety as DHFR and quorum sensing inhibitors: Synthesis, antimicrobial, and antibiofilm activities with molecular modelling study. *Bioorg. Chem.* **2022**, *119*, 105571. [CrossRef]
28. Srikanth, D.; Joshi, S.V.; Shaik, M.G.; Pawar, G.; Bujji, S.; Kanchupalli, V.; Chopra, S.; Nanduri, S. A comprehensive review on potential therapeutic inhibitors of nosocomial *Acinetobacter baumannii* superbugs. *Bioorg. Chem.* **2022**, *124*, 105849. [CrossRef]
29. Raorane, C.J.; Lee, J.H.; Lee, J. Rapid Killing and Biofilm Inhibition of Multidrug-Resistant *Acinetobacter baumannii* Strains and Other Microbes by Iodoindoles. *Biomolecules* **2020**, *10*, 1186. [CrossRef]
30. Kim, Y.G.; Lee, J.H.; Park, S.; Lee, J. The Anticancer Agent 3,3′-Diindolylmethane Inhibits Multispecies Biofilm Formation by Acne-Causing Bacteria and *Candida albicans*. *Microbiol. Spectr.* **2022**, *10*, e0205621. [CrossRef]
31. Tatta, E.R.; Kumavath, R. Attenuation of *Enterococcus faecalis* biofilm formation by Rhodethrin: A combinatorial study with an antibiotic. *Microb. Pathog.* **2022**, *163*, 105401. [CrossRef]
32. Amer, M.A.; Ramadan, M.A.; Attia, A.S.; Wasfi, R. Silicone Foley catheter simpregnated with microbial indole derivatives inhibit crystalline biofilm formation by *Proteus mirabilis*. *Front. Cell. Infect. Microbiol.* **2022**, *12*, 1010625. [CrossRef] [PubMed]
33. Boya, B.R.; Lee, J.H.; Lee, J. Antibiofilm and Antimicrobial Activities of Chloroindoles Against Uropathogenic *Escherichia coli*. *Front. Microbiol.* **2022**, *13*, 872943. [CrossRef]
34. Cernicchi, G.; Felicetti, T.; Sabatini, S. Microbial Efflux Pump Inhibitors: A Journey around Quinoline and Indole Derivatives. *Molecules* **2021**, *26*, 6996. [CrossRef]
35. Ahmed, B.; Jailani, A.; Lee, J.H.; Lee, J. Effect of halogenated indoles on biofilm formation, virulence, and root surface colonization by *Agrobacterium tumefaciens*. *Chemosphere* **2022**, *293*, 133603. [CrossRef] [PubMed]

36. Zhang, S.; Yang, Q.; Fu, S.; Janssen, C.; Eggermont, M.; Defoirdt, T. Indole decreases the virulence of the bivalve model pathogens *Vibrio tasmaniensis* LGP32 and *Vibrio crassostreae* J2-9. *Sci. Rep.* **2022**, *12*, 5749. [CrossRef]
37. Sathiyamoorthi, E.; Faleye, O.S.; Lee, J.H.; Raj, V.; Lee, J. Antibacterial and Antibiofilm Activities of Chloroindoles Against *Vibrio parahaemolyticus*. *Front. Microbiol.* **2021**, *12*, 714371. [CrossRef]
38. Li, Z.; Sun, F.; Fu, X.; Chen, Y. 5-Methylindole kills various bacterial pathogens and potentiates aminoglycoside against methicillin-resistant *Staphylococcus aureus*. *PeerJ* **2022**, *10*, e14010. [CrossRef]
39. Nobre, L.S.; Todorovic, S.; Tavares, A.F.; Oldfield, E.; Hildebrandt, P.; Teixeira, M.; Saraiva, L.M. Binding of azole antibiotics to *Staphylococcus aureus* flavohemoglobin increases intracellular oxidative stress. *J. Bacteriol.* **2010**, *192*, 1527–1533. [CrossRef] [PubMed]
40. Olaifa, K.; Ajunwa, O.; Marsili, E. Electroanalytic evaluation of antagonistic effect of azole fungicides on *Acinetobacter baumannii* biofilms. *Electrochim. Acta* **2022**, *405*, 139837. [CrossRef]
41. Qiu, W.; Ren, B.; Dai, H.; Zhang, L.; Zhang, Q.; Zhou, X.; Li, Y. Clotrimazole and econazole inhibit *Streptococcus mutans* biofilm and virulence in vitro. *Arch. Oral. Biol.* **2017**, *73*, 113–120. [CrossRef] [PubMed]
42. Nasr, M.; Bondock, S.; Eid, S. Design, synthesis, antimicrobial evaluation and molecular docking studies of some new thiophene, pyrazole and pyridone derivatives bearing sulfisoxazole moiety. *Eur. J. Med. Chem.* **2014**, *84*, 491–504. [CrossRef]
43. Gomes, M.P.; Correia, E.M.; Gomes, M.W.L.; Santos, C.C.C.; Barros, C.S.; Abreu, F.V.; de Antunes, L.S.; Ferreira, V.F.; Gonçalves, M.C.; Pinto, C.E.C.; et al. Antibacterial profile in vitro and in vivo of new 1,4-naphthoquinones tethered to 1,2,3-1h-triazoles against the planktonic growth of *Streptococcus mutans*. *J. Braz. Chem. Soc.* **2022**, *33*, 1028–1040. [CrossRef]
44. Sapijanskaite-Banevic, B.; Palskys, V.; Vaickelioniene, R.; Šiugždaite, J.; Kavaliauskas, P.; Grybaite, B.; Mickevicius, V. Synthesis and Antibacterial Activity of New Azole, Diazole and Triazole Derivatives Based on p-Aminobenzoic Acid. *Molecules* **2021**, *26*, 2597. [CrossRef]
45. Nechaeva, O.V.; Tikhomirova, E.I.; Zayarsky, D.A.; Bespalova, N.V.; Glinskaya, E.V.; Shurshalova, N.F.; Al Bayati, B.M.; Babailova, A.I. AntiBiofilm Activity of Polyazolidinammonium Modified with Iodine Hydrate Ions against Microbial Biofilms of Uropathogenic Coliform Bacteria. *Bull. Exp. Biol. Med.* **2017**, *162*, 781–783. [CrossRef] [PubMed]
46. Dawoud, N.T.A.; El-Fakharany, E.M.; Abdallah, A.E.; El-Gendi, H.; Lotfy, D.R. Synthesis, and docking studies of novel heterocycles incorporating the indazolyl thiazole moiety as antimicrobial and anticancer agents. *Sci. Rep.* **2022**, *12*, 3424. [CrossRef]
47. Rando, D.G.; Doriguetto, A.C.; Tomich de Paula da Silva, C.H.; Ellena, J.; Sato, D.N.; Leite, C.Q.; Varanda, E.A.; Ferreira, E.I. A duplicated nitrotienyl derivative with antimycobacterial activity: Synthesis, X-ray crystallography, biological and mutagenic activity tests. *Eur. J. Med. Chem.* **2006**, *41*, 1196–1200. [CrossRef]
48. Scotti, L.; Oliveira Lima, E.; da Silva, M.S.; Ishiki, H.; Oliveira Lima, I.; Oliveira Pereira, F.; Mendonça Junior, F.J.; Scotti, M.T. Docking and PLS studies on a set of thiophenes RNA polymerase inhibitors against *Staphylococcus aureus*. *Curr. Top. Med. Chem.* **2014**, *14*, 64–80. [CrossRef]
49. Ramalingam, A.; Sarvanan, J. Synthesis, Docking and Antimicrobial Activity Studies of Some Novel Fused Thiophenes of Biological Interest. *J. Young Pharm.* **2020**, *12*, 118–124. [CrossRef]
50. Metwally, H.M.; Khalaf, N.A.; Abdel-Latif, E. Synthesis, DFT investigations, antioxidant, antibacterial activity and SAR-study of novel thiophene-2-carboxamide derivatives. *BMC Chem.* **2023**, *17*, 6. [CrossRef]
51. Kavanagh, F.; Hervey, A.; Robbins, W.J. Antibiotic substances from basidiomycetes. *Proc. Natl. Acad. Sci. USA* **1951**, *37*, 570–574. [CrossRef]
52. Li, B.; Zhang, Z.; Zhang, J.F.; Liu, J.; Zuo, X.Y.; Chen, F.; Zhang, G.Y.; Fang, H.Q.; Jin, Z.; Tang, Y.Z. Design, synthesis and biological evaluation of pleuromutilin-Schiff base hybrids as potent anti-MRSA agents in vitro and in vivo. *Eur. J. Med. Chem.* **2021**, *223*, 113624. [CrossRef] [PubMed]
53. Hogenauer, G. The mode of action of pleuromutilin derivatives: Location and properties of pleuromutilin binding site on *Escherichia coli* ribosomes. *Eur. J. Biochem.* **1975**, *52*, 93–98. [CrossRef]
54. Paukner, S.; Riedl, R. Pleuromutilins: Potent drugs for resistant bugs-mode of action and resistance. *Cold Spring Harb. Perspect. Med.* **2017**, *7*, a027110. [CrossRef] [PubMed]
55. Poulsen, S.M.; Karlsson, M.; Johansson, L.B.; Vester, B. The pleuromutilin drugs tiamulin and valnemulin bind to the RNA at the peptidyl transferase centre on the ribosome. *Mol. Microbiol.* **2001**, *41*, 1091–1099. [CrossRef] [PubMed]
56. Hodgin, L.A.; Högenauer, G. The mode of action of pleuromutilin derivatives. Effect on cell-free polypeptide synthesis. *Eur. J. Biochem.* **1974**, *47*, 527–533. [CrossRef]
57. Gürel, G.; Blaha, G.; Moore, P.B.; Steitz, T.A. U2504 determines the species specificity of the A-site cleft antibiotics: The structures of tiamulin, homoharringtonine, and bruceantin bound to the ribosome. *J. Mol. Biol.* **2009**, *389*, 146–156. [CrossRef]
58. Adhikary, S.; Duggal, M.K.; Nagendran, S.; Chintamaneni, M.; Tuli, H.S.; Kaur, G. Lefamulin: A new hope in the field of community-acquired bacterial pneumonia. *Cur. Pharm. Rep.* **2022**, *8*, 418–426. [CrossRef]
59. Veve, M.P.; Wagner, J.L. Lefamulin: Review of a promising novel pleuromutilin antibiotic. *Pharmacotherapy* **2018**, *38*, 935–946. [CrossRef]
60. Yi, Y.; Zhang, J.; Zuo, J.; Zhang, M.; Yang, S.; Huang, Z.; Li, G.; Shang, R.; Lin, S. Novel pyridinium cationic pleuromutilin analogues overcoming bacterial multidrug resistance. *Eur. J. Med. Chem.* **2023**, *251*, 115269. [CrossRef]
61. Deng, Y.; Tang, D.; Wang, Q.R.; Huang, S.; Fu, L.Z.; Li, C.H. Semi-synthesis, antibacterial activity, and molecular docking study of novel pleuromutilin derivatives bearing cinnamic acids moieties. *Arch. Pharm.* **2019**, *352*, e1800266. [CrossRef]

62. Farney, E.P.; Feng, S.S.; Schafers, F.; Reisman, S.E. Total synthesis of (+)-pleuromutilin. *J. Am. Chem. Soc.* **2018**, *140*, 1267–1270. [CrossRef]
63. Alberti, F.; Khairudin, K.; Venegas, E.R.; Davies, J.A.; Hayes, P.M.; Willis, C.L.; Bailey, A.M.; Foster, G.D. Heterologous expression reveals the biosynthesis of the antibiotic pleuromutilin and generates bioactive semi-synthetic derivatives. *Nat. Commun.* **2017**, *8*, 1831. [CrossRef] [PubMed]
64. Yi, Y.; Yang, S.; Liu, Y.; Yin, B.; Zhao, Z.; Li, G.; Huang, Z.; Chen, L.; Liu, F.; Shang, R.; et al. Antibiotic resistance and drug modification: Synthesis, characterization and bioactivity of newly modified potent pleuromutilin derivatives with a substituted piperazine moiety. *Bioorg. Chem.* **2023**, *132*, 106353. [CrossRef]
65. Novak, R. Are pleuromutilin antibiotics finally fit for human use? *Ann. N. Y. Acad. Sci.* **2011**, *1241*, 71–81. [CrossRef] [PubMed]
66. Waites, K.B.; Crabb, D.M.; Duffy, L.B.; Jensen, J.S.; Liu, Y.; Paukner, S. In vitro activities of lefamulin and other antimicrobial agents against macrolidesusceptible and macrolide-resistant Mycoplasma pneumoniae from the United States, Europe, and China. *Antimicrob. Agents Chemother.* **2017**, *61*, e02008-16. [CrossRef]
67. Sader, H.S.; Biedenbach, D.J.; Paukner, S.; Ivezic-Schoenfeld, Z.; Jones, R.N. Antimicrobial activity of the investigational pleuromutilin compound BC3781 tested against Gram-positive organisms commonly associated with acute bacterial skin and skin structure infections. *Antimicrob. Agents Chemother.* **2012**, *56*, 1619–1623. [CrossRef]
68. Afshari, A.; Taheri, S.; Hashemi, M.; Norouzy, A.; Nematy, M.; Mohamadi, S. Methicillin- and Vancomycin-Resistant *Staphylococcus aureus* and Vancomycin-Resistant Enterococci Isolated from Hospital Foods: Prevalence and Antimicrobial Resistance Patterns. *Curr. Microbiol.* **2022**, *79*, 326. [CrossRef] [PubMed]
69. Tang, Y.Z.; Liu, Y.H.; Chen, J.X. Pleuromutilin and its derivatives-the lead compounds for novel antibiotics. *Mini Rev. Med. Chem.* **2012**, *12*, 53–61. [CrossRef] [PubMed]
70. Killeavy, E.E.; Jogl, G.; Gregory, S.T. Tiamulin-Resistant Mutants of the Thermophilic Bacterium *Thermus thermophilus*. *Antibiotics* **2020**, *9*, 313. [CrossRef]
71. Klitgaard, R.N.; Ntokou, E.; Norgaard, K.; Biltoft, D.; Hansen, L.H.; Traedholm, N.M.; Kongsted, J.; Vester, B. Mutations in the bacterial ribosomal protein l3 and their association with antibiotic resistance. *Antimicrob. Agents Chemother.* **2015**, *59*, 3518–3528. [CrossRef]
72. Patel, A.B.; Lighter, J.; Fulmer, Y.; Copin, R.; Ratner, A.J.; Shopsin, B. Retapamulin Activity Against Pediatric Strains of Mupirocin-resistant Methicillin-resistant *Staphylococcus aureus*. *Pediatr. Infect. Dis. J.* **2021**, *40*, 637–638. [CrossRef]
73. Singh, R.; Gombosev, A.; Dutciuc, T.; Evans, K.; Portillo, L.M.; Hayden, M.K.; Gillen, D.; Peterson, E.; Tjoa, T.; Cao, C.; et al. Randomized Double-Blinded Placebo-Controlled Trial to Assess the Effect of Retapamulin for Nasal Decolonization of Mupirocin-Resistant Methicillin-Resistant *Staphylococcus aureus* Nasal Carriers. *Open Forum. Infect. Dis.* **2016**, *3* (Suppl. S1), 301. [CrossRef]
74. Surowiak, A.K.; Balcerzak, L.; Lochyński, S.; Strub, D.J. Biological Activity of Selected Natural and Synthetic Terpenoid Lactones. *Int. J. Mol. Sci.* **2021**, *22*, 5036. [CrossRef] [PubMed]
75. Sartori, S.K.; Diaz, M.A.N.; Diaz-Muñoz, G. Lactones: Classification, Synthesis, Biological Activities, and Industrial Applications. *Tetrahedron* **2021**, *84*, 132001. [CrossRef]
76. Fan, B.Z.; Hiasa, H.; Lv, W.; Brody, S.; Yang, Z.Y.; Aldrich, C.; Cushman, M.; Liang, J.H. Design, Synthesis and Structure-Activity Relationships of Novel 15-Membered Macrolides: Quinolone/Quinoline-Containing Sidechains Tethered to the C-6 Position of Azithromycin Acylides. *Eur. J. Med. Chem.* **2020**, *193*, 112222. [CrossRef]
77. Mazur, M.; Masłowiec, D. Antimicrobial Activity of Lactones. *Antibiotics* **2022**, *11*, 1327. [CrossRef] [PubMed]
78. Kowalczyk, P.; Gawdzik, B.; Trzepizur, D.; Szymczak, M.; Skiba, G.; Raj, S.; Kramkowski, K.; Lizut, R.; Ostaszewski, R. δ-Lactones-A New Class of Compounds That Are Toxic to *E. coli* K12 and R2-R4 Strains. *Materials* **2021**, *14*, 2956. [CrossRef]
79. Yokoe, H.; Yoshida, M.; Shishido, K. Total synthesis of (-)-Xanthatin. *Tetrahedron Lett.* **2008**, *49*, 3504–3506. [CrossRef]
80. Matsuo, K.; Ohtsuki, K.; Yoshikawa, T.; Shisho, K.; Yokotani-Tomita, K.; Shinto, M. Total synthesis of xanthanolides. *Tetrahedron* **2010**, *66*, 8407–8419. [CrossRef]
81. Nagahama, N.; Suzuki, M.; Awataguc, S.; Okuda, T. Studies on a new antibiotic, albocycline. I. isolation, purification and properties. *J. Antibiot.* **1967**, *20*, 261–266.
82. Koyama, N.; Yotsumoto, M.; Onaka, H.; Tomoda, H. New structural scaffold 14-membered macrocyclic lactone ring for selective inhibitors of cell wall peptidoglycan biosynthesis in *Staphylococcus aureus*. *J. Antibiot.* **2013**, *66*, 303–304. [CrossRef]
83. Daher, S.S.; Franklin, K.P.; Scherzi, T.; Dunman, P.M.; Andrade, R.B. Synthesis and biological evaluation of semi-synthetic albocycline analogs. *Bioorg. Med. Chem. Lett.* **2020**, *30*, 127509. [CrossRef]
84. Wilson, D.N. The A-Z of bacterial translation inhibitors. *Crit. Rev. Biochem. Mol. Biol.* **2009**, *44*, 393. [CrossRef] [PubMed]
85. Liang, H.; Zhou, G.; Ge, Y.; D'Ambrosio, E.A.; Eidem, T.M.; Blanchard, C.; Shehatou, C.; Chatare, V.K.; Dunman, P.M.; Valentine, A.M.; et al. Elucidating the inhibition of peptidoglycan biosynthesis in *Staphylococcus aureus* by albocycline, a macrolactone isolated from *Streptomyces maizeus*. *Bioorg. Med. Chem.* **2018**, *26*, 3453–3460. [CrossRef] [PubMed]
86. Barna, J.C.J.; Williams, D.H. The structure and mode of action of glycopeptide antibiotics of the vancomycin group. *Annu. Rev. Microbiol.* **1984**, *38*, 339–357. [CrossRef] [PubMed]
87. Nagarajan, R. Glycopeptide antibiotics. In *Drugs and the Pharmaceutical Sciences*; Marcel Dekker: New York, NY, USA, 1994; Volume 63.
88. Zeng, D.; Debabov, D.; Hartsell, T.L.; Cano, R.J.; Adams, S.; Schuyler, J.A.; McMillan, R.; Pace, J.L. Approved Glycopeptide Antibacterial Drugs: Mechanism of Action and Resistance. *Cold Spring Harb. Perspect Med.* **2016**, *6*, a026989. [CrossRef]

89. Singh, M.; Chang, J.; Coffman, L.; Kim, S.J. Hidden mode of action of glycopeptide antibiotics: Inhibition of wall teichoic acid biosynthesis. *J. Phys. Chem. B* **2017**, *121*, 3925–3932. [CrossRef] [PubMed]
90. Brown, S.; Santa Maria, J.P.; Walker, S. Wall teichoic acids of gram-positive bacteria. *Annu. Rev. Microbiol.* **2013**, *67*, 313–336. [CrossRef]
91. Cegelski, L.; Kim, S.J.; Hing, A.W.; Studelska, D.R.; O'Connor, R.D.; Mehta, A.K.; Schaefer, J. Rotational-echo double resonance characterization of the effects of vancomycin on cell wall synthesis in *Staphylococcus aureus*. *Biochemistry* **2002**, *41*, 13053–13058. [CrossRef]
92. Muller, A.; Klockner, A.; Schneider, T. Targeting a cell wall biosynthesis hot spot. *Nat. Prod. Rep.* **2017**, *34*, 909–932. [CrossRef] [PubMed]
93. Olademehin, O.P.; Shuford, K.L.; Kim, S.J. Molecular dynamics simulations of the secondary-binding site in disaccharide-modified glycopeptide antibiotics. *Sci. Rep.* **2022**, *12*, 7087. [CrossRef]
94. Brotz, H.; Bierbaum, G.; Reynolds, P.E.; Sahl, H.G. The lantibiotic mersacidin inhibits peptidoglycan biosynthesis at the level of transglycosylation. *Eur. J. Biochem.* **1997**, *246*, 193–199. [CrossRef]
95. Arthur, M.; Molinas, C.; Bugg, T.D.; Wright, G.D.; Walsh, C.T.; Courvalin, P. Evidence for in vivo incorporation of D-lactate into peptidoglycan precursors of vancomycin-resistant enterococci. *Antimicrob. Agents Chemother.* **1992**, *36*, 867–869. [CrossRef]
96. Nicas, T.I.; Mullen, D.L.; Flokowitsch, J.E.; Preston, D.A.; Snyder, N.J.; Zweifel, M.J.; Wilkie, S.C.; Rodriguez, M.J.; Thompson, R.C.; Cooper, R.D. Semisynthetic glycopeptide antibiotics derived from LY264826 active against vancomycin-resistant enterococci. *Antimicrob. Agents Chemother.* **1996**, *40*, 2194–2199. [CrossRef] [PubMed]
97. Sweeney, D.; Stoneburner, A.; Shinabarger, D.L.; Arhin, F.F.; Belley, A.; Moeck, G.; Pillar, C.M. Comparative in vitro activity of oritavancin and other agents against vancomycin-susceptible and -resistant enterococci. *J. Antimicrob. Chemother.* **2016**, *72*, 622–624. [CrossRef] [PubMed]
98. Kim, S.J.; Tanaka, K.S.; Dietrich, E.; Far, A.R.; Schaefer, J. Locations of the hydrophobic side chains of lipoglycopeptides bound to the peptidoglycan of *Staphylococcus aureus*. *Biochemistry* **2013**, *52*, 3405–3414. [CrossRef] [PubMed]
99. Patti, G.J.; Kim, S.J.; Yu, T.Y.; Dietrich, E.; Tanaka, K.S.; Parr, T.R., Jr.; Far, A.R.; Schaefer, J. Vancomycin and oritavancin have different modes of action in *Enterococcus faecium*. *J. Mol. Biol.* **2009**, *392*, 1178–1191. [CrossRef]
100. Kim, S.J.; Matsuoka, S.; Patti, G.J.; Schaefer, J. Vancomycin derivative with damaged D-Ala-D-Ala binding cleft binds to cross-linked peptidoglycan in the cell wall of *Staphylococcus aureus*. *Biochemistry* **2008**, *47*, 3822–3831. [CrossRef]
101. Kim, S.J.; Cegelski, L.; Stueber, D.; Singh, M.; Dietrich, E.; Tanaka, K.S.; Parr, T.R.; Far, A.R.; Schaefer, J. Oritavancin exhibits dual mode of action to inhibit cell-wall biosynthesis in *Staphylococcus aureus*. *J. Mol. Biol.* **2008**, *377*, 281–293. [CrossRef]
102. Chun, T.; Pattem, J.; Gillis, R.B.; Dinu, V.T.; Yakubov, G.E.; Corfield, A.P.; Harding, S.E. Self-association of the glycopeptide antibiotic teicoplanin A2 in aqueous solution studied by molecular hydrodynamics. *Sci. Rep.* **2023**, *13*, 1969. [CrossRef] [PubMed]
103. Parenti, F.; Beretta, G.; Berti, M.; Arioli, V. Teichomycins, new antibiotics from actinoplanes teichomyceticus nov. sp. *J. Antibiot.* **2006**, *31*, 276–283. [CrossRef] [PubMed]
104. Reynolds, P.E. Structure, biochemistry and mechanism of action of glycopeptide antibiotics. *Eur. J. Clin. Microbiol. Infect. Dis.* **1989**, *8*, 943–950. [CrossRef]
105. Vimberg, V.; Gazak, R.; Szűcs, Z.; Borbás, A.; Herczegh, P.; Cavanagh, J.P.; Zieglerova, L.; Závora, J.; Adámková, V.; Novotna, G.B. Fluorescence assay to predict activity of the glycopeptide antibiotics. *J. Antibiot.* **2019**, *72*, 114–117. [CrossRef]
106. Pintér, G.; Batta, G.; Kéki, S.; Mándi, A.; Komáromi, I.; Takács-Novák, K.; Sztaricskai, F.; Röth, E.; Ostorházi, E.; Rozgonyi, F.; et al. Diazo transfer–click reaction route to new, lipophilic teicoplanin and ristocetin aglycon derivatives with high antibacterial and anti-influenza virus activity: An aggregation and receptor binding study. *J. Med. Chem.* **2009**, *52*, 6053–6061. [CrossRef] [PubMed]
107. Tollas, S.; Bereczki, I.; Sipos, A.; Rőth, E.; Batta, G.; Daróczi, L.; Kéki, S.; Ostorházi, E.; Rozgonyi, F.; Herczegh, P. Nano-sized clusters of a teicoplanin ψ-aglycon-fullerene conjugate. Synthesis, antibacterial activity and aggregation studies. *Eur. J. Med. Chem.* **2012**, *54*, 943–948. [CrossRef]
108. Corno, G.; Coci, M.; Giardina, M.; Plechuk, S.; Campanile, F.; Stefani, S. Antibiotics promote aggregation within aquatic bacterial communities. *Front. Microbiol.* **2014**, *5*, 297. [CrossRef]
109. Higgins, D.L.; Chang, R.; Debabov, D.V.; Leung, J.; Wu, T.; Krause, K.M.; Sandvik, E.; Hubbard, J.M.; Kaniga, K.; Schmidt, D.E., Jr.; et al. Telavancin, a multifunctional lipoglycopeptide, disrupts both cell wall synthesis and cell membrane integrity in methicillin-resistant *Staphylococcus aureus*. *Antimicrob. Agents Chemother.* **2005**, *49*, 1127–1134. [CrossRef]
110. Draghi, D.C.; Benton, B.M.; Krause, K.M.; Thornsberry, C.; Pillar, C.; Sahm, D.F. Comparative surveillance study of telavancin activity against recently collected gram-positive clinical isolates from across the United States. *Antimicrob. Agents Chemother.* **2008**, *52*, 2383–2388. [CrossRef]
111. Food and Drug Administration. FDA Labelling Information. 2009. Available online: https://www.fda.gov/files/food/published/Food-Labeling-Guide-%28PDF%29.pdf (accessed on 15 November 2010).
112. Das, B.; Sarkar, C.; Das, D.; Gupta, A.; Kalra, A.; Sahni, S. Telavancin: A novel semisynthetic lipoglycopeptide agent to counter the challenge of resistant Gram-positive pathogens. *Ther. Adv. Infect. Dis.* **2017**, *2*, 49–73. [CrossRef]
113. Breukink, E.J.; Humphrey, P.P.A.; Benton, B.M.; Visscher, I. Evidence for a multivalent interaction between telavancin and membrane-bound lipid II. In Proceedings of the 46th Annual Interscience Conference on Antimicrobial Agents and Chemotherapy, San Francisco, CA, USA, 27–30 September 2006.

114. Benton, B.; Breukink, E.; Visscher, I.; Debabov, D.; Lunde, C.; Janc, J.; Humphrey, P. Telavancin inhibits peptidoglycan biosynthesis through preferential targeting of transglycosylation: Evidence for a multivalent interaction between telavancin and lipid II. *Int. J. Antimicrob. Agents* **2007**, *29*, 51–52. [CrossRef]
115. Lunde, C.S.; Hartouni, S.R.; Janc, J.W.; Mammen, M.; Humphrey, P.P.; Benton, B.M. Telavancin disrupts the functional integrity of the bacterial membrane through targeted interaction with the cell wall precursor lipid II. *Antimicrob. Agents Chemother.* **2009**, *53*, 3375–3383. [CrossRef] [PubMed]
116. Dunne, M.W.; Puttagunta, S.; Sprenger, C.R.; Rubino, C.; Van Wart, S.; Baldassarre, J. Extended –duration dosing and distribution of dalbavancin into bone and artic ular tissue. *Antimicrob. Agents Chemother.* **2015**, *59*, 1849–1855. [CrossRef]
117. Fazili, T.; Bansal, E.; Garner, D.; Gomez, M.; Stornelli, N. Dalbavancin as sequential therapy for infective endocarditis due to Gram-positive organisms: A review. *Int. J. Antimicrob. Agents* **2023**, *61*, 106749. [CrossRef]
118. Zhang, Y.; Sass, A.; Van Acker, H.; Wille, J.; Verhasselt, B.; Van Nieuwerburgh, F.; Kaever, V.; Crabbé, A.; Coenye, T. Coumarin Reduces Virulence and Biofilm Formation in *Pseudomonas aeruginosa* by Affecting Quorum Sensing, Type III Secretion and C-di-GMP Levels. *Front. Microbiol.* **2018**, *9*, 1952. [CrossRef] [PubMed]
119. Ušjak, D.; Ivković, B.; Božić, D.D.; Bošković, L.; Milenković, M. Antimicrobial activity of novel chalcones and modulation of virulence factors in hospital strains of *Acinetobacter baumannii* and *Pseudomonas aeruginosa*. *Microb. Pathog.* **2019**, *131*, 186–196. [CrossRef] [PubMed]
120. Ušjak, D.; Dinić, M.; Novović, K.; Ivković, B.; Filipović, N.; Stevanović, M.; Milenković, M.T. Methoxy-Substituted Hydroxychalcone Reduces Biofilm Production, Adhesion and Surface Motility of *Acinetobacter baumannii* by Inhibiting ompA Gene Expression. *Chem. Biodivers.* **2021**, *18*, e2000786. [CrossRef]
121. Qi, P.; Wang, N.; Zhang, T.; Feng, Y.; Zhou, X.; Zeng, D.; Meng, J.; Liu, L.; Jin, L.; Yang, S. Anti-Virulence Strategy of Novel Dehydroabietic Acid Derivatives: Design, Synthesis, and Antibacterial Evaluation. *Int. J. Mol. Sci.* **2023**, *24*, 2897. [CrossRef] [PubMed]
122. Zhou, J.W.; Ruan, L.Y.; Chen, H.J.; Luo, H.Z.; Jiang, H.; Wang, J.S.; Jia, A.Q. Inhibition of Quorum Sensing and Virulence in *Serratia marcescens* by Hordenine. *J. Agric. Food Chem.* **2019**, *67*, 784–795. [CrossRef]
123. Du, Y.; Sun, J.; Gong, Q.; Wang, Y.; Fu, P.; Zhu, W. New α-Pyridones with Quorum-Sensing Inhibitory Activity from Diversity-Enhanced Extracts of a *Streptomyces* sp. Derived from Marine Algae. *J. Agric. Food Chem.* **2018**, *66*, 1807–1812. [CrossRef]

MDPI AG
Grosspeteranlage 5
4052 Basel
Switzerland
Tel.: +41 61 683 77 34

Antibiotics Editorial Office
E-mail: antibiotics@mdpi.com
www.mdpi.com/journal/antibiotics

www.ingramcontent.com/pod-product-compliance
Lightning Source LLC
Chambersburg PA
CBHW061629210926
51850CB00009B/2480
9783725853779